Simon Y. Mills

Out of the Earth

The Essential Book of Herbal Medicine

VIKING ARKANA

VIKING

Published by the Penguin Group
Penguin Books Ltd, 27 Wrights Lane, London W8 5TZ, England
Penguin Books USA Inc., 375 Hudson Street, New York, New York 10014, USA
Penguin Books Australia Ltd, Ringwood, Victoria, Australia
Penguin Books Canada Ltd, 10 Alcorn Avenue, Toronto, Ontario, Canada M4V 3B2
Penguin Books (NZ) Ltd, 182–190 Wairau Road, Auckland 10, New Zealand

Penguin Books Ltd, Registered Offices: Harmondsworth, Middlesex, England

First published in 1991
10 9 8 7 6 5 4 3 2 1

Set in 12/14 pt Lasercomp Sabon
Printed in England by Clays Ltd, St Ives plc

A CIP catalogue record for this book is available from the British Library

ISBN 0-670-83565X

Library of Congress Catalog Card Number: 91–66419

for Rachel

The Lord hath created medicines out of the earth; and
he that is wise will not abhor them

Ecclesiasticus 38:4

Contents

xi   Contents

xv   Contents

Preface

Part I: ROOTS

In the first part of this book an attempt is made to draw together the many strands of practice and belief that appear to underlie the use of herbal medicine around the world and through history.

The thesis pursued is that in spite of diverse cultural and historical differences there are clear themes that recur repeatedly whenever humans have explained how they use plants for medicines.

The implication is that to get the most benefit from medicinal plants today we should be prepared to absorb these themes ourselves, and then adapt them to our own circumstances. Most that is written today about herbs suffers from not making the necessary shift of perspective away from conventional views of medicines.

Although plants are the major source of medicine for most of the world's population even today, and have provided the sole source since prehistory, their use has not often been clearly articulated. The following text is an attempt to understand the herbal practitioner, from classic texts, anthropological accounts, and from personal clinical experience over many years as a member of the National Institute of Medical Herbalists in Britain.

The viewpoint is obviously partisan, but hopefully not excessively so. Some traditional practice was, after all, born of parochialism, prejudice and a proven inability to adapt to changing circumstances. Assumptions have turned out to be simplistic and inaccurate; certainly many are not appropriate to modern times.

There is, however, a very rich tapestry to select from: it is hoped that the golden threads can be picked out. What we will concentrate on are the most distilled products of traditional beliefs, those most able to stand the test of time.

There is one urgent requirement before herbal medicine can be assessed fairly: it needs a coherent base in medical science, one that can allow fair assessment for a strategy that is fundamentally based on:

> the paramount importance of the individual's many levels of experience of health and disease;
>
> recognizing the powerful self-correcting forces in the body;
>
> the subsequent emphasis in practice on influencing the body's recuperative functions rather than only treating symptoms or pathologies.

Medical science has so far developed in line with the conventional approach to illness. It still inhabits a Newtonian-Cartesian world in which the whole is understood by reference to the behaviour of its parts, and supports a therapeutic approach that values precise expert interventions against pathologies.

An attempt will be made in this part to represent the medical sciences so that the particular qualities and claims of herbal medicine can be more fairly assessed. There needs to be another, more qualitative and experiential view of human body function (*physiology*), of illness (*pathology*), of the action of medicines (*pharmacology*) and of their practical application (*therapeutics*). There are indeed very old approaches to these subjects, of surprising sophistication, and these will be rehearsed in modern terms as a suggested basis for a broader realignment.

In line with scientific tradition, we will also be generating hypotheses, fundamental axioms on which the whole edifice is founded, that are submitted for assessment (they are inserted in the text under the title **Propositions**). Future inquiry may validate these or prove them unacceptable. The fate of this whole enterprise will ultimately depend on such verdicts.

The image of roots is of many strands converging to give nourishment to the whole. It may be seen as a most appropriate metaphor for this first part.

Part II: BRANCHES

The second half of the book is concerned primarily with the practical consequences of choosing to apply herbal remedies as medicines. Whereas the first part was concerned with setting up the scientific and therapeutic framework by which to judge the potential role of herbal medicine, to create a herbal medical science, so to speak, this is devoted to pursuing the details of that therapy.

Attention is given to specific modern and practical issues. What is the state of research into the efficacy and safety of herbal medicines? How does one select a herb sample of good quality and how does one interpret the definitions used to identify such standards? What are the best ways to prepare herbs for specific applications?

Above all, and this is a major theme in this part, *how do herbal remedies work?* It is now possible to piece together from a diversity of sources an account of the pharmacological activity of the prominent plant constituents. This exercise helps to dispel the mystery that might otherwise surround the subject and provides strong circumstantial evidence for clinical effectiveness. There is no doubt that the subject of herbal pharmacology will develop rapidly in the coming years and this is one part of the book that will be most updated in later editions. It will still be obvious though that the parts of the herb will never adequately explain the whole and such a pursuit will always be secondary to the experience of the remedies themselves.

Thus it is that a large part of the book is given to a discussion of individual remedies, emphasizing depth of description rather than numbers, so as to set up a basic palette of remedies. My own experience has been the prime factor in selecting the remedies, in the hope that their underlying qualities may be better conveyed by reflecting personal encounters with their performance in real clinical settings. It is implied that themes and archetypes emerge that might be equally applied by those who do not wish to use Anglo-American herbs.

The final part of the book is a clinical index. It is a recurrent theme in both these parts that the herbalist does not primarily apply the remedies to symptoms, but hopefully to underlying disturbances of function and homoeostasis. Nevertheless, it is obvious that symptoms remain the usual language of illness, and for those who might otherwise risk losing the trees for the forest, I have appended a clinical index, providing pointers to possible herbal strategies for common illnesses.

The image of branches is of diverging movements away from a core, in contrast to the convergent imagery of the first part. There is, however, an obvious connection between the branches and the trunk. The challenge in adapting herbal medicine to the modern world is in keeping sight of the core principles of the discipline.

Simon Y. Mills
Exeter, June 1990.

NOTE: In the following pages the author has drawn on a number of different cultural sources and on his own clinical experience to distil common themes in the use of herbal medicine so that something of the essential nature of the therapy may emerge. It is therefore not the aim of this book to represent any particular tradition of practice, such as that developed by the National Institute of Medical Herbalists since 1864, or to describe the widespread medical application of phytotherapy across Europe (as manifested by the formation in 1989 of the European Scientific Cooperative for Phytotherapy). Nor does the book reflect the curriculum of the School of Phytotherapy in Sussex, the major training programme for professional herbal medicine in Europe.

With Many Thanks

There are many who help keep the practice of herbal medicine as a living tradition whose influence in the framing of this work needs special acknowledgement.

Notable are the many members of the National Institute of Medical Herbalists in Britain who have been generous in their support and encouragement over the years. They are the major group of practitioners in the developed world pursuing a new role for professional medical herbalists as a speciality complementary to, but separate from, conventional medicine.

Special appreciation is due to Hein Zeylstra, who has blazed a path for the profession into the modern world in providing at The School of Herbal Medicine (Phytotherapy) near Hailsham in Sussex, a training programme of unparalleled depth. He originally commissioned from me a pharmacology course which for the first time enabled the material in Part II to be assembled. His own detailed course on pharmacy also helped provide the framework and some of the material for that section in the same part.

Mr Fred Fletcher Hyde almost single-handedly carried the torch of professional medical herbalism in Britain through its darkest times in the 1960s, and in the negotiations with Government over the Medicines Act of 1968, helping to ensure that herbalism emerged with heightened legal protection and on a course that was to see it become ever stronger. He has been a positive beacon for those who followed him, standing firm by the need to combine the highest professional standards in the use of herbal remedies with the application of the best scientific and technical skills.

The cause of professional medical herbalism in Britain is also in debt to the founding members of the British Herbal Medicine Association (BHMA), leading figures from the herbal industry who still clearly value loyalty to the tradition of herbal medicines above narrow commercial interests. They have been sound and effective negotiators with Government over the fate of herbal remedies in Britain. I am especially grateful to Hugh Mitchell and Vic Perfitt for their warm support over many years.

The BHMA has produced two completely separate editions of the *British Herbal Pharmacopoeia*, the latest (with therapeutic Compendium) published in 1990. I have been privileged to have been able to serve on the therapeutics revision committee, along with Fred and Hein, and have received and been able to read a number of the papers cited in Part II. The *BHP* is a world leader in setting standards for herbal remedies and Peter Bradley is to be congratulated for getting the 1990 edition together.

In collating, distilling and developing the material in this book I owe most to my students in New York. For six years they have generated the fertile conditions where these ideas could be worked and re-worked. They often had considerable clinical experience themselves, representing a number of disciplines, and they gave as much as they ever received, putting the notions to work in frequent case conferences as well as in classroom conditions. Particular thanks go to those in my first New York intake, who have become good friends and colleagues, especially Paulette Pettorino, Jason Elias, and Janice MacKenzie.

The Americans figure large in this work, albeit invisibly. Mark Seem combines being an inspiring advocate of a practical hands-on acupuncture and a vigorous academic in his own right with making my trips to New York possible. Bob Duggan shared the big vision and showed that it could be turned into reality; somewhere out there is Bryan Manuele who once made three: in one moment in 1983 they showed that it was possible to bring together different cultural traditions and mould them into something appropriate for modern times.

I shared many ideas with Jan Resnick over the years. He instilled a healthy resistance to the easy dogma that so bedevils any discussion of health care.

Final thanks go to the islanders of Skiathos.

List of Abbreviations

Agr. Biol. Chem.: *Agricultural and Biological Chemistry* (Tokyo)

Amer. J. Chin. Med.: *American Journal of Chinese Medicine* (New York)

Amer. J. Clin. Nutr.: *American Journal of Clinical Nutrition* (Los Angeles)

Amer. J. Gastroenterol.: *American Journal of Gastroenterology* (New York)

Ann. Allergy: *Annals of Allergy* (Bloomington, Minnesota)

Ann. Rev. Pharmacol.: *Annual Review of Pharmacology* (Palo Alto, California)

BMJ: *British Medical Journal* (London)

Brit. J. Dermatol.: *British Journal of Dermatology* (London)

Brit. J. Pharm. Practice: *British Journal of Pharmaceutical Practice* (London)

Brit. J. Rheumatol.: *British Journal of Rheumatology* (London)

Bull. Nat. Form. Comm.: *Bulletin of the National Formulary Committee* (Washington DC)

Canad. Pharm. J.: *Canadian Pharmaceutical Journal* (Toronto)

Carbohyd. Res.: *Carbohydrate Research* (Amsterdam)

Chem. Comm.: *Chemical Communications* (Chemistry Society, London)

Chem. Pharm. Bull.: *Chemical and Pharmaceutical Bulletin* (Tokyo)

Chin. J. Cardiol.: *Chinese Journal of Cardiology* (Beijing)

Clin. and Exp. Pharmacol. and Physiol.: *Clinical and Experimental Pharmacology and Physiology* (Melbourne)

Clin. and Exp. Rheumatol.: *Clinical and Experimental Rheumatology* (Pisa)

Fed. Proc.: *Federation Proceedings* (Federation of American Societies for Experimental Biology, Washington DC)

Hum. Toxicol.: Human Toxicology (Basel, Switzerland)

J. Allergy Clin. Immunol.: Journal of Allergy and Clinical Immunology (St Louis, Louisiana)

JAMA: Journal of the American Medical Association (New York)

J. Amer. Chem. Soc.: Journal of the American Chemical Society

J. Antibio.: Journal of Antibiotics (Tokyo)

J. Asthma: Journal of Asthma (New York)

J. Bio. Sci.: Journal of Biological Sciences (Bombay)

J. Clin. Endocrinol. Metab.: Journal of Clinical Endocrinology and Metabolism (Philadelphia)

J. Ethnopharmacol.: Journal of Ethnopharmacology (Limerick)

J. Med.: Journal of Medicine (Westbury, New York)

J. Med. Chem.: Journal of Medical Chemistry (Washington DC)

J. Nat. Cancer Inst.: Journal of the National Cancer Institute (Bethesda, Maryland)

J. Pharmacol. Dyn.: Journal of Pharmacological Dynamics (Washington DC)

J. Pharm. Pharmacol.: Journal of Pharmacy and Pharmacology (London)

J. Pharm. Sci.: Journal of Pharmaceutical Sciences (Washington DC)

J. Psych. Dr.: Journal of Psychoactive Drugs (San Francisco)

Nut. Res.: Nutrition Research (New York)

Ohio St. Med. J.: Ohio State Medical Journal (Columbus, Ohio)

Pharm. J.: Pharmaceutical Journal (London)

Pharmacol. Biochem. and Behav.: Pharmacology, Biochemistry and Behaviour (New York)

Phytother. Res.: Phytotherapy Research (London)

Proc. Soc. Exp. Biol. Med.: Proceedings of the Society for Experimental Biology and Medicine (New York)

Prog. Lip. Res.: Progress in Lipid Research (Oxford)

Prog. Med. Econ. Pl. Res.: Progress in Medical and Economic Plant Research (London)

Q. J. Crude Drug Res.: Quarterly Journal of Crude Drug Research (Amsterdam)

S. Afr. Med. J.: South African Medical Journal (Cape Town)

Scan. J. Rheumatol.: Scandinavian Journal of Rheumatology (Stockholm)

Soc. Sci. & Med.: Social Science and Medicine (Elmsford, New York)

33rd Ann. Rep. Bur. Amer. Ethn.: 33rd Annual Report of the Bureau of American Ethnography (Washington DC)

Trans. Assoc. Amer. Physicians: Transactions of the Association of American Physicians (Philadelphia)

Trop. Geogr. Med.: Tropical and Geographical Medicine (Haarlem, Holland)

Part I
ROOTS

1 Introduction

Up to three-quarters of medicines taken around the world today will be herbal remedies. The people taking them will usually be following approaches to their illnesses that are older than civilization itself.

So far medical science has ignored this vast collective tradition. It is an astonishing oversight and there may now be a feeling that it has gone far enough. If the modern world is to learn more about the old ways, however, these have to be made more understandable.

This book is a belated attempt to review traditional medicine for the twentieth century. The surprise is that it can look remarkably modern, even providing useful tips for future health care. It may follow that the 'primitive' world has not been so deprived after all.

An obvious starting point for the reconsideration of the role of traditional medicine is where it still survives and even prospers alongside conventional medicine, in an affluent Western community. In Britain there is once again a growing profession of herbal practitioners, members of a body founded in 1864, the National Institute of Medical Herbalists. They are trained in all the medical sciences, as well as botany and analytical techniques, and work in what look like conventional general medical practices. The difference is that they are not in the orthodox health care system and they only prescribe herbal medicines.

Although what follows is not confined to the approaches of members of the Institute – and may even be disputed by them – their legacy forms the basis of this story. I have been happy to count myself among their number.

Several years ago the husband of one of my patients was sitting in the waiting room while I prepared his wife's prescription. Striking up conversation, he asked, in faultless Devon dialect: *'These 'erbs then – they're fairly new are they?'*

As I happened at the time to be including in the prescription a tincture of a herb, dandelion, that had been equally familiar to the Greeks and to the Chinese 3,000 years ago, among others, I was delighted by the question. Yet he and his wife had known no other form of medicine than that provided through the British National Health Service. This ancient therapy they had turned to, out of desperation as it happened, was genuinely new to them and to many others as well.

They were among many turning again to other approaches, hoping to find a new answer to their question. That the new answer was really very old was merely ironic. They had stumbled on a completely different medical approach and it fitted their needs.

It is often argued that early medicine was flawed by its inadequacies in performance, and that at best it is not relevant to modern problems and priorities. Such arguments hold that if there is anything of value in crude plant drugs at all, it is as a source of potentially effective new drugs, and there is no advantage in dredging up archaic and dubious concepts of pharmacology as well.

The new popularity of the herbal option is one reason, however, why there might be value in looking again at the rationale of traditional medicine. The archaeological and anthropological evidence moreover supports the view that, where food was adequate and suitably diverse, human beings have lived to a considerable age and have done so in reasonable health, with good bone structures and with few of the modern signs of ageing. A number of these primitive societies have been associated with considerable longevity[1] and in a contemporary account a James Easton in 1799 recorded cases of a considerable number of individuals who had lived longer than a century.[2] While this is as much an argument for healthy, active lifestyles freed from modern stresses, it is also a suitable testimonial for health care to set against the usual historical archetype. The effectiveness of the local herbal treatments has also featured in several accounts of travels by early European settlers in North America and Asia.

5   Introduction

It has even been claimed that the poor state of health of many rural populations in developing countries today is not only the obvious result of poverty but also of European and other outsider contact which has been intensified by modernization and external as well as internal 'colonial' economic development.[3] To discredit the value of local medical practices and traditional therapies for their inability to deal with current mortality and morbidity patterns in such situations would therefore be particularly inaccurate and misleading.

Life was almost certainly 'nasty, brutish and short' in the ghastly squalor and crowding of early town and city life. Epidemics of infectious diseases were associated with such lifestyle as early as the Han dynasty in China 2,000 years ago. Modern experience of the conditions rife in the vast conurbations in much of the developing world today suggests that no system of medicine can completely cope with the diseases that follow lack of a clean water supply and inadequate nourishment.

Of course, not all ill health was in the cities. Parasitic infestation was almost universal and killer febrile diseases were common enough in even the most Arcadian rural habitat. There was certainly a persistent decimation among infants and mothers that affected social and family policy the world over, at least until Semmelweis launched his courageous attack on the hygienic standards of obstetricians in nineteenth-century Europe. But these and other causes of mortality were reduced more by such public endeavours than by any miracle discovery in medicine. (The city and borough councillors who oversaw improvements in water supply and waste disposal have deserved their re-evaluation as major contributors to the abolition of medieval plagues in western Europe.)

Throughout all the turbulent history of health care and the lack of it in Western cultures however, the 'wise woman' and the village herbalist plied their craft in the countryside, with what appears to be a reasonable effect. Where, in China and other countries, support has been given to traditional healers, there has been little doubt that they perform moderately well. When, as seems likely, they apply principles that are almost universally common to traditional healers everywhere, such principles merit attention.

There is, however, another more positive reason for looking

again at health care as our ancestors did. The possibility is that it may teach us something. Apart from the obvious clues they might give us to the development of new treatments,* we shall see how their perspective was essentially a whole-world view, with each part irreplaceably contributing to a pattern: diseases were seen as imbalances to be corrected rather than as alien invasions to be attacked. Herbal remedies were judged by their ability to adjust patterns of disorder, not by any conventional 'antidisease' or allopathic activity. In times when germs and the other usual 'bad guys' of disease are proving harder and harder to attack, we may be ready to look again at medicines that treat illness differently.

Part of this difference is the observation that herbs behave as more than just assemblages of chemicals. Again and again, when a herbal remedy is examined experimentally it is found to have activity that is apparently more than the sum of that of its active constituents. Their combination gives it unique properties, properties that are often hard to mimic with any single isolated drug. We shall see many examples of this in Part II. Given that these properties are often interesting, that they are traditionally seen as a different sort of medicine anyway, with vitalistic, supportive action on the body's recuperative powers, then it makes sense to try to see them as they once were used rather than merely gutting them for interesting chemical titbits.

Any attempt to review such a different type of medicine in modern terms will mean also attempting to establish a new system of therapeutics to set against convention. This is particularly difficult.

Unlike other more academic disciplines, medical science has constantly to prove itself against nasty realities. Illness can be a frightening experience and often involves a sense of hopelessness. The sufferer usually finds comfort in turning to the expert, who is then handed the burden of making good out of an unwellness that is sometimes beyond understanding.

Faced with the daily job of shouldering another's fear and

*As V. Vogel writes in *American Indian Medicine* (University of Oklahoma Press, 1970, on p. 267): 'In 1970 a study of the drugs in the *U.S. Formulary* listed about 170 vegetal drugs which were derived from the Indians north of Mexico and fifty more were used by the natives of the West Indies, Mexico, Central and South America.'

7   Introduction

confusion, it is not surprising that physicians are less patient with grand theories than most. It is not surprising either that they prefer to reduce the emotional load, to concentrate on that which is most tangible, most amenable to treatment, and that their comfort in the consulting room is in direct proportion to the clarity with which the diagnosis and treatment can be worked out.

Thus medicine strives in any illness to find an identifiable 'bad guy' (now so often a 'virus', even when the validity of that diagnosis is almost non-existent). It specializes in surgery and, dramatically, in replacement surgery. Its pharmacological ideal is to target its drugs better: monoclonal antibodies are the answer to a medical prayer. Even a more 'holistic' approach is often little more than making stress or mental strain the new 'bad guy'.

But this caution, though understandable, is not inevitable. There are other ways to react to the vagaries of nature. One can strive for the illusion of control and protection by building a stronger and more sophisticated citadel, or one can respond to nature in the way a sailor does.

The seafarer first respects nature as essentially unfathomable, yet he also tries to learn some of its tricks, and then sets out to share his life with it, sufficiently well to make a living himself.

He learns to read the elements, the ways of weather and tides. He sees adversity, not to be controlled, let alone attacked, but to be sailed out of and even turned to advantage. The skill with which this can be done is a combination of good boat design and trained seamanship. As Buckminster Fuller used to point out, the skipper of a ship has to know as much as possible about as much as possible to have a truly comprehensive view of the world he chooses to work in and to read, understand and act on the broadest pattern of events possible.

In medicine it is also possible to see the living being as a cosmos, subjected to vagaries of weather and tides, which lead in turn to predisposition to illness, the illness having identifiable patterns as a result. With the recognition of these patterns one can look for treatment that emphasizes the return to homoeostatic balance rather than attacks symptoms or external agents.

This means seeing illness as more 'soil' than 'seed', more disposition than pathogen (the old nature-cure pioneers used to see germs as saprophytic organisms, like forest fungi, taking advantage of dead or decaying matter, thus emphasizing that they have little place in healthy living tissues).

These are the underlying, often unwritten assumptions of the ancient ways of medicine, of every healing tradition the world over, whether American Indian, early European, Islamic Middle Eastern, or rooted in the Ayurvedic medicine of the Indian sub-continent or the richness of the Chinese and Japanese systems. Such assumptions comply with what is known of the medical practices of the wandering hunter-nomads and pastoralists from Africa.

They seem, however, not to apply to one system: that of modern technological medicine! Only our conventional medicine has dared to control nature, to ignore the wider ecological pattern in favour of manipulating the outward symptom or sign of disorder. Its scorching progress has been undeniable, but it has often been remote from what patients really feel about their illness. Every other tradition has sought to work from within nature, to find the pattern of disharmony, *to make sense of what we feel*.

There is in fact a great thrill in seeing our internal affairs in such a context – and also a powerful, even primal, recognition. Much of what is in this book is felt and understood by everyone. It is a matter of rediscovering each patient's *story*. Demonstrating that the disease is part of one's whole life pattern is almost always to see a revelation dawn, as the illness becomes meaningful, perhaps for the first time.

Only a minority of ailments are simple and specific. As we pause after the first triumph of public health care and the virtual disappearance of the old killer diseases, we are faced with different health problems for which, ironically, the old discarded health concepts have renewed relevance.

Modern scientific technology has already forced a rethink. New computer-based studies of those physical phenomena at the edge of what is measured and measurable: weather problems, turbulence in fluids, economic cycles, under the heading of what is now termed 'chaos' studies, have shown that the natural world is essentially chaotic, but that *there are powerful patterns in this chaos*. These patterns are of a different order to the ones we learnt in school science, but they are not soft, vague or woolly options. (In fact, they involve the most rigorous mathematics and physics.) They insist on a general re-orientation of all other sciences, and especially those concerned with the study of humankind.[4]

One already widely accepted means of understanding complex phenomena in other scientific disciplines is to look at them in terms of their interactions, so that not only is the whole pattern of events more than the sum of its parts but it actually determines them.[5] This approach has been proved in the hard economic arena as well: the managing director of any large modern corporation would now consider as dangerously incomplete any information about the business that was not based on the most comprehensive possible assessment of the interactions occurring between individual departments: the *systems analysis*.

That we have come so far without applying the principles of the systems view to our understanding of the most complex corporation of all – the human being – can only be understood if there are deep aversions to the approach in medical science.

Apart from the instinct of the physician to find the best way simply to cope, mentioned earlier, another anxiety must lie in considering the question of therapeutics. If we try to understand diseases as disorders of patterns in the functions of the body, mind and spirit, then conventional drugs and interventions are at best only partially appropriate, and at worst they contribute further to the disruption.

If we see the body, mind and spirit as a complex whole, applying a constant self-corrective force to maintain a homoeostatic balance in spite of wildly varying environmental pressures, then we should use different medicines, and even redefine the term. The search is on for those agents that support homoeostatic efforts, which help the body help itself.

This would be an awesome task if it had to be tackled fresh, but fortunately there are still medicines and approaches developed and applied around the world, and over the centuries, along intuitive lines of pattern and system.

Herbal medicines have not enjoyed a good scholastic press: like most rural skills they have been applied very much more in the practice than the theory. Most modern texts on the subject in

English are appallingly devoid of academic rigour, substituting lazy simplicities instead. Herbs do not shine on such a stage.

The fact is, however, that herbs are not historical remnants but, on World Health Organization figures, they are still used around the world three to four times as much as conventional drugs. In reassessing the best course for improving health care for the world's population, a meeting of the WHO was presented with a report prepared jointly with UNICEF which showed that of the 80 per cent of the world's population living in developing countries, only 15 per cent had access to modern scientific medicine: the rest depended mainly on their traditional and indigenous systems of health care in which herbal remedies played the prominent part.[6]

In response the WHO at its 1976 conference at Alma Alta on Primary Health Care launched its programme for the 'Promotion and Development of Traditional Medicine', with the following objectives:

(i) to foster a realistic approach to traditional medicine in order to promote and further contribute to health care;

(ii) to explore the merits of traditional medicine in the light of modern science in order to maximize useful and effective practices and discourage harmful ones;

(iii) to promote the integration of proven valuable knowledge and skills in traditional and Western medicine.[7]

In countries that have again taken herbal remedies seriously in recent times they have shown themselves to have remarkable relevance to modern problems,[8] and to be very popular.[9]

If one looks at the herbal approaches and therapeutics of the many sophisticated cultures that have applied them comprehensively, one finds exciting evidence of common principles of pattern, process and system that would delight a modern natural scientist. We shall be attempting to point in that direction in this book.

We do not have to abandon the achievements of medical science to date. Rather we need a different way of organizing our knowledge, to bring it in line with ancient truths, and strive for a grand synthesis of the new and the old, a hybrid that vigorously does justice to both.

2 Physiology

Setting the Scene – an introduction to another medical science

One of the most frequent complaints made about doctors by patients turning to alternatives, at least in Britain, is that they do not take enough notice of the patients' stories.

It is not just the usual argument that the doctor has so little time: it really seems as though the doctor is not interested in the details of the story. Even more disquieting, and this is a complaint most often made by women patients, the doctor will actually discount features of the story that do not accord with the expected presentation. The following example might not seem unfamiliar:

PATIENT: *My stomach swells up straight after eating, especially after eating acid foods . . . I feel as though I cannot lose this weight even though I eat only a tiny amount . . . I also get a lot of headaches and feel very tired all the time . . .*

DOCTOR: *The blood tests show there is nothing wrong with you; it is probably your nerves . . . the only real way to lose weight is to cut back on your calories – of course, you could also try and do a little more exercise . . . I can give you something to help you relax better . . .*

Apart from the obvious slight to the patient, in such conversations the implication is that the doctor knows what goes on in the patient's body better than the patient. This is not surprising.

Medicine is only rational

Medical science has grown, like science as a whole, on the premise that the neutral observer, by isolating any phenomenon from all those around it, is better able to see and understand what is going on. Rationalist scientific method has insisted that only 'objective' observations can reveal the absolute truth, anything else might be

14 Physiology

personal bias, a view distorted by deceptive incidentals, at most a relative truth that is not generally applicable.

Rationalism is a system of thought that seeks to minimize the influence of the senses, that works with a priori concepts rather than empirical observations. It also refers particularly to the legacy of the European rationalists, notably Spinoza, Leibniz and Descartes, the latter of whom has given his name to the adjective Cartesian, used for classical scientific method.

Non-rationalist thought, that which dominated all human perception throughout human history up to the modern age, was positively rejected by science. Subjectivity, feelings and personal experience are all suspect, confusing, casting a web of illusion over the truth.

The rejection of the evidence of the senses had one of its earliest and most dramatic effects on human consciousness when Copernicus showed conclusively that almost every human in history had got it wrong by assuming that the sun and stars moved round a flat earth. It most certainly looked and felt like that, but it was not an objective truth.* *Adhering to it and other such illusions stood in the way of real understanding.*

Rationalism has been an immense success for humanity. It provided the essential basis for the development of natural sciences, of physics, astronomy, meteorology. It gave birth to the Industrial Revolution and so to cars, refrigerators, washing machines, TV, and summer holidays in Greece. It led to the major reduction of starvation and mass diseases over large parts of the globe, and improved the everyday expectations of the common people so that they exceeded those of medieval royalty.

It also entered into a private conspiracy with its adherents. It reinforced the natural but selfish instinct that says that each person is an individual alone, someone who can be a neutral observer of the rest of creation. It justified the forbidden notion that it might be possible to stand outside nature, dissect it (without bias, of course!), and thus dominate it. In short it helped to remove the

---

* In fact a recent survey (see Jowell, R., Witherspoon, S., Brook, L., eds. (1989) *British Social Attitudes: Special International Report*, Gower Press, Aldershot, UK) has shown a surprising number of people in the developed West (27 per cent in the USA and 37 per cent in Britain) still think the sun moves round the earth!

primal fear of a capricious and possibly cruel world, and provided a way to turn it to apparent security, comfort and material advantage.

It has further accorded with the dominant instinct of the Western world, the Judaeo-Christian assumption of a controlling influence in all phenomena, not only that of a controlling deity, but within the birthright of each individual human being as well. This is the instinct that also sees nature as something that needs to be transcended, improved upon, not immersed in in some primitive fashion.

Rationalism is rarely seen, however, as an alien creed. The evidence from around the world outside its birthplace in Europe is that when cultures are introduced to it they grasp it eagerly. We who profit from its material benefits should not be too hasty in reviling it.

But the success of rational thought is success at a price, perhaps a price that may yet be too much to bear. Obsessive concentration on fragments of the whole prevents one from seeing the whole itself. It should have been expected that technological progress would be at the expense of the ecosystem; that pollution, the break-up of the family, tribal and village community and an increasing sense of personal alienation would follow from denying that the whole of nature is as important as the bit you are concentrating on.

Faced with the implications of our technological success, the ecological and new-consciousness movements press for a change in attitude. Yet it really is hard for us to shift our faith towards a systems view that says that the whole is more than the sum of its parts and is therefore worth the personal sacrifice (even the remnants of that widespread view of the past, loyalty to country or community, are derided and under threat in modern society). The prize of a comfortable lifestyle dissuades most from even trying.

The benefits to the consumer of rationalist medicine have perhaps been the most impressive, the hardest to deny. Massive reduction of suffering has followed rational observations such as those made by John Snow in 1849 when he showed that an outbreak in London of the hitherto mysterious disease cholera could be traced to one supply of drinking water, or of Semmelweis, who survived the fury of his obstetrician colleagues to show conclusively that their own unwashed hands were the primary cause of the death of mothers after labour. Rational science has produced drugs and surgical techniques that can assault diseased tissues with increasing precision. Life expectancy has never been higher.

Yet in spite of these advances, it is also accepted that diseases still exact their toll on us. We might live longer, but the arthritic deterioration, heart disease, cancer and pneumonia that are most likely to plague our final years increase accordingly and still elude isolation and elimination. Bacterial diseases may be largely gone but low-grade debilitating viral and immuno-deficient conditions are on the increase. And patient after patient turns away from their doctors and goes towards practitioners of alternative therapies because they say that the priest of rationalist scientific medicine either is no longer effective or does not even seem to be able to understand their story any more.

An irrational truth?

Herbalists have always survived in modern times through the support of their patients. The primitive, irrational notion that messy, crude and variable plant drugs might compete with the latest razor-sharp chemical agent clearly has had little support from the medical or scientific community. Yet the history of herbalism outlined in this book shows how stubbornly it has survived in rural and other self-sufficient communities. Its renaissance in the modern world points to its filling a new need in its consumers. Herbalists have rarely viewed the human being through the eyes of the modern scientist. They have rarely gone out to attack fragmented diseases or even been particularly interested in them. At times when herbal therapy has been articulated, in the Greece of Hippocrates or the Roman world of Galen, in the Islamic revival of Avicenna or El-Rhazes, throughout the written history of China, Japan, or India, the approach adopted has definitely been non-rationalist.

The personal experience of modern medical herbalists with their patients suggests that there may be value still in an alternative to rationalist scientific explanations of human illness: it might actually be possible to accept that for most of us, so to speak, it still feels as though the sun is going round the earth, and that there are meaning and poetry and truth in such movement.

There are of course many dangers in embracing the non-rational. The traditional system has not readily lent itself to experiment, to innovation, to development. It has been allowed to perpetuate much that is simply counter-productive in health care as well as such other essential areas as agriculture. Its many small errors on the small scale of the village or tribe were perhaps acceptable, its large errors in the medieval city life of Europe quite horrendous. No one would want to turn the clock back towards Nineveh.

Yet there may be a middle way, a way of illuminating one tradition with the other to transcend both.

The philosophical tradition of phenomenology works with the assumption that the most scientific pursuit is to rigorously investigate one's own 'being-in-the-world'.[1] Nietzsche stated earlier: '*We others who thirst for reason want to look our experiences in the eye as severely as at a scientific experiment!*'[2]

This approach has been increasingly accepted by other scientific theoreticians, notably modern physicists[3] and social scientists,[4] but strangely not by scientists in medicine. The suggestion that there might be a phenomenological version of physiology and the other medical sciences seems hardly to have registered. A tentative move towards such a goal will be attempted in what follows. In fact, it is suggested that there may be a wider truth in accepting and trying to understand what our patients feel as the truth for themselves.

In this review, however, we will not dare to follow completely Robert Pirsig's example in *Zen and the Art of Motorcycle Maintenance*.[5] He looked for and found the ghost of rationality and 'thrashed him good', subjecting both this ghost and that of romanticism to a higher truth, that facet of the Godhead he called 'Quality'. It will take as rigorous a philosophical and personal exploration as he pursued in that extraordinary book to subject both rationalist and romantic medicine to the higher truth, that facet of the Godhead we would call 'Health'. This more humble attempt will simply aim to provide some substance to the intuitive approach of herbalists through history, and some support for anyone who suspected that what they felt about themselves might

18 Physiology

not be untrue simply because it could not be independently proved.

Carving up the cadaver

To provide a new scientific explanation for the processes of health it is necessary to focus on the existing science of physiology. This has so far been almost entirely shaped by rationalist, reductionist observations.

Physiology is the study of normal functions. It has developed as a science in close association with anatomy (which the Chinese call 'dissection science') and pathology (the study of diseases). Most medical students are introduced to a dead human body within the first weeks of starting their studies, while they are still barely school-children. This is a suitably harrowing entry to their future calling, but it quickly becomes routine. They will return to their body every few days for the next two years until every cubic inch of tissue has been explored and recorded.

They will go through the body piece by piece, maybe the arms and hands first, then the legs and feet, then perhaps the thorax, with its skin and tissue coverings, its muscles, ribcage, then the pleural cavity and the lungs, the pericardial sac and the heart, noting as they go the displacement of the aortic arch and its branches, the vagal and phrenic nerve trunks, and so on. Then they might tackle the abdominal cavity, tease out the stomach, intestines and bowel, dissect the liver, the pancreas, the kidneys, the ureters, the bladder, and look at their relationship to the structures of the internal reproductive organs (requiring those teams dissecting males to swap with those working on females). Finally, they will turn to the spine, the neck, the face and head, with particularly close attention to the brain.

Given the practicalities of this exercise it is inevitable that theory will follow practice. Anatomy lectures will refer to work being done in the dissection room at the time. Not surprisingly they will try to integrate other work as well. The physiology of respiration will be best taught while the lungs are being explored and will also accompany microscopic studies of detailed lung tissues. The liver will be looked at as a unit, with particular relevance to its bile function; the kidneys will provide a fascinating exercise in fluid dynamics, and so on. In practice, *physiology is primarily geared to teaching medical students about how different anatomical structures work.*

Later the subject of pathology will be introduced. This study of diseases, along with the study of drugs to treat them (pharmacology), will increasingly dominate the curriculum. By the time he or she graduates, the young doctor will be a specialist in the detection (diagnosis) and treatment of disease, and will have learnt to see patients as human beings with potential diseases. If they opt for surgery they will specialize further in their anatomy. Very few doctors will go back and pursue their physiology again.

The ability of modern doctors to target disease is a historical breakthrough. Modern patients with a life-threatening pathology are in much better hands with a modern physician than they could have been with any from earlier generations. However, the ability to isolate, identify and treat a pathology does not often involve the doctor in an interpretation of normal body function. Any memory of physiology the doctor retains will tend to be subservient to the primary duty of tackling the 'bad guy'.

'What about me?'

While a patient with a clear disease will have an excellent chance of effective treatment, this satisfaction diminishes if the problem is less identifiable. Often there are symptoms without evidence of disease (on X-ray, blood test, or other investigation). More often the problem is low-grade and chronic, either resisting drug treatment or being only temporarily relieved by it. In all these cases the most usual reaction from the doctor is one of slight frustration. The problem becomes 'psychosomatic' or 'all in the mind' if there is no measurable damage done, the patient put on indefinite repeat prescriptions if little progress is being made.

Even when the problem is classifiable, like the myriad skin diseases, the patient often feels left out of the discussion. An arcane diagnosis of pityriasis alba ('or is it seborrhoeic eczema?') will seem rather distant from the question 'What is wrong with me?', especially if the treatment is superficial or absent.

One of the most telling critiques of non-conventional, alternative or complementary medicine by physicians has been that its new popularity owes much more to its ability to provide a 'better story' of the patient's illness, than to any efficacy. These views were aired notably by one or two participants at the Royal Society of Medicine Colloquia on complementary medicine.[6] (One implicit charge is that it is merely massaging modern middle-class neuroses, or even creating a new amoral romantic escapism.)[7]

The implication is that modern doctors have relinquished the shamanistic or priestly role of addressing the patient's whole world and have sought a specialist job as body mechanics. Alternative or complementary medicine has clearly claimed to provide more time for patients, a listening service, and then offered them imagery and models of their illness that they can relate to. In this context it is almost immaterial that some of these ideas are half-baked or even medically outrageous, or that they are almost certainly unverifiable: their very popularity, at least as a salve for modern metropolitan neurosis, is a simple reflection of the poverty of the modern medical story.

It is genuinely arguable whether herbal medicine really belongs in the category of 'alternative medicine'. It is too close to the heart of history for that. But it clearly does have an excellent story to share with its participants, and one that could more widely be used today if an appropriate review of medical science could be accepted.

A subjective science

One thing is very clear when the traditional uses of herbal remedies are examined: the early human view of health and disease was very different from modern conventional ideas. There were no investigative scientists to probe and peer into the deep recesses of the remedies' functions. Traditional herbalists had only their intuitions, their own subjective impressions of health and illness and of the workings of the natural world around them.

The latter was important because all early concepts of the world were cosmic ones: each level of nature was a microcosm of the whole; the same natural laws applied throughout, to the weather and the land and sea as much as to the human body. *You could understand the inner workings of the human being by linking your own experience with what you knew of the way things behaved in nature.*

This led to very different views of the way the body works. Unfortunately, when systematized these ancient approaches tended to become less flexible. Traditional herbalists were prone to a dangerous mix of dogma and empiricism. They were paradoxically less able to adapt their precepts to accommodate the unique data of the individual experience or even to subject themselves to rigorous scrutiny.

In many cases their observations were misleading and their conclusions were actually wrong. Nevertheless the remarkable fact that emerges, when this primitive physiology is examined, is that much of it is actually still relevant.

It would be most interesting to develop a new approach to modern medical science that addressed growing modern needs yet was able to accommodate a realistic assessment of these older, intuitive ways of understanding health and disease.

What seems to be required is:

> a way of charting the whole pattern of human illnesses, before they became pathologies;
>
> a working physiology that could help a physician really interpret disorders as disturbances of homoeostasis, or diseases as manifestations of a long story of difficulty;
>
> an approach to human functions that could actually be understood by ordinary humans themselves, and thus perhaps the beginning of an answer to the patient's most pressing question about his or her illness: 'Why me?'

This is where early physiology comes in. It may also be where a new physiology takes off.

A Herbal Physiology – Physiology as if feelings mattered

If herbalism is to sustain a consistent argument, it is essential that it takes it into the court of medical science.

Though it may have been the instinctive choice of the great majority of the population who are not interested in academic issues, this is not the forum in which it will progress into any new role. Herbal medicine will never have a future unless it comes to terms with changes in medicine in the last century and provides its own coherent and credible perspective on them. However, the herbal perspective on medical science has not so far been developed.

This is an astonishing position. On one hand there is the overwhelming experience of billions of human encounters with herbal medicine leading right up to the present day; on the other the extraordinary hybrid of science and medicine that has so transformed human expectations of health and life in the last century; and the two have never really met! A tentative step will be made towards such a meeting here.

In some ways the particular herbal interest in medical sciences is actually quite limited. Anatomy and histology, the structure of the body and its tissues are not in contention, pathology, the study of disease processes, is safer in the hands of those for whom it is a speciality; it is the study of body *function* that captures the herbalist's imagination. Herbal remedies are prescribed specifically with the aim of affecting the *behaviour* of the body and mind, much more than with the intent of attacking a disease. If herbal medicine is to develop its own perspective on the medical sciences, it will be physiology and its associated disciplines that need appraisal.

A new and better story

It is possible to develop a new approach to the subject of physiology from several convergent directions.

One can distil the essential features of the traditional viewpoint by analysing what survives of traditional therapeutics and notably that which is recorded at considerable length in the texts of Galenic, Chinese, Islamic and other ancient systems of medicine.

Or, it is possible to look at modern medical science with the eyes of the postgraduate, someone past the stage of having to learn the fragments by rote. Science in general has come a long way from the days of Newton and Descartes. Physics has lived with the Uncertainty Principle since the 1930s, and systems analysis has been a part of engineering and business planning since the 1950s. Although medical sciences are certainly the most conservative in tackling the broad shifts of paradigm, there has nevertheless been an explosion of physiological and biochemical research effort in the last two decades, notably covering immune, cardiovascular, and metabolic functions. This proliferation has led to the blurring of boundaries, so that neuropeptide science is completely multi-disciplinary, and the new subject of psychoneuroimmunology is a hot favourite of the intellectually adventurous, particularly in North America. Such new prospects, coupled with insights from embryology and the other natural sciences, mean that it is possible to redraft the boundaries and suggest new patterns.

In the outline that follows we shall be starting with a modern version of the microcosm, the living cell, and developing the notion of integrated fundamental vital processes that might apply equally to all living systems.

Each of these processes can be understood, even *felt*, by most people, and would be recognized by the traditional practitioner: the explanations that follow are designed to expand, with modern discoveries and analytical approaches, the traditional observations and interpretations for each process, linking functions together in ways that are meaningful to modern clinical experience.

Such a return to the cosmic view of life and to the tenets of vitalism is not familiar to the modern physiologist. However, they have been implicit in systems theory for some time[8] and the approach developed here should prove itself to be hard-nosed enough for the most pragmatic scientist.

Modern physiological data will still form the basis of this review. The section headings, however, and the arrangement of material will follow cues distilled from a variety of human experiences of health and illness.

To start a new process of integration of physiological science with traditional concepts of health and disease, it is necessary to summarize what the latter are:

> the human is a wilful vibrant idiosyncratic wonderful being, not to be divided into compartments, whether these are of 'body', 'mind' or 'spirit', or separate functional fragments;
>
> all living beings are inherently self-regulating; and in health their functions are totally integrated and barely identifiable; disorders, however, manifest as patterns of dysfunction that can be recognized, charted and interpreted, to the benefit of any healing intervention.

These are axioms that have formed the basis of philosophical doctrine for centuries. They are not accepted by all today. However, they are a cornerstone for pre-rationalist views of life and health and will be posited as the foundation of this realignment of physiology.

Such an approach to physiology will demand that one looks at overall *processes* within the living being rather than at discrete mechanical functions. It is possible to develop propositions to create the necessary infrastructure for the concept.

Propositions:

all living things, from the simplest to the most complex, engage in essentially the same fundamental processes;

in health these processes are relatively indistinguishable, but become increasingly distinct in disease states, very often assuming largely predictable patterns of disturbance;

these processes are reflected as much in human psychological, emotional, social and even spiritual

25   A Herbal Physiology

dimensions as in the somatic sphere;

each process involves the co-ordination of all physiological functions contributing to it;

any disturbance in a process will affect all such physiological functions, but may also be corrected at any level;

all these processes are yoked to the perpetuation of the whole being, the ecosystem.

In providing a different explanation of physiology, of how the body works, there will be many risks. Many of those nurtured on rational scientific and medical assumptions will find the process either outrageous or unnecessary. There will be inevitable inconsistencies until the associations are better honed by experience. But the ideas themselves are not new, they are common to most human experience through history and simply need the chance to adapt to the modern medical climate.

Patterns of process

We shall start this review of physiology by making a systems analysis of the living organism, identifying key features of both its performance and its organization.

The resulting framework can be set out in the form of a systems flowchart, with the main processes linked sequentially or functionally.

The role of each process in the organism and its relationship with other processes are essentially the same whether the organism is a single cell or a human being, or even the planet Earth. These processes, and the pattern that binds them, are thus genuinely universal.

We take as our starting point a highly schematized living being, best expressed diagrammatically. We can then identify these essential vital processes. They are as follows, arranged in two complementary groups:

Organization	Performance
Managing vital rhythms	Perception
Balancing activity and rest	Response: Accommodation
Integration of all other processes	Reaction
Reproduction	Ingestion: Assimilation
	Rejection
	Processing
	Circulation
	Removal

This is clearly not a physiology textbook.[9] The concepts presented will not be elaborated too far. The choice of examples will be biased in favour of the herbalist's perspective. Those familiar with physiology will be able to insert the appropriate material into the framework provided; those unfamiliar with the subject need not do so here. The comprehensive integration of medical science that is eventually required can await another opportunity.

The position can be summarized by reference to our representative embryonic life form illustrated schematically in the following diagram (see Fig. 1). It is important to be reminded that the explanations that follow will range freely through all life forms from the single cell to the social unit, on the assumption that all manifest the same essential processes.

A body language

There are many places to start from. It is only a convenience to begin with the relationship of living things with events in the world around them. However, an essential requirement is that the organism should *perceive* what these are, and make appropriate *responses* to them. Even amoebas, as every schoolchild knows, will move away from acid dropped into their locality: they are in fact perceiving the presence of hydrogen ions, finding them harmful, and taking avoiding action. Conversely, the same amoebas will move towards light or in the direction of nutrient-rich fluids. The basis of this primal

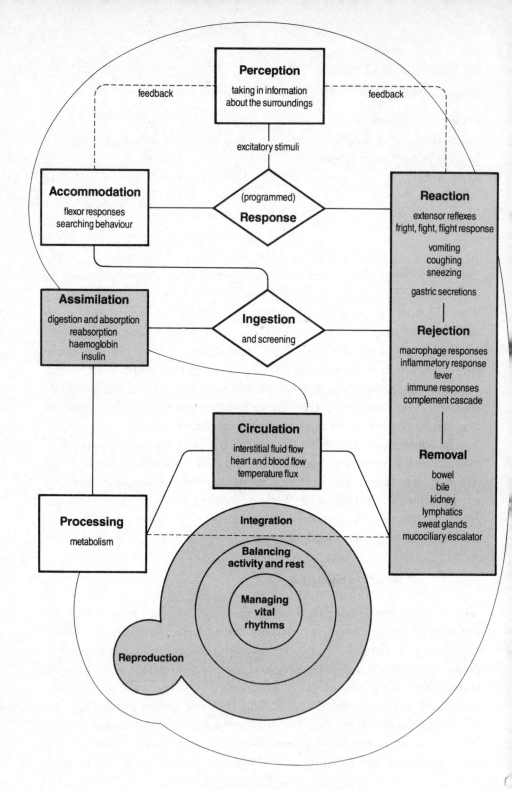

Fig. 1 Essential living processes

function is a sensory cell membrane, scaling up in complexity, but not in nature, to the higher senses of animals and humans.

The sensory device is linked to some form of effector mechanism, initially mediated by an intracellular enzyme change and leading either to contraction of cellular microfilaments or release of cellular secretions (such as neurotransmitters) and most obviously, to the complex neuromuscular apparatus that is the basis of all movement.

All these processes will be explored further in later pages, but before moving on it is important to note that the fact of perceiving and responding entails an immediate *discrimination*: a choice between what is helpful and what is potentially harmful. If the latter, avoidance responses (*reaction*) are invoked; if the former, there is *accommodation*: responses may include moving so close as to actually seek to incorporate the influence in some way. *Ingestion* thus becomes the next possibility.

Taking in external influences, whether they be food, fluid, oxygen or something less material like light or other cosmic radiations, entails a large element of risk. This is reduced by vigilant discrimination as already mentioned, but immediately after ingestion, a further process of selection is necessary. The result of this will determine what material is actually *assimilated* into the inner functions, and what is *rejected*.

Rejection at this level, which might be referred to as *secondary discrimination*, is most usefully seen in the physiological functions of higher creatures, from vomiting to the secretion of stomach acid and digestive enzymes (that sterilize and denature harmful material), through the activity of the phagocytes (the prowling scavenger/policing forces in the body fluids), the inflammatory processes, fever mechanism and as a back-up, the vast immune system. The role of these systems in maintaining the integrity of the organism will form a key part of the discussion of herbal treatment to follow.

The reciprocal process of *assimilation* is equally significant in the context of herbal therapeutics. In all traditional views of human health, vital energy is seen as arising from two sources. The first is one's inherited constitutional reserves with their catalytic potential, harboured in most traditions in the kidneys and gonads (a concept to be explored when we look at Chinese tradition), and the second is one's acquired energy, assimilated via the digestive system and via the lungs.

In this view, all growth, development, repair and the simple maintenance of vital functions depend on an efficient assimilation of energy and raw materials from outside. It is hardly a contentious idea. It does however imply that lack of energy, fatigue and debility arise as a result of demands on body reserves exceeding supplies. It also implies that convalescent strategies should concentrate on improving the efficiency of assimilation as the only practicable way of restoring vitality (the fact that debilitating illness is often marked by diminution in digestive and absorptive functions only supports the point). The herbal 'tonic' is a concept that needs scrutinizing: it will be seen that the notion of improving assimilation will be a key to explaining it.

Assimilation, of course, is a process that covers more than food and oxygen, or just conventional physiological entities. We shall see how such various phenomena as shopping at the supermarket, one's relationship with one's mother, sweet craving and the ability to give, to accept and to love are in human terms all equally part of the process.

External material that has been assimilated, and that has therefore passed successfully through the first two stages of discrimination, is then *processed*, to be rendered available for use by the organism. In physiological terms this encompasses the metabolic pathways explored in the science of biochemistry. It stretches to cover the processes of initial digestion, the breakdown of large molecules into smaller, more portable building blocks for new development. It includes those which we understand as liver functions, and the activities of the endoplasmic reticulum and microsomes in each individual cell. It is the all-pervasive process of making good of that which is assimilated.

Linked, as we shall see, with processing are the final two vegetative functions of *circulation* and *removal*:

Circulation covers the distribution of material and other energies around the organism, through diffusion and transpiration on the small scale, through to the massive hydraulic miracle of the circulatory system in mobile creatures. The minutiae of circulatory functions will provide an insight into some of the claims made for herbal remedies in a later section.

The process of *removal* is the final act of clearing up metabolic wastes and other debris remaining after cellular and tissue activity. It involves the eliminative functions of lymph, bile, bowel, kidney, lungs and sweat glands, and represents what to the traditional practitioner was the most accessible route to improving health in illness. Most herbal strategies began with the task of improving deficient eliminatory functions, and a majority of herbal remedies were classified in this way. In terms of what has gone before, the process of removal represents the third stage of rejection and resistance against undesirable influences that have either been internally generated, or found their way from outside after all.

Running through all these day-to-day processes there are essential co-ordinating and regulating functions without which they would be inconceivable. They represent a single spectrum of activity but for convenience they will be classified into three.

The first is hardly a function at all. *Managing vital rhythms* is a process intrinsic to all life forms. The very cell matter, its protoplasmic contents, is subjected to a tidal pulse of varying physical consistency and to repeating cycles of change in the structure of intracellular organelles. Its intracellular consistency is maintained in an age-old homoeostasis, at a life-generating tension relative to the fluids surrounding it, by a sodium pump. This is a mechanism pumping sodium ions out of the cell and potassium ions in, both against their relative concentration gradients, that proceeds constantly, using up to two-thirds of all the cell's energy, as long as there is life in the cell.

This essential vital pulse permeates upwards through higher forms. Every tissue is engaged in a tidal rhythm of function, alternating activity and rest. Every muscle cell maintains a constant background tone. This is a phenomenon best seen in the isolated heart muscle, where, if suitably nurtured, each part will contract at its own pace, without nervous impulse, for a considerable time. Spontaneous contractions of 'smooth muscle' cells also form the basis of the activity of the gut, so that, as we shall see, it runs essentially to its own tune, and the movement of material through it is largely automatic.

31   A Herbal Physiology

All these phenomena, and others, have been used to support the notion of a Vital Force, an essential vitality, in living things. One need not stray into philosophical debate to see them as evidence of an essential vital 'hum' that underpins all other living functions.

In therapeutic terms the obvious implication is that, like the Hippocratic physician, one learns to be humble in the face of *vis medicatrix naturae*, the healing power of life, and seeks only to help it on its way. Disturbances in vital rhythms, like arrhythmias, irritable bowel syndrome, insomnia, menstrual disorders and so on, are seen as indications for remedies that will relax excesses but leave essential vitality intact. There is an inbuilt caution about the whole concept of 'sedative' that will be developed here.

An immediate and linked manifestation of managing vital rhythms is the *balancing of activity and rest*, a function that involves in the animal, for example, switching between a resting and an exercising economy, between parasympathetic and sympathetic regulation, between arousal and resting, waking and sleeping. It includes the interesting concept of posture, of cerebellar and basal nuclear function in the central nervous system, the use of caffeine and Valium as drugs, and much more.

Providing an all-permeating influence through all else is the most complex process of all, that of *integration*. Closely connected to it, in a number of ways, is that of *reproduction*: the demanding function of perpetuating the life form through the generations.

As we develop these ideas it is hoped that the point of the exercise may emerge:

These processes can be understood, even felt, by anyone. They might thus once again form the basis of a common language allowing patient and physician to understand each other better.

They will certainly provide a better way to understand the potential benefits of herbal medicines.

Perception and Response

As 'no man is an island', so no living thing could conceivably prosper – apart from short periods of dormancy – without being able to interact closely with its environment. Its immediate surroundings provide both sustenance and potential danger. An ability to detect all meaningful events, to discriminate between them and to respond appropriately is essential to all life.

Perception

The cell membrane

In the individual cell, communication with external events is largely mediated by the extraordinary structure of the cell membrane. So thin that if the cell was the size of Earth it would be only three feet thick, it nevertheless maintains its integrity and successfully divides the environment inside the cell from that outside.

The internal cell environment is significantly different from external fluids. Cells in the body are bathed in fluid that is relatively high in sodium compared with potassium (similar in this way to sea-water). By contrast the interior of all cells is relatively higher in potassium. Since both ions diffuse freely through the semipermeable cell membrane, the difference in concentrations has to be maintained by continuous work: a constant pump pushing sodium ions out and potassium ions in and incidentally maintaining a vital electrical difference between inside and outside as well. The mechanism of this *sodium pump* is a type of protein molecule in the cell membrane, acting as both pump structure and its enzymatic catalyst.

Other proteins act as 'gates' or 'pores', either permitting small molecules, like water, oxygen and carbon dioxide, to diffuse through the membrane, or acting as carrier mechanisms for specific larger ones, such as nutrient building blocks like glucose and amino-acids.

This combination of electrical pump activity within, and selective passage through, cell membranes allows many cells to respond to certain stimuli with a self-propagating *electrical pulse*, the basis among other results of the nerve impulse and muscle contraction. In higher animals the senses of *touch*, *heat*, *cold* and *pain* arise as nerve impulses from specialized nerve structures whose cell membranes have been suitably provoked.

The membrane receptor

For larger molecules still, easy passage through the cell membrane is denied. Some, however, may have structures that can act as 'keys' to fit in 'locks' present on the surface of the cell membrane. These 'locks', also protein molecules, are called *receptors*. The cell membrane is covered with them. Each receptor is specific to certain structural shapes. If engaged, the structure of the receptor is itself changed ('the key has turned the lock') and acts as an enzyme to catalyse a reaction on the inside of the surface, inside the cell.

This reaction can lead to a change in the behaviour of the whole cell. It may be encouraged to induce contraction of filamentous structures, so changing the cell shape. This may eventually lead to the cell moving away from the stimulus (like the schoolchild's amoeba and its pseudopod), or moving towards and engulfing it as in phagocytosis.

More often it will activate genetic material to provide a different mix of enzymes or other agents, to thus change the internal functions of the cell, and possibly to package and secrete them into the fluid in turn. As some of the substances that triggered the receptor may have been produced by other cell secretions themselves, this provides a basis for *cell-to-cell communication*.

Smell – the first sense

Simple cells, like other aquatic organisms, are surrounded by a fluid environment. Their primal sense is their ability to respond to small quantities of substances in the water. The more complex organisms, like fishes, however, devolve their sensory surfaces to small areas on their bodies covered with specialized olfactory cells, cells particularly covered with receptors, whose responses are transmitted by nerve fibres to the controlling centres in the nervous system. Their size and complexity mitigate a general sensory surface but the ease of reception means that they lose nothing in acuity: the ability of sharks to trace the source of blood over many miles is not just something out of adventure stories.

In animals that no longer live in water, the opportunity to detect water-borne material is limited to a tiny pocket of fluid most often located at the top corner of the nasal cavity. Here inhaled air is drawn in and some of its constituents dissolved. Just as in the fish, specialized olfactory cells are found, particularly able to respond to different volatile principles. Again their responses are transferred to the central nervous system, so that the whole body can interpret them and react.

This sense of *smell* is still the most powerful of the senses in higher creatures and, although attenuated, even in humans. Similarly to the sense of touch it most simply elaborates the qualities of cellular perception. Unlike touch it maintains its direct links with central control. The olfactory lobe, the mass of nervous tissue that serves the olfactory cells, is actually an extension of the limbic system.

The limbic system is effectively a self-contained inner brain underlying and underpinning the cerebral cortex in the human, and the highest centre in more primitive forms of life. Within the human it acts with the hypothalamus as the seat of emotion and affect; it has been shown that a major role is to put experiences into context and give them meaning. It has been linked by some with the attainment of higher contemplative insights.

In aquatic creatures the sense of smell provides the essential capacity to differentiate vital changes in the environment. Clearly, this sensibility is a most direct affair, there being no need to conceptualize the sensation. Olfaction is thus not only the most primitive of all the senses, it has the most direct line to the higher centres; in short olfaction is the ability of an animal to *feel its environment directly*. Even in the human, the direct access to our deepest consciousness remains intact, and it is the case that a scent can still move directly, deeply, in a way that owes nothing to rationalization or conceptualization. The most direct of senses is still associated with that part of consciousness that provides the ability to make immediate experience meaningful.

The discovery that some aromatic constituents are found to have travelled through the olfactory system to lodge in parts of the limbic system[10] only reinforces the common experience that the sense of smell is both the most primitive and the most powerful of the higher sensations. It literally 'touches' us at our core.

In herbal medicine, especially in Mediterranean cultures, there is a common tradition of using *aromatic herbs* in ways that accentuate this quality, as, for example, with steaming decoctions and infusions for inhaling, and volatile oil preparations. The recently popular practice of aromatherapy, originating in France, has capitalized on the obvious attraction of using strong pleasant plant aromas in massage treatments and other applications. In addition, however, it has been claimed that these volatile oils can influence emotional states in predictable ways and they have been directed to that end. In a few cases there is some possible support for this claim (volatile oils have also been used internally for their powerful antiseptic and occasional anti-inflammatory properties – see later).

Taste

Almost as direct as the sense of smell is that of taste. This depends on the presence of four groups of specialized receptors in the mouth: different types of cells responding to various chemical constituents in food to register tastes of sweet, sour, bitter and salty. These cells connect to cranial nerves so that the message is passed to the lower levels of the brain.

As will be elaborated elsewhere (see 'Chinese Pharmacology', on pp. 183–94), a number of activities in the body are influenced by these messages, a fact of some significance to the herbalist.

Sight and sound

The higher senses of vision and hearing involve very complex nerve networks analysing and *making sense* of the data arising from the retina, and from the organs of Corti in the inner ear. Even this extraordinary perception originates, however, in a simple stimulation of cell membranes. Specialized cells in the retina generate electrical impulses on being stimulated by photons, the infinitesimally tiny 'packets' of light radiation. In the inner ear other cells respond to sound vibrations in their surrounding fluid like very sensitive touch receptors.

A common process

So far we have seen how even complex processes of perception share common underlying mechanisms in stimulation of the cell membrane. This is a convenient start. It illustrates the principle that such primal processes are common to all life.

It is not, however, a typical example. In others to follow the scaling up of the function from single cell to the human being will involve different mechanisms, and if psychological, emotional, or even spiritual processes are involved, different modalities as well. The principle pursued is rather that *the role and implications of each process are the same for all creatures.*

The development of the *theme* of perception, rather than just its literal continuity, may become clearer in looking at other aspects of the process in human beings.

Perception beyond the cell

The process of perception in human beings involves other physiological functions. It must include the transmission of messages from sensor to higher centres in the brain: the passage of impulses through the neural pathways running from sensory nerves in the body through the dorsal roots of the spinal cord, up through the brain stem to the thalamus, the reticular activating system, and the sensory cortex; the 'gate' and other selective mechanisms that begin the task of filtering out the sensory barrage and 'making sense' of it.

37   Perception and Response

The latter are particularly well developed in the 'higher senses', in which sensory input from eye and ear is passed through a series of analytic relay stations for progressive reconstruction, so that by the time it reaches the appropriate area of the cortex in the brain it has been processed to match the data patterns with templates that the brain can 'make sense of'.

Further relating these patterns of sensation to those of other senses and to previous experience so that they are put into context is another cortical function, carried out in so-called *association areas*. These also link to the limbic system and thus to the affective functions, the many hormones, neuropeptides and other humoral elements which are collated in the limbic system of the brain and perceived as *feeling* – the perception of the inner state. This in turn affects what we 'see' externally, what sense is made of our perceptions.

Also to be included as part of the perception process are its fine mechanics, the *nerve fibres*, and the *synapses* and *neurotransmitters* that separate and connect them and provide the basis for the sorting and analysis of messages. The central nervous system is a vast data-processing network with each of the millions of neural fibres entering a plexus of other fibres, collateral branches and interneural connections. By selective use of excitatory and in-hibitory neurotransmitters at the synapses between the fibres an elaborate system of check and counter-check is set up. As the nervous system scales in complexity, assessment scales into *memory* and *learning*: each sensory input can be graded against precedent, evaluated, prioritized, and the whole result stored for better co-ordination the next time.

Intelligence

This discussion of perception is followed by a look at the process of response. This reflects an obvious linkage in all organisms: one makes sense of one's surroundings so that one can then respond to changes and gain advantage from them as far as possible, by either moving in on some useful feature or taking evasive action. It means, of course, that perception must involve an immediate *discrimination*, a distinction made between good and ill.

The mysterious concept of *intelligence* must now be invoked. All living things, even the most simple, can figure their world out to some extent. Their survival in their habitat depends on it. The ability to succeed in life is dependent on the ability to make sense of the maximum range of vagaries, to adapt.

This ability to choose the right survival options is incidentally irrelevant of size and sophistication. A complex nervous system means that more complex analyses of incoming data can be made – the overall intelligence activity is greater – but this complexity is very often tied to a more sophisticated piece of machinery that limits the scope for making real choices. The tiger and the dolphin have both boxed themselves into a corner; by contrast the humble rat and sparrow have kept more options open, the insects and scorpions will survive a nuclear or 'greenhouse' Armageddon and the blue-green algae have made better sense of their environment and thus prospered longer than any other life form!

The ability to adapt will be discussed at the end of this review of physiology as part of the process of integration, but it may already be possible to see that *the capacity to discriminate is the rationale for perception*, and that this capacity is *an essential aspect of the organism's identity*.

Response

The reflex

Such considerations clearly also underpin the way that the organism responds to its sensory input. At the cellular level the response to stimuli affecting the cell membrane can include electrical pulses and enzymatic activity. The first can lead in turn to stimulation of contractile elements in the cell so that the cell moves, contracts or squeezes a sac of secretory material back out through the cell membrane. The second can change cell behaviour in any number of other ways.

In the larger animal such responses can lead to neural conduction, to muscle contraction, to the release of neurotransmitters, hormones or other chemical communications between cells. The behaviour of the creature is altered, whether through observable action or through internal metabolic changes.

The nature of the response is interesting. Because the organism acts as an integrated whole its reactions to events are also co-ordinated. *Responses are not arbitrary or haphazard; they occur in organized patterns.* Even a cell's response to a stimulus, like fibril contraction or enzyme secretion, is an intricate performance that must not become unco-ordinated; the simple knee-jerk reflex is even more so.

Most are familiar with the story of Pavlov and his unfortunate dogs who were observed to salivate at the thought of food as much as at its materialization. He trained them to link a dinner bell with the expectation of food, thus evoking what he termed a 'conditioned reflex', in contrast to the 'unconditioned reflex' that has all dogs (and other mammals) secreting digestive juices when they eat. What Pavlov did was to change the trigger for digestive activity; he did nothing at all to affect the pattern of response itself. The perception had changed, the marvellously complex programme of events that followed had not.

The closer one looks at reflex responses the more it is apparent that all involve such complexity and that most seem programmed before, at, or soon after, birth. Conditioned reflexes, as with Pavlov's dogs, are most often elaborations of previous unconditioned reflexes.

The healing reflex

The programmed reflex is of fundamental therapeutic importance.

Most alternatives to conventional modern medical technology emphasize their role in helping the body's own recuperative powers. In essence they seek to trigger healing responses rather than control any particular physiological function directly. One obvious such trigger is the acupuncture point (which loses some of its mystery if seen in this light), but there are other such principles in much of osteopathy, chiropractic and therapeutic massage, and, to the extent that words and thoughts are triggers, in psychotherapy.

It is certainly a principle in herbal medicine. Many remedies are provocative in action, leading to a range of potentially useful responses. A clear example is the bitter remedy, switching on the upper digestive system almost entirely through stimulating taste buds in the mouth. Other examples include the acrid remedies, the emetics and sub-emetic expectorants, the stimulating laxatives, the mucilages and tannins, the volatile oils and carminatives. Most of these, as shall be illustrated later, act as triggers on the gut wall. It is the 'perception' of this highly sensory structure that is involved: the reflex response in gut, lung, liver, bladder function or blood circulation is already programmed in.

There is in all this an implicit *trust* that innate responses effect healing more than any man-made intervention, a respect for Hippocrates' healing power of life, *vis medicatrix naturae*.

This remedial approach is in stark contrast to the effects of most conventional strategies. The antibiotic, anti-inflammatory, anti-thrombotic, hypotensive, analgesic and sedative, among others, all act directly on their target function, with little regard for the rest of the physiology. A possible fundamental cause of side-effects is this disregard for the vital domain. The side-effects of herbal remedies usually involve excessive or inappropriate stimulation of reflex responses (e.g. more bowel or bladder excretion, intestinal colic, nausea), these being at once more obvious and, except in the very debilitated, less damaging.

> **Proposition:**
> **most herbal remedies contain constituents that provoke reflex reaction from the gut wall; this is an essential factor in explaining the effects of herbs on the body.**

Choice

In general living beings have two types of response. The stimulus may be perceived as potentially harmful, necessitating avoiding action, *reaction*; or as potentially beneficial, as useful to the organism, in which case it will *accommodate* it.

Both types of response involve either innate unconditioned reflexes or acquired, conditioned reflexes that result from an organism learning from its experiences. In either case there is a basic choice, a process of discrimination, involved. It is an abiding feature of life that this choice is exercised: it is more than just simple flow dynamics, following the path of least resistance, to which all material is subject. Living things have the power to transcend physical forces to a degree, to move against the current of gravity, to fuse with other matter or to repel it, to resist entropy, and eventually to divide and replicate. Each such response involves constant decision between at least two responses to every change in circumstances. This is one of life's mysteries.

Reaction

A reactive response can take many forms. In all organisms a simple reaction to a stimulus is to move away, and aversion behaviour is very speedy if necessary or appropriate (the reflex involved in withdrawing a limb from pain is a good example). In the human being overt reactive responses of this type include such flexion reflexes and, on a broader scale, the sympathetic response that mobilizes adrenaline and extraordinary muscle power to get out of trouble fast. However, within the body, reaction often has to take different forms – most cells and tissues have to stay *in situ*. Reactive responses may thus include secretion of bacteriostatic substances and interferon and its like, the production of saliva and particularly gastric secretions, the function of the mucociliary escalator that keeps the lungs clean, and the cough. Failure at the immediate portals of entry might well involve a signal to call in the phagocytes, or even lymphocytes to produce certain antibodies (notably of the IgE, IgA and IgD classes). However, these responses and those connected with them, like inflammation and fever, are generally reserved for deeper penetration of pathogenic influences and will be referred to later.

The therapeutic implication of all this is that *immediate aversion to harmful influences is much better than letting them penetrate.* Any remedial measure that can improve the capacity of the body to take quick evasive action, that *enhances its primary defences*, is to be preferred. This is a persistent theme in traditional herbal therapeutics and in this text.

There are herbal strategies that increase upper digestive secretions (the *bitter* and *sour* remedies, and the *aromatic digestives*), the action of the mucociliary escalator and the productivity of the cough (the *expectorants*) and the phagocyte response (the *volatile oils* and *resins*). There are also strategies to shore up the mechanical defences of skin and mucosa (such as the *tannins* and other *astringents*), and these will be discussed in full later.

Accommodation

Accommodative responses steer the organism towards the stimulus for its potential enhancing effects. All photosynthesizing green plants and algae, as well as most other creatures, will move towards light; aquatic organisms will move towards sources of oxygen (unless they are anaerobic, in which case oxygen will provoke reactive responses). All creatures will gravitate towards sources of nourishment. Any behaviour that leads towards the *ingestion* of food comes under the category of accommodative response. In the case of the cell this involves either diffusion through the cell membrane or its pores, or phagocytosis or pinocytosis, the invagination of the cell to envelop solid or fluid material respectively. (Although phagocytes are involved in the body's reactive response, their own behaviour is accommodative.)

In a complex creature like a human being accommodative responses include all feeding and food-searching behaviour, up to and including shopping at the supermarket and choosing a restaurant; they also include orienting towards light, heat, sunshine, refreshment, company, affection, love, music, bright lights and laughter. All these phenomena are linked by the fact that they lead to an increase in the accommodation of new stimuli.

There might be the suggestion that in some ways the reactive responses are more vigorous than the accommodative. This could be a consequence of living in an affluent society, where food and nurture are less threatened. Observations of other creatures and even of humans in more natural environments show clearly that accommodative responses are very vigorous indeed, perhaps symbolized by the powerful grasping of a suckling infant: taking in that which is essential for life is not a passive process.

Most of this, however, is a prelude to the discussion of the next process, *assimilation*, and it will be elaborated further there.

Summary

The process of perception, the registering of information about the surroundings, and the choice and commission of the appropriate response include aspects of such cellular and human physiology as:

cell membrane receptors
the synapse – inhibitory and excitatory neurotransmitters
nerve and muscle
motor control – the cerebellum and basal ganglia
smell and taste and the limbic system
the tactile senses
hearing and vision
sensory associations – thought and feeling
pain
the reflex patterned response
learning and memory
communication

Assimilation and Rejection

Taking in – cautiously

The process of *assimilation* is the making good of the ingestion of foreign influence or material.

In the energetic perspectives of Eastern medicine acquired energy (as opposed to the constitutional energy harboured in the 'kidneys' or gonads) arises from two sources, the essence of inspired air through the lungs (*prana* or *ta qi*) and the essence of food distilled by the 'spleen' (*gu qi*). Linking the spleen with digestion sounds like lousy anatomy, but ancients were doubtlessly aware that the spleen is only palpable in certain serious digestive disorders, notably those which we now know as liver diseases.

In these terms the availability of acquired, nutrient energies depends on an effective process of assimilation. In modern Western terms this process is implicit in the functions of the digestive system and liver, and in the blood in the lungs. It is also likely, given the wide remit of this review, that assimilation will be found to underpin other aspects of cellular function and human behaviour.

Assimilation is also coupled with an extended, and more powerful, form of the reactive process discussed earlier, termed *rejection* for the purpose of this text. It is as though continued vigilance is necessary to monitor the value of that which has been allowed to slip into the organism. The defence functions, like inflammation, fever response, and the phagocyte and immune system are included within this role; it is particularly associated with the surveillance of food. We now realize how many challenges ordinary food contains, including pathogenic organisms, undesirable chemical constituents, both natural and synthetic, and the potentially immunological challenge of whole protein and other large food molecules. An ability to reject that which may yet prove to be harmful is essential. In practice it is difficult to demarcate between rejection and the processes of *reaction* referred to earlier, a point reflected in the design of Fig. 1, on p. 28. Some of what follows could also be thought of as reactive responses.

Digestion

The physiological processes of both assimilation and rejection, at the cellular level and beyond, start in the action of the *digestive secretions*. These are enzymes with the effect of splitting large organic molecules and rendering them into smaller components, like simple sugars, and amino and fatty acids, that are more readily absorbed and used. In the cell these enzymes are contained, in the form of benign precursors, in specialized vacuoles called lysosomes.

In the larger body like the human body they are produced by cells in the lining of the stomach and upper alimentary canal, and in the pancreas. The more powerful enzymes at least are also stored in precursor forms: in general they are not converted into their formidable destructive version until safely in the lumen of the gut. This is an astonishing feat – the cell produces within itself substances that could dissolve its own contents, yet manages to find ways of protecting itself from auto-digestion. (In fact, cells regularly auto-destruct when they reach the end of their healthy lifespan, a phenomenon of importance to what follows.)

As a result of successful digestion, food is largely converted into safe, useful pabulum. However, this is only the beginning of the process. It has then to be assimilated into the body.

Assimilation

Absorption

Many small molecules, like water and the simple solutes, especially if these are fat-soluble, pass readily enough through the semi-permeable cell membrane, by *simple diffusion*. All that is required is a concentration gradient and they will move from one fluid to the other without any energy being needed by the cells involved. Other materials however, notably glucose, the simple sugars and the amino-acids, are not intrinsically absorbable. Energy needs to be expended and specialist *carrier mechanisms* provided to transfer them across the intestinal wall into the circulation, and from the circulation into the destination cell. This energy may be completely essential (*active transfer*) or partially so (*facilitated diffusion*).

The energy-consuming carrier mechanisms are an intrinsic part of the process of assimilation and the presence and efficiency of their components are an important measure of the health of the process.

The mechanism is often linked to the sodium pump that maintains the electrolytic difference between cells and their surroundings, and the fluid integrity of the tissues themselves. It is remarkable therefore that in Chinese medicine the same function, the *Spleen*, (see 'A Traditional Physiology', on pp. 618–19) is seen to be responsible for assimilation and for maintaining the shape of the tissues, as well as the integrity of the circulation of fluids and *qi*.

Glucose

Other factors play their part in the assimilative process. There are several humoral influences on the availability to the tissues of key nutrients. The major unit of nutrient currency is glucose, used widely as a raw material of calorific energy by the body's tissues and as the sole such source by the nervous tissues and some others. Many of the body's hormones affect the rate of uptake of glucose from and supply to the blood circulation. Notable is *insulin*, whose production by the pancreas is largely in response to raised glucose levels in the blood, and whose major effect is to increase the entry of glucose into the cells, especially the glucose stores of fat, liver and muscle cell.

If there is too little insulin, glucose cannot easily be absorbed into tissues, it banks up in the blood and spills over into the urine: the result is diabetes mellitus. If insulin is relatively excessive in its response (perhaps because glucose levels rise too fast as in a diet of refined carbohydrates like sugar and white flour), then low blood-sugar levels may result (reactive hypoglycaemia). Either event is a disorder of assimilation in the context of this discussion and *its treatment will be found to link with treatments of other such disorders.*

Many other hormones influence blood-sugar levels, but most act to mobilize reserves from the tissue, and are thus hyperglycaemic. They have less relevance to the topic of assimilation except in as much as they compensate for that action of insulin. Glucagon, growth hormone and the stress hormones produced by the adrenal cortex are notable in their contribution to the overall balance of blood-sugar levels.

Fats

Another area of interest is the fascinating story of fat assimilation. Although fats, or lipids, dissolve through cell membranes and are thus absorbed entirely by simple diffusion, they are of course moving through the body in a watery (aqueous) environment. Fat and water mix no better in the body than they do anywhere else, so elaborate mechanisms are invoked to facilitate their transfer to the body's tissues. Various emulsifying strategies are adopted, using cholesterol and lecithins to form complexes with the lipids. After the fat is absorbed in crude emulsion (with the bile) from the gut, these complexes are formed in the liver and act to carry the fats safely round the body. As the fats are taken up by the tissues the complexes become increasingly cholesterol-, and then protein-rich, moving from what are termed very-low-density lipoproteins (VLDLs) through to LDLs and to high-density-lipoproteins (HDLs). The relative quantity of the latter in the blood is a fair measure of the efficiency with which fat transfer has occurred and is thus a positive factor in the prevention of fat deposition in the blood vessels, arteriosclerosis and other cardiovascular diseases.

The ability of the body both to produce appropriate levels of cholesterol and the lecithins, and to successfully reduce the relative concentrations of VLDLs and LDLs is an important part of good assimilation. Disorders in the mechanism, perhaps provoked by excessive fat, alcohol or carbohydrate consumption and inadequate exercise, can likewise be considered as part of a greater assimilative disorder, referred to later.

The liver

The role of the liver in assimilation should be emphasized. It acts as a gateway through which portal blood draining the digestive system is introduced to the rest of the body. All such blood actually percolates through the liver cells and is subjected to initial preparation by them (see 'Processing', on pp. 80–85). Nutrient material is rendered down to be more suitable for assimilation and utilization by the tissues. The liver's secretion, bile, is an emulsifier, essential for the assimilation of fats from the gut, and also contains ingredients that affect digestion and assimilation in the lower intestines. Disorders in liver function have significant effects on assimilation in the wider context. They are one possible problem the herbalist looks closely for, especially given the increased toxic and nutrient load the organ has so often to bear.

Minerals

An immediate concern in discussing assimilation is the degree of absorption of certain nutrients, notably the relatively insoluble mineral ions like iron, calcium and zinc. These are at best only partially assimilated (in the case of iron about 90 per cent of that found in food passes unabsorbed through the gut). Rates of absorption are often determined by the type of food present in the gut at the time and by the types of complexes formed by the minerals. Most are chelated in more readily absorbable complexes when provided in the form of animal tissues or products (like eggs and dairy foods). Conversely, certain cereal carbohydrates, notably complexes of phytic acid, tend to bind such minerals in unassimilable forms. For those adjusted to a high-cereal diet, bacteria in the bowel usually produce enzymes and phytases that split the phytate complexes, so absorption of minerals is less of a problem. However, for those new to wholemeal cereal consumption there is a significant risk of mineral deficiency. They join those with intestinal disease, pernicious anaemia and other causes of malabsorption, as requiring help in assimilating minerals.

Vitamins

The problem is intrinsically less likely to occur with vitamins, most of which, if present in the diet, are readily absorbed. There is, however, a notable problem affecting fat-soluble vitamins (vitamins A, D, E and K) and all other lipids: intestinal damage resulting from damage by the cereal protein gluten in those who are sensitive to it. Coeliac disease and sprue, for centuries undiagnosed and often fatal, can be treated by the elimination of wheat, oats, rye and barley from the diet. The classic symptoms of the disease start with the appearance of undigested fat in the stool (steatorrhoea): the peptide fragment of gluten, α-gliadin, which is actually always slightly irritating to the intestinal wall, leads to severe damage in those who are allergic to it. The damage particularly affects the lymphatic absorption mechanism for fats and lipid-soluble substances.

Reabsorption

A further aspect of assimilation is provided by the various forms of reabsorption that occur in the body. This usually involves the excretory channels and the retrieval from the initial elimination of water and solutes that the body needs to retain. The major examples are in the bowel, the tubules of the kidney, the sweat glands and the gall-bladder. Lipid-soluble materials usually move back and forth on the principle of simple diffusion, i.e. down concentration gradients. Sodium, potassium, calcium, the amino-acids and glucose are among many solutes that need a form of active transfer for their reabsorption. Water is primarily retained on the back of sodium reabsorption, but, in fact, water follows all reabsorbed solutes through osmotic pressure. Reabsorption can thus be thought of as *secondary assimilation*, but an aspect quantitatively at least as important as the original. There will be clinical advantages in linking the two phenomena as well.

The desire for assimilation

Assimilation also has its behavioural and its uniquely human aspect. In early thought the archetypal nutrient was widely considered to be mother's milk: warm, easily assimilable and *sweet* pabulum. In Chinese medicine, at least, sweetness was a metaphor for nourishment. It is important to recall that sweetness to our forebears was not the sweetness of sugar, and that only very rarely would honey have been consumed (the land flowing with milk and honey was the biblical version of heaven on earth).

To the ancients sweetness was the natural sweetness of cereals, vegetables (e.g. cooked carrots, peas and parsnips) and fruit, in other words the main components of their diet. Sweetness was food, and the search for sweetness was the effective corollary for the need for nourishment.

In such a context the human preoccupation with sweetness has a new perspective. The Chinese view was that although sweetness was nourishing, and intrinsically tonifying and supportive of homoeostatic balance, excessive sweetness was dangerous, damaging the roots of the constitution (the *kidneys*) and leading to premature ageing. The modern orgy of consumption of sugar and refined carbohydrates followed industrialization of food production a hundred years ago. From that time sugar ceased to be an expensive spice (the provender of the rich only) and the populace could get off their rough diet of wholemeal bread. Since then, recourse to such easy nourishment, the infantile love of the sweet, has been widespread. In developed countries consumption of refined carbohydrates has reached astonishing levels. The symptoms predicted by the Chinese are, coincidentally or otherwise, also prominent. In the context of human history this development can only be seen as a disorder.

It is also a disorder of assimilation. Having undue recourse to such instant nourishment distorts and undermines the normal demanding and complex processes of assimilation. Some recognized consequences of this distortion, like diabetes and reactive hypoglycaemia, and cholesterol and lipid disorders (which include obesity), have already been touched on. More widely, a bias towards excessive sweetness, implicitly predicted by the ancients as a consequence of an alienation from the mother lode, the wider family and *the earth itself*, draws its own connotations. The title of this book may serve as a metaphor for the ultimate need to return to this broader base of health.

The traditional herbal view

The main focus of activity for herbal remedies in the human body is the digestive system, so it is not surprising that questions of assimilation are high on the herbalist's therapeutic agenda. There are many remedies used to affect the process but they mostly fall into two main categories, the 'cooling and drying' *bitters* and the 'warming and drying' *aromatic digestives*, chosen according to the wider needs of the body.

The emphasis on drying is interesting. In Chinese physiology the function of the *Spleen* is particularly vulnerable to 'damp', a quality described later in this text but essentially similar to the naturopathic concept of *catarrh*: a congestion, an accumulation of toxicity, a sluggish flow. Most assimilative disorders were seen in the past to be associated either with a phlegmatic 'cold-damp' disorder (with congestive dyspepsia, lack of appetite, bloating and retention after eating and other signs discussed later); or with 'damp-heat', approximating to Western notions of liver strain or disease (with intolerance to fats and alcohol, biliary disorders, associated lack of appetite and bowel irregularities and other signs of 'heat' and 'damp'). There will be opportunities later in this text to see how modern insights into the action of herbal remedies and these primitive therapeutic concepts have a bearing on some of the details of assimilative disorders discussed earlier.

The lungs

Assimilation also occurs in the very different context of oxygenated blood. Aerated blood leaving the lungs is saturated with oxygen well beyond its ability as a fluid to dissolve it. The secret of its extraordinary capacity is the presence of *haemoglobin* in the red corpuscles. Haemoglobin, a porphyrin molecule, like the equally pivotal *chlorophyll* in plants, has the unusual property of taking in oxygen molecules when there are a lot of them around, and letting them go when there are not. It incidentally does the same with carbon dioxide on the return journey. It enables a relatively small blood circulation to provide sufficient oxygen for a very large mass of active tissue. (One only needs to think of the elephant to see how much! The somewhat less demanding tissues of cold-blooded creatures like fish, lizards and dinosaurs are serviced by a similar porphyrin, haemocyanin.)

The assimilation of oxygen is less vulnerable to functional variation. However, lack of haemoglobin, anaemia, or damage to the aerating surface, lung disease, can reduce the ability of the body to assimilate sufficient oxygen. Similarly, interference in circulation such as arteriosclerosis or other vascular disease can hamper the assimilation of oxygen at the tissues.

In many such disorders remedies are chosen that are warming *circulatory stimulants* or *peripheral vasodilators*, though anaemia will also dictate nutritional treatments. Pathological lung damage is not treatable although obstructive disorders can sometimes be mitigated by the warming *expectorants* (sometimes the same remedies as the circulatory stimulants), and other pulmonary remedies.

Rejection

The precautions that the living being takes against damage from ingested material are astonishingly powerful. By their very nature they have to be carefully constrained and in ill health can readily lead to damage.

The symptoms of many conventional diseases are in fact rejective mechanisms, either working vigorously, or malfunctioning. One of the most important diagnostic requirements for the herbal practitioner and for others concerned to help rather than attack the body, is to differentiate between the two.

The importance of the subject justifies a closer look at its main features, even if some of the following material appears rather technical.

INFECTION

Bugs and germs

Herbalists do not on the whole now claim to have pre-eminence in the treatment of infections. There are two main reasons for this.

The first is that herbal antibiotics are less active than their conventional counterparts. There are many plant constituents with antiseptic action, notably volatile oils and some phenol derivatives, but in practice such effects are relatively mild.

Most direct antiseptic action follows the topical application of resinous plant tinctures like myrrh (*Commiphora mol-mol*) and marigold flowers (*Calendula officinalis*), preparations with volatile oils (such as those of thyme), and strong tannin decoctions. These have potential benefits for infections of the mouth, throat and upper digestive tract, and tannins can disinfect open wounds.

Several plants contain constituents that are antifungal, amoebicidal and anthelmintic (destroying worms), and they have been used in the past as vigorous treatments for worm and amoebic gut infections (see the chapter 'Traditional Pharmacology', and 'Alteratives' on p. 486 for more information on all these). Such heroic measures are now less suitable for gentle society.

Two other remedies, garlic (*Allium sativum*) and echinacea (*Echinacea angustifolia*), have genuinely systemic antibiotic-like activities, and both are discussed at length in Part II, but even their effects are more complex than that. This point will become clearer below.

The second reason for reducing an emphasis on infection is that the herbalist arises from a tradition that sees the role of the germ as rather less important than it is seen by most in modern times. It is easy to conclude that herbalists might have little choice, or that they hark back to a less enlightened age, but the principles involved are important to this discussion.

The fungus on the forest floor

There is an ecological view of bacteria, viruses and other disease-causing organisms that is rarely explored. In any balanced eco-system all living things have to find a niche that fits with the whole.

here is only temporary room for any organism that runs rampant through the biosphere: such a creature would find itself cutting its life-support. Plagues of aphids or locusts quickly burn themselves out as they strip their food supply and destroy their habitat. The human species, allowing for a longer generation time, shows disturbing signs of a similar cataclysmic population disruption.

It is almost inconceivable that bacterial populations, potentially doubling every twenty minutes or so, multiplying a millionfold every five or six hours, could survive at all if they were not held in severe check by their environment. If their effect was to destroy their host then these checks have to be even more stringent: it does not further any organism to destroy its residence.

Even more important than the rather negative factor of stepping warily through life to avoid spoiling one's chances is the positive role every organism must have in order to play its part in the ecosystem. There is in nature no room for passengers or free-loaders. All actions have their consequences and their implications for the whole ecosystem. Every creature is part of a food cycle; every excretion, every demise, creates a source of nutrients for some other organism; every act of predation creates an opportunity for more of the prey to fill the gap.

Thus, all bacteria, fungi, viruses, every form of mosquito, fly and other pest, must have their positive roles in the balance of life. An attitude that says that any of these life forms is always evil, always to be attacked, is as unimaginative and counter-productive as any jingoistic nationalism.

What possible role can a pathogenic organism have? One image used by naturopathic practitioners is the fungus on the forest floor. As trees die and fall they leave large carcasses of relatively tough wood that would potentially litter the forest floor; the mineral and other nutrients that they contain would be locked up and unobtainable for other plants; life would be choked off. It is thus essential that organisms exist that act to rot hard wooden logs. Fungi and wood-boring insects between them can recirculate the material in a dead tree and bring it back into the ecocycle. They may marginally affect, but they do not damage, healthy living trees. Their survival depends on finding dead wood; the forest's survival also depends on them doing so.

Such organisms are termed 'saprophytic'. The naturopathic view is that most so-called pathogens are in fact saprophytes. Germs do not arrive 'out of the blue' to strike down an unwary victim. Rather, they exploit a gap in the tissues and colonize only where there is tissue unhealthy enough to provide them with nourishment. Having arrived they actually produce benefits! To illustrate such a puzzling conclusion let us look at one example.

The common cold is the cause of considerable misery. Searches for its cure are like searches for the Holy Grail. Much is known about the rhinoviruses, coxsackieviruses, coronaviruses and paramyxoviruses that cause the condition, but anti-infective treatments are hampered by the fact that they shift their characteristics almost endlessly. Antibiotics, of course, have no effect on any viral infections.† The judgement is almost universal: these viruses are bad and should be attacked and resisted at all costs.

It may be, however, that they have a beneficial role. It is an obvious point that not everyone catches colds that pass around a group. The lucky ones may be blessed with an alert and primed immune system, or, just as likely, with a healthy and vigorous respiratory mucous membrane (and mucociliary escalator – see 'The Respiratory System', on pp. 114–17). Either way, those that are not lucky, for whatever reason, do not have such a healthy defence and may need both informing of that fact and a chance to correct the situation.

The common cold can be seen as an excellent alerting mechanism. It precipitates both inflammatory and febrile responses that in most cases are resolved completely, with protection against further colds that lasts for several months or even years (see 'Inflammation', on pp. 58–63 and 'Fever', on pp. 63–7). At the very least it

---

† This does not stop many doctors trying. In an extraordinary comment on a survey that showed that fewer than half the patients in Britain trust that their doctor knows what is wrong with them the spokesman for the 32,000 general practitioner members of the British Medical Association was reported as saying: *'If I am prescribing antibiotics for somebody with flu, I will tell them to complete the full course, but I would not launch into an explanation of how the medicine affects the bacteria. I don't think patients want that level of information.'* (Durham, M. and Rafferty, F., *Sunday Times*, 10 Dec. 1989). Flu is of course a viral infection, a fact highlighted by the headlines on the current flu epidemic on the same front page!

acts as a forcible reminder that one's health at the time is not something to be taken for granted!

The balance of odds

There are, of course, always exceptions to such a benign course, and there will always be casualties. It may be that the role of medicine is to protect those that are genuinely vulnerable to infections and are likely to be more severely harmed by them. It would be quite irresponsible to discount the need for antibiotics (where appropriate), or for vaccinations against dangerous infections for those vulnerable to them.

But the main point is that there are no rampant killer germs ravaging humankind. For every infectious disease it is possible to follow a route of intrusion that shows that at all stages there is a balance between host and pathogen. Respiratory infections tend to be associated with conditions that adversely affect the health of the airways; most cases of polio are simply diagnosed as influenza and only 10 per cent go on to become systemic infection; the cholera vibrio can barely survive a healthy stomach secretion, and this is a formidable defence against most other stomach 'bugs'. The majority of infectious disease today, as in the past, is associated with conditions of environmental or social adversity. Even Aids, for all the suburban alarm that greeted its arrival, and while still a most serious prospect for humankind, has, after its initial attacks, turned out to be a disease most at home among the urban and Third World deprived.

In gardening terms, the soil is at least as important as the seed. A healthy body coexists quite comfortably with a host of pathogenic organisms, on the skin, or in the mouth or gut. Although Pasteur did the world a great favour in isolating the germ as a causative factor in disease, and thus cleared a vast backlog of medieval medical malpractice, he himself always recognized that germs were never the sole problem (and is reported as saying so on his deathbed). It was only his successors that encouraged that view.

The herbal approach to infections

A herbal approach to infectious diseases can thus be glimpsed. The first step is to assess the extent and severity of infection. In a proportion of acute infections a treatment with conventional antibiotics will be the only choice. In the majority of cases, however, the condition is relatively mild and self-limiting, or involves viral infection and thus cannot be treated with antibiotics. Here first principles of nursing care, bedrest and fever management are still the most appropriate techniques. The herbal prescription might be to service a fever management, or might attempt in other specific ways to improve body defences (see 'The Immune System', on pp. 67–79).

For chronic infections the potential benefit of conservative and supportive measures is even more clear. As most chronic infections involve 'slow' viruses, antipathogenic measures are almost completely useless. Every emphasis is on encouraging a more robust defence of the body using techniques that are elaborated further below, when discussing inflammatory and immunological diseases.

Herbal remedies that have a particular reputation in supporting these defensive measures include echinacea and wild indigo (*Baptisia tinctoria*) from North America, and garlic.

INFLAMMATION

Definition

Inflammation is the response of living tissue to injury. It involves a relatively predictable sequence of changes first classified by Celsus, a writer from the time of Christ, as *rubor, tumor, calor* and *dolor* (redness, swelling, heat and pain). If the injury is containable, the end result is healing, either resolution or repair.

The initial stages of inflammation are as follows:

1 dilation of blood vessels in the area with consequent greatly increased blood flow (*rubor, calor*);

2 increased permeability of the capillaries in the area allowing fluid, or exudate, to leak into the tissues (*tumor*);

3 migration of leucocytes (and later macrophages) through the leaky capillary wall into the tissues.

All these stages, along with the associated pain (*dolor*), are brought about by the activity of chemical mediators of inflammation, including histamine, bradykinin, complement, plasmin and the prostaglandins and leukotrienes.

The total effect is to lead to the breakdown of damaged tissue and foreign material with sufficient pain and immobility, so that the area is protected by the body from further damage. If this is completely successful, resolution can occur: buds of regenerating blood vessels and other replacement tissues move into the site and healing is eventually completed. If regeneration is not adequate to seal the wound, then a fibrous plug is also formed and a scar results.

Chronic inflammation

If, on the other hand, regeneration cannot keep pace with the rate of damage, the inflammation becomes chronic, and inflammatory and repair processes occur simultaneously. The inflammation becomes increasingly counter-productive. Such a scenario can result from:

1 persistence of some foreign material at the site (the 'foreign body reaction'), such as dirt, chemicals, metabolites (like uric acid), insoluble particles like silica and asbestos, or accident debris, shrapnel, etc.;

2 infection by certain pathogens, notably tuberculosis, syphilis, brucellosis and leprosy, where phagocytic activity is compromised and hypersensitivity develops to persistent antigens;

3 autoimmune diseases, also marked by hypersensitivity to persistent antigens, in this case intracellular protein.

Specific examples of chronic inflammation include chronic suppuration, where a fibrous capsule or foreign material prevents healing of an abscess and extended fibrous scarring results (examples are osteomyelitis and empyema, in the bones and lungs lining respectively), and chronic ulceration, such as is seen in stomach, duodenum, or following severe varicose veins.

In all cases of chronic inflammation there is a shift in the population of phagocytes. The neutrophil leucocytes that are the first on the scene and are largely responsible for resolving acute inflammation are progressively replaced by macrophages, and also by eosinophil leucocytes and, often, lymphocytes as well. The macrophages can coalesce to form 'giant cells', when phagocytic demands are high, to such an extent that they can be visible to the naked eye as granulomas, such as in tuberculosis (the 'tubercle'), sarcoidosis, brucellosis and leprosy.

Most cases of chronic inflammation are not as dramatic as some of the examples described. *The condition is in fact very common.* Any condition whose name ends in '-itis' is one theoretically marked by inflammation, either acute or chronic. Chronic versions of arthritis, bronchitis, sinusitis, pharyngitis, rhinitis, colitis, gastritis, hepatitis, dermatitis, and so on, provide the most common problems in clinical medicine. Their acute versions, and such other examples as appendicitis and peritonitis, are a very common cause of emergency medical treatment.

All this leads to a fundamental issue differentiating conventional medicine from its traditional origins, including herbal medicine.

Inflammation – good and bad

The modern physician is primarily concerned with treating '-itises' and their unpleasant sequelae. His or her orientation to matters pathological will in any case mean a preoccupation with any causative pathogen and with the details of the damage done. In short, *inflammation is a problem*, it is 'the backbone of pathology'.

In traditional herbal medicine by contrast, *inflammation is an opportunity*. It is a sign that the body has recognized a problem and is engaging it. It is a call for support of the active participants in inflammation, those mediators responsible for increasing blood flow and the phagocytes responsible for resolving the damage. It is a recognition that the body is mobilizing forces that are otherwise dormant and thus providing a new opportunity to resolve what is possibly a long-standing malady.

The two approaches each have their place. Where inflammation is life-threatening, emergency measures are called for. There are heroic strategies in herbal medicine, and some survive in places like China where they can still merit a role in a modern rural economy (there are modern accounts of the treatment of acute appendicitis by Chinese herbs, for example, and garlic is credited with the treatment there of acute cryptococcal meningitis). However, in modern developed economies there is rarely a valid substitute for hospitalization or other conventional intervention.

On the other hand, chronic inflammatory conditions are sometimes notoriously resistant to conventional drug treatments. With the increasing likelihood that viral or immunological factors will be implicated, the role of the antibiotic diminishes. Anti-inflammatories, whether steroids or aspirin-derived, can alleviate the symptoms while they are being taken but have possibly negative long-term effects. Thus the prospects for the sufferer from chronic arthritis, salpingitis, ulcerative colitis, eczema or sinusitis are not improved by conventional treatment, although they are likely to be more comfortable, and patch-up surgery may repair damage after a certain point.

The herbalist's approach to inflammation

Herbal medicines have properties that encourage a number of constructive approaches to chronic inflammations. These are not always conventional anti-inflammatory effects. The traditional 'nature cure' view of unresolved inflammation is that it is a sign of a persisting toxicity or damage in the tissues affected. The initial provocation to inflammation is not removed and the inflammatory process is inadequate to contain it. The notion might be simplistic but its implications are constructive. Notable is the idea that the best way to help such a situation is to *support the inflammatory response*. If mobilization of the body's eliminative and resolutive agents is the aim of the exercise, then, so the idea goes, those remedies that increase circulation, phagocyte activity, elimination and tissue repair should be sought. The very notion of the 'anti-inflammatory' is a dubious one.

Thus it is that if herbal remedies traditionally used for inflammatory diseases are examined they are found to possess *circulatory stimulant, diuretic, laxative, choleretic* (bile stimulating), *digestive stimulant*, or other eliminative effect. There is a growing body of research that suggests that several chronic inflammatory diseases, often by definition with an autoimmunological element, are linked to low-grade chronic infections in separate parts of the body, and that either a cross-sensitivity is being set up to certain pathogenic antigens, or some toxic factor is being introduced. Many traditional approaches to such conditions, like rheumatoid arthritis and ankylosing spondylitis, have antiseptic or eliminative action in such suspect areas as the lungs, bowel or urinary system (see 'Auto-immune disease', on pp. 73–4).

Another strategy might involve reducing intake of dietary antigen or other contaminants with *bitter* or *aromatic digestive* tonics (often coupled with dietary exclusions or reform) or, through the same techniques, effectively altering the bowel environment.

Alternatively, herbs may possess some locally provocative or healing action. The role of counter-irritation, for example, figures large in the traditional treatment of inflammation. The technique involves applying a heating influence to the inflamed site, in effect increasing the inflammatory effect by promoting extra circulation to the area. The measures may simply involve massaging *rubefacient* ('redness-forming') volatile oils in the form of liniments or embrocations, or they may scale up through the mustard family: cabbage-leaf poultices were popular for chest inflammations, mustard plasters or baths for arthritic joints, or, for dramatic effect, the cayenne plaster or even acrid blistering agents were used.

The widespread reputation these techniques had for producing rapid relief (sometimes dramatic in the case of the old blistering techniques) in the case of incapacitating inflammations, perhaps permitting an early return to working in the days when there was no welfare support, is undeniable. The impression that even cumulative benefits can be gained from using the less drastic approaches supports the idea that inflammation can indeed be reduced by mimicking some of its processes. A further user-advantage is that all such counter-irritation is painless, suggesting that the effect is not mediated by pain-producing histamines and other agents.

Inflammation involving mucosal surfaces or open wounds may also be reduced with other topical effects. *Tannins* and some *mucilages* reduce irritation and promote temporary healing, an effect seen notably in the upper intestinal tract. Inflammation may also be affected by administering remedies containing *resins* or *volatile oils*

62 Physiology

close to the site, a technique often employed in mouth and throat washes, and in pessaries and inhalations. The explanation proffered is that these provoke phagocyte activity in the region.

FEVER

An ancient plague

The notion that inflammation is a healthy vital response to be supported where necessary and possible is seen again in the traditional approaches to fevers. The febrile response is in some ways inflammation writ large, a whole-body rather than a tissue response to adversity.

The key symptom of fever is raised body temperature, or pyrexia. This is accompanied by a broad array of other symptoms of varying degrees of discomfort. Fevers have always been one of the most common causes of death, and some, like plague, smallpox, typhoid and cholera, have been notoriously destructive. In the cramped unhygienic conditions of pre-twentieth-century European cities and towns epidemics of fevers, or pestilences, have decimated populations and caused untold personal hardship. It is not surprising therefore that desperate measures have often been sought to attack the fever and reduce the risk of mortality from it.

Coincident with the rise of urban culture was the development of the use of mineral medicines as medicaments. Preparations of compounds of arsenic, mercury, sulphur and other toxic elements were increasingly used to suppress the febrile and other symptoms of severe infections. As poisons, their use was far more dangerous than plant remedies, and the rise of the apothecary-physician relatively skilled in the delicate art of dosage, posology, was an essential result of the switch. (To this day registered medical practitioners are the only persons effectively licensed to administer poisons to others!) The effect of these new mineral treatments was hopefully to suppress unpleasant and dangerous symptoms, in doses small enough not to damage the patient as well. It was an obviously risky strategy and side-effects, some of which were appalling, became an intrinsic part of the medical scene for the first time. A new tradition of allopathy, of symptomatic prescribing, was born.

An extraordinary response

The older, rural traditions barely understood such concepts. To them, fever was a raising of the vital stakes, a sign of extraordinary vital rejective activity: the heat generated was an obvious marker of that fact. Fevers were to be managed, not aborted, the better to help the body come to terms with the adversity. The physiological events in fever lend some support to this view.

Fever typically (but not always) follows a generalized infection of the bloodstream or other body fluids. Many pathogenic organisms either produce metabolites, or present surface antigens, triggers, referred to as exogenous pyrogens, that effect changes in the temperature control mechanism in the hypothalamus in the brain. They 'set the thermostat higher'. The result is a stimulus to the heat-generating and heat-conserving mechanisms of the body, so that body temperature can rise to match the new setting in the hypothalamus. Such mechanisms include the shutting down of the blood flow to the surface (pallor), shivering, and seeking warmth. In short the person *feels cold*.

This, the 'chill' phase of fever, indicates that the body temperature is rising. When it reaches that set by the hypothalamus, a new stability with balance of heat gain and loss returns. The symptoms of chill recede and a less uncomfortable phase commences.

With the rise in body temperature, blood flows through the tissues and the activity of the phagocytes increases. The body's defences are alerted and mobilized. The intruder's chances of prosperity are much reduced, as is its production of exogenous pyrogen. The upward stimulus on the hypothalamus is reduced. The thermostat setting falls. The outward sign of this change could be predicted from knowing that the body temperature will now be higher than that set in the thermostat: heat has to be lost. The circulation to the periphery opens up again, the sweat glands operate, coverings are thrown off. The patient *feels hot*. In traditional terms the fever has 'broken', 'crisis' has been reached, and 'lysis', or resolution, intervenes. With luck the invasion has been successfully repelled and recovery can commence.

64 Physiology

This is a most simplistic account. Yet it provides an acceptable basis for a policy of fever management in which basic principles of nursing can be augmented by herbal remedies. *The successful and safe conduct through a fever requires more than academic knowledge, so the following should not be used by those without clinical skills.* For this reason details of nursing care have been omitted.

Fever management

The essential priority in handling fevers is to accept them as potentially useful rather than seeking to abort them at all costs. There are, of course, dangers, and some practical medical knowledge is required to spot them, but the moderate rise in body temperature itself is not dangerous provided due care is observed.

At a temperature of about 38–39°C (approx. 101–102°F) the body's defences are operating at peak levels: the circulatory system is highly charged and the phagocytes are positively frenetic. This is a level that can be set as the ideal fever temperature. Fever management can be defined as nurturing that temperature and minimizing discomfort and risk until crisis is reached, and then providing support through lysis and convalescence.

The first requirement is for some means of monitoring the situation. A clinical thermometer is obviously central, but its usefulness is greatly enhanced by knowing how to interpret its findings. Referring to the account of fever above will explain the following points:

1 feeling cold, having a pale cyanosed skin and shivering means that the body temperature is lower than the thermostat setting in the hypothalamus, and is most likely to be *still rising*;

2 feeling hot, having a flushed skin and sweating means that the body temperature is higher than the thermostat setting, and is most likely to be *coming down*;

3 having no dominant feeling of being hot or cold suggests relative equilibrium between thermostat and body temperature.

65   Assimilation and Rejection

With these clues and a clinical thermometer it is generally possible to assess progress through the fever. If, for example, the temperature was 40°C (104°F) its importance would depend on whether the patient was feeling hot or cold. In the former case one would expect the temperature to fall, in the latter case some quick treatment would be called for.

Apart from the usual techniques for bringing temperature down, such as cold wet face flannels or tepid baths, there is conventional aspirin. This, however, simply switches the thermostat controls down without attending to any other aspects of the fever: the risk of an unresolved conflict is high. Herbal remedies by contrast appear to be otherwise useful.

As a gentle coolant the *peripheral vasodilators* or *diaphoretics*, remedies 'hot in the first degree' (see 'The Temperaments of Plant Remedies', on pp. 174–83), such as yarrow (*Achillea millefolium*), elderflower (*Sambucus nigra*), catmint (*Nepeta cataria*), and boneset (*Eupatorium perfoliatum*) are ideal. Their effect is to encourage perspiration and they also have a variety of other useful benefits for the digestion, mucous membranes and neuromuscular system.

For more significant cooling the *bitters* are favoured: they have the additional advantage of switching on the otherwise dormant digestive system, thus helping to counter fermentation or infection arising from the gut.

As well as containing excessive body temperature there might be a need to keep it up. If it is clear that the fever is prolonged or low-key, and that the body temperature is not reaching 38°C (approx. 101°F), it is possible that warming remedies might be chosen. This is a rather unusual choice in conventional terms, but a review of the discussion about the legacy of Samuel Thomson later in this text will put it in better context. If the benefits of a good fever are accepted, then the disadvantage of not having the resources to run one are also apparent. This is a widespread problem among adults in affluent societies. In practice fevers are rare after childhood. Unresolved low-grade chronic infections, often classified as viral, are not. In a case of persistent catarrh, for example, it is often useful to take advantage of a partial attempt by the body to raise the stakes, a cold or sore throat perhaps, and set a therapeutic fever into train.

66 Physiology

The patient should be strongly advised to prepare properly. Bedrest, a minimal fresh diet and plenty of fluid are basic requirements. It is then possible to take one of the many *circulatory stimulants*, such as cinnamon (*Cinnamomum* spp.), angelica (*Angelica archangelica*), ginger, garlic or even, if practised, cayenne (*Capsicum minimum*). The febrile process can then be nudged through, often to considerable advantage.

Apart from monitoring body temperature there are other symptoms of fever that need to be watched. Many such as nausea, vomiting, diarrhoea, headaches, coughing, pains and spasms, can usually be controlled by the appropriate herbal remedy. Accepting the potential value of the febrile reaction does not mean consigning the patient to unnecessary discomfort. There are, of course, danger signs as well (a pulse that does not rise with temperature as expected might herald meningitis; convulsions, although common enough in children, can disguise and exacerbate polio; the dry cough of measles is similar to that of pneumonia, and so on); the untrained must not attempt to take full responsibility for any such treatment.

As important as any other part of the treatment is to allow for adequate convalescence after it is all over. The need for this, and the consequences of the current tendency to ignore it, are discussed at greater length in 'Convalescence' on pp. 217–23.

THE IMMUNE SYSTEM

In conventional terms the immune system is thought of as the most specialized, but not the most potent, defence mechanism in higher animals.

The body's protection against intrusion from the outside may usefully be compared to concentric defensive fortifications in that each level needs to be penetrated before those deeper need to be involved. The further in the trouble penetrates, the more involved and specific the defences and the more complex the issues for the body. Healthy defences are superficial defences.

This is a recurrent theme in traditional herbal therapeutics and throughout this work. An important feature of the herbal approach to many infective and inflammatory diseases lies in supporting those defence functions that reduce potential long-term complications. The following lists each defence in order, from the most superficial to the most profound.

1 the body's physical barriers (skin and mucous membranes), supported by indigenous products that suppress and kill pathogens (unsaturated fatty acid, metabolites, lactic acid on the skin, secretions containing enzymes and lysosymes from mucous membranes). Resident 'commensural' bacteria also have a protective effect against unwelcome infections. The acid and digestive secretions in the stomach complete these primary defences.

2 a number of *non-specific humoral* (blood-borne) responses including lysosyme, the properdin-complement pathway, interferons and lactic acid.

3 the *non-specific cellular* mechanisms, the *phagocytes*, principally in two classes: macrophages (including the Kuppfer cells and osteoclasts in the liver and bone respectively) and polymorphonuclear leucocytes (neutrophils). These cells are the most active agents of defence in the body, and in fact form the teeth of the next type of defence.

4 the *specific* defence mechanism: the immune response, which consists of the following axes:

a The *cellular* axis of specific immunity comprises 'T' (or thymus-derived) lymphocytes, the lymphokines that they secrete, and macrophages. This system is activated when T-lymphocytes recognize a foreign protein (antigen) or another cell membrane, release lymphokines and activate macrophages to ingest the offending cell vigorously; it is typically localized in the affected tissue.

b The *humoral* axis of specific defence comprises 'B' lymphocytes, secreted antibodies, complement and neutrophils. B-lymphocytes were originally found to be derived from, and were named for, the bursa of Fabricius in birds: they are thought to originate from bone marrow and gut-associated lymphatic tissue in humans. They are far fewer than T-lymphocytes. When a B-lymphocyte recognizes an antigen, specific antibodies are secreted that combine with the antigen to form a complex: complement is thereby activated, or 'opsonization' occurs and neutrophils phagocytize the whole lot. The antibodies are sometimes referred to as immunoglobulins: there are several types. The most common is the IgG group, but IgA and IgE are clinically very significant, and IgM and IgD are also found.

The B-lymphocyte response is extensively controlled by certain T-lymphocytes, some the 'helper T-cells' which stimulate antibody production, and others, the 'suppressor T-cells', which reduce it. It is incidentally the T-lymphocytes which are the victims of the HIV virus in Aids.

The mechanisms of immunity

In both the above cases the lymphocyte response is similar. Every protein molecule in nature has a portion that is matched by a membrane receptor somewhere on one of the vast array of different lymphocytes in the bloodstream (i.e. all proteins are antigens). The result of any such encounter, via a very complicated mechanism, is a stimulation to cell division. Thus the initially small population of lymphocytes bearing the relevant receptor rapidly increases ('antigen-driven clonal expansion'), with the production of large populations of both 'effector' lymphocytes ('plasma cells' in the case of the B-lymphocytes), and 'memory' lymphocytes. The first group effects the defensive response, either by producing an antibody or through direct (T-cell) contact.

As it can be several days before the population of effector lymphocytes is large enough to make a significant difference to the problem at first exposure, the population of memory cells is left to circulate in the blood for years, ready to provide an immediate response to any repetition of the same trouble. This is the rationale behind vaccination: the early injection of detoxified versions of specific dangerous antigens so that the body can have memory cells in place ready to respond instantly should it later be exposed to a real infection.

A phenomenon of some importance to later discussion is that of the hapten response. Haptens are molecules too small to provoke an immune response (and as explained below they may even block one). Combined with a 'carrier', however, an anti-hapten response (involving both B- and T-cells) is initiated which can then be invoked by the hapten alone.

Although a distinction has been made so far between the T- and B-cell responses, this latest example actually illustrates a general principle: every immune response requires both T- and B-lymphocyte involvement. Stimulation and control of immunity depend on their interaction.

Allergy

There are other types of immunological response. Notable is the immediate allergic response resulting from the combination of certain types of antigens with type IgE antibody, on the surface of a cell referred to as a mast cell or basophil.

The combination provokes the mast cell into secreting inflammatory mediators, especially histamine and serotonin, that produce such symptoms as hay fever, asthma and allergic eczema. This dubious response does in fact seem linked to a specialist defence against infestation with parasites such as intestinal worms and amoebas. In the modern context, however, it has mostly an adverse effect and it can front a general disruption of immunological function. Certain individuals are born with particularly large quantities of IgE antibodies and mast cells and are thus more prone to the disabling effects of allergies.

Autoimmunity

All the mechanisms mentioned until now were uncovered in pursuit of an explanation and treatment for serious diseases. Initially, the priority was the protection, through vaccination, against the killer infections. Then the need was to explain the sometimes fatal and always destructive allergic disorders. Lastly, the search has been on to understand the even more widespread, just as dangerous, but much more mysterious problem of autoimmune disease. The last attempt may suggest that all the previous concepts of immunity are upturned.

The obvious question is why does the immune system not attack the body's own tissues? If antibodies to any protein can be produced, why are there no antibodies to 'self', to one's own proteins: why are there no autoantibodies?

There are two apparently contradictory answers to this question:

1 autoantibodies are in fact common, even in health, and appear to do no harm;

2 immunity against self is also the key pathology in a considerable number of serious diseases. These include rheumatoid arthritis, psoriasis, ulcerative colitis, diabetes mellitus, chronic active hepatitis, myasthenia gravis, multiple sclerosis, glomerulonephritis, among many more, perhaps even most, degenerative diseases. It is clear that in health the immune system lays off attacking the body's own tissues, but that in certain circumstances it does not.

Any interpretation of the role of the immune system must be able to accommodate both answers.

Developing tolerance to oneself

As explained earlier, the current wisdom is that immune attack involves an active co-ordination between macrophages, and B- and T-cells. 'Tolerance' to any protein can thus involve a neutralizing of any one of the three participants.

In trying to explain tolerance of self proteins most attention has been paid to the 'clonal elimination' hypothesis of Burnet, dating from 1959, which suggests that at an early stage in foetal development, exposure to antigen leads not to the usual stimulus to lymphocyte division, but to elimination of the lymphocyte involved. By definition the proteins involved will be those native to the body, so all lymphocytes that could mount an attack on the body tissues should thus be removed. The experimental support for this model is now very strong and it is generally accepted as providing the main basis for protection against autoimmune attack.

The immune system is, however, very complicated. Many of the body's proteins are found within its cells, and thus do not generally reach the body fluids. When they do, a long time after Burnet's elimination could occur, as in major tissue injury, there need to be different mechanisms to prevent immune attack against them. There also needs to be protection against disruptive immune responses to dietary antigens, and also, in the pregnant mother, against the foreign proteins from the child in her womb (or for that matter against the foreign spermatozoa necessary for its conception).

In other words, there need to be mechanisms of tolerance that can operate continuously throughout adult life.

It is known that such mechanisms exist. Understanding them may make it easier to see what happens when things go wrong. The following are available clues:

> exposure to very low levels of an antigen can induce tolerance in the relevant T-cells. This could be seen as a form of 'vaccination', allowing tolerance to protein entered in tiny amounts over a long period to develop;

> exposure to very high levels can 'tolerize' both B- and T-cells. This might be important in reinforcing Burnet's mechanism in the foetus and in preventing gross immunological destruction in serious injury;

> the 'suppressor' T-cells limit excessive immunological responses at many levels, and most probably encourage tolerization. A healthy liver is known to be important for their function (supporting liver health has a high priority in herbal medicine);

> the enzymatic digestion of proteins is also likely to yield breakdown particles that induce tolerance to the parent protein, at least up to a certain level. This would allow the immune system to maintain a relatively benevolent attitude to intracellular and dietary antigens, assuming that under normal circumstances they would effectively be accompanied by their own breakdown products (through digestive and lysosomal enzymes respectively).

This last mechanism points to an important role for healthy digestion and phagocytosis in preventing autoimmunity.

Autoantibodies – a good thing?

Even with the protections listed above, it is still the case that if tolerance to one's own proteins breaks down, one's own lymphocytes will produce antibodies to them, that is will produce autoantibodies.

However, these in themselves do not automatically mean trouble. The quantity of antibodies is actually known to increase naturally with age, and to be not necessarily linked to disease. It is indeed possible that autoantibodies have a positive role.

Up until his death in 1986 at 88, the notable Parisian immunologist, Pierre Grabar, championed such a view. He saw *the levels of autoantibodies as a measure of the extent of tissue damage due to any cause*; he saw their primary role as opsonins, to identify and clutch on to protein molecules that should not be wandering around the body fluids, and present them to the active scavenger-defenders, the phagocytes, for destruction.[11]

This leads to the broader suggestion that *the whole immune system is primarily designed for opsonization*, that it is the body's ultimate specialist surveillance system, and that its primal duties would have been directed more towards the most substantial sources of antigen, the contents of its own cells, and food, and perhaps only secondarily towards defence against foreign intruders. This is not a radical departure for immunology: it simply reverses the usual order of priorities. Yet it provides, as we shall see, an intriguingly constructive new framework for assessing what happens when things really start to go wrong.

Autoimmune disease

Unfortunately they do. Autoantibodies and cell-mediated attacks can become uncontrollable and produce serious inflammatory diseases (such as those listed earlier). Of the many models to explain autoimmunity, two predominate.

The first suggests that slight distortions of the structure of body proteins, through viral or toxic action, might lead to a *breakdown of normal tolerance*. Many tolerances are T-cell-based only: B-cell capabilities for autoantibody production often remain through life. A slight variation in antigen could lead to a new population of 'helper' T-cells to switch on B-cell activity and flood the tissues with autoantibody.

The second explanation is that of *cross-reactivity*, especially with bacterial antigens. It is suggested that certain bacterial proteins are sufficiently like host protein that the immune response to the former backfires on to the latter. It has long been known that *Streptococcus pyogenes* infections can lead to endocarditis, and this is now known to be due to the antigenic similarity between the bacteria and the cell membranes of the heart lining. Recently it has been realized that other cross-reactions occur between infective organisms and inflammatory diseases. Examples include *Proteus* and rheumatoid arthritis, *Klebsiella* and ankylosing spondylitis, *Escherichia coli* and ulcerative colitis. Associating ankylosing spondylitis with urinary infections and with changes in gut flora is a long tradition, and a similar link is made between rheumatoid arthritis and chronic or early lung infection.

Both associations, and several others like them, have been supported in modern clinical medicine.[12]

The view is growing in medical circles that arthritic diseases at least may involve, in effect, an 'allergy' to a separate long-standing infection.

Developing tolerance to food

Tolerance to food proteins was first demonstrated by H. G. Wells, in a pre-artistic career, when he showed that guinea pigs which had eaten egg white were less sensitized to its injection into their body fluids. Mechanisms for the phenomenon have been further elucidated.

There are special lymphocytes found in patches in the gut wall (Peyer's patches), and separated from the gut contents by extremely fine membranes called M-plates, which actively sample the antigens in the gut. They in turn promote secretion by B-cells of non-inflammatory antibodies called IgAs into the gut and elsewhere through the body. The effect of IgA is to painlessly mop up most antigens in the gut that might threaten the body's integrity. These Peyer's patch lymphocytes also probably lead to more suppressor T-cells being produced for any food antigen that does breach the walls.

The combination of these cells and high levels of specialized IgAs probably accounts for most of the tolerance in the body to food protein. However, the sheer pressure of antigens in the gut means that an enormous proportion of the immune system's attention is directed there: the stakes are high and it would be very surprising indeed if there were not many more defences against trouble from that quarter. That they are necessary is evident in reviewing the food threat.

The challenge of food

The popular and conventional medical concern with food tends to focus on the risks of contamination and infection. The presence of *Salmonella* in eggs or chicken or *Listeria* in soft cheeses and pâtés are recent examples of public concern. Other types of food poisoning also merit attention. Yet the most common dietary assault on the body is usually overlooked. If bacterial antigens might cause problems, then the potential for disruption from the ingestion of massive quantities of dietary antigen is overwhelming. Yet, incredibly, the topic is almost completely ignored in standard references on the immune system.

Hardly any general immunology texts even mention the prospect facing the body of all the foreign protein it has to ingest.[13] This is in spite of the fact that the gut is associated with intense lymphatic activity, and that it is the site of unusual types of antibody.

All this has meant that the subject of food intolerance has had very little credibility in medical circles. Many doctors still find it unbelievable that foods might cause upsets to patients, or might even be sources of illness. This has had the most unfortunate effect that the growing number of people who become convinced that foods are causing trouble have few places to turn within orthodox medicine. Their concerns are often left to a band of practitioners touting possibly the most inconsistent and potentially damaging strategies in the field of alternative medicine.

The term 'food allergy' is widely used to describe the problem. An astonishing range of methods are used to establish such a diagnosis, including cytological challenge, dowsing, hair analyses and 'muscle testing'. Most have shown themselves to be inconsistent, misleading and incorrect in application.[14] The typical patient comes away from such an encounter with a long list of foods to which he or she is said to be 'allergic' and with strict instructions to avoid them. Apart from the dangers of encouraging dietary 'neurosis', sometimes with a disabling self-perpetuating cycle of food aversions, the simple truth is that the basis of such a diagnosis is fundamentally flawed.

Genuine food intolerances or sensitivities do occur. There is only one sure way of establishing the fact: to undertake a rigorous programme of selective elimination of the suspect foods alternating with challenges of the same foods.

The mechanisms for food intolerance are not well understood, but in any individual case there is likely to be at least one of the following problems:

1 the classic allergy reaction with IgE production and the release of histamine, serotonin, prostaglandins and other inflammatory mediators, either locally, to damage the gut wall, or systemically;

2 the formation of different types of antibody complexes with food antigens, so that they are less effective opsonins, and the phagocytes do not deal with them as effectively;

3 deficient enzymes leading to inadequate metabolism of certain food or chemical substances and various sensitivities or reactions to them; this could be made worse by an increased consumption of some chemicals in food: at least one metabolic enzyme, PST-P, is known to be selectively depressed by artificial food colourings;

4 the production of peptides called lymphokines by affected lymphocytes that can produce subjective symptoms like malaise and fatigue;

5 the production of mood-altering peptides, known as exorphins, by incomplete digestion of certain foods, leading to stimulation by or craving for the foods involved (wheat, milk and maize are known to produce these under some circumstances); this effect would be stronger in those with unusually leaky gut walls;

6 disturbed gut flora, especially after antibiotic administration,

leading to the colonization by strains of bacteria living only off certain foods and then producing toxins or peptides;

7 invasion of the gut by an aggressive version of thrush or *Candida albicans*, increasing the leakiness of the gut wall and further disturbing the gut flora.

Two factors seem to be common to many of the mechanisms mentioned: *inadequate digestion* is more likely to leave undigested antigens or other disruptive agents, and a *damaged* or *leaky gut wall* will lead to increased penetration into the bloodstream of such materials.

How can herbal medicine help in immune disturbances?

At first glance it might be concluded that using crude plant drugs could have little impact on the bewildering complexity and mechanistic interactions of the immune system, in health or disease. All that we know about the subject has been learnt long after the traditional approach held sway: it appears that the agenda has been set entirely by those immersed in the conventional reductionist approach to medicine.

There are, however, some most interesting approaches that herbal medicine does suggest. The evidence of history and clinical experience is that herbal treatment can help with autoimmune diseases and allergies. It will be interesting to suggest ways in which that might happen.

In the first place traditional practice lends emphasis to the view that the immune system has a position relative to other defensive mechanisms. This would suggest that anything but the simplest involvement of the immune system in defence is itself an indication for treatment, that a useful strategy is to support defensive measures that do not involve the immune response. In the concentric arrangement mentioned earlier, obvious advantage is to be had in enhancing primary defences, and possible benefit in stimulating the second level. This might apply even after the immune system has been involved, if reducing further assaults on it is a priority.

Thus healing and protecting open wounds on the skin is an obvious precaution. Correcting gum and dental disease, inflamed throats, gastritis and intestinal disease is not usually considered so important, yet the potential breach in defences may be very much greater. The use in such cases of remedies rich in *tannins*, *resins* and other *astringent* principles may be justified solely in reducing absorption of antigenic material and reducing immune complications. The potential role of a leaky gut has already been highlighted: it is not generally realized that even hay fever implies a degree of mucosal damage sufficient to allow allergens to penetrate and is a possible indication for mucosal (*anticatarrhal*) herbal remedies.

Stimulating other primary defences may be equally beneficial. Remedies (like *bitters* and *aromatic digestives*) that stimulate digestive secretions can markedly improve the condition of those suffering from an immune disorder following food intolerance or other intrusion from the gut. Alternatively the priority might be to enhance eliminative defences: promoting expectoration, bile flow or bowel movement (with *expectorants*, *cholagogues* and *laxatives* respectively) may help reduce toxic antigenic pressure (see 'Removal', on pp. 95–117).

Reaching the secondary level is not as clear a strategy. There are occasional suggestions that *volatile oils*, *resins*, *bitters* and *acrid* remedies provoke increased phagocytic activity. The *lymphatics* seem to relieve inflammatory pressures in the lymphatic system and are indicated where there are persistent low-grade infections. Either strategy might provide potentially a dramatic sparing effect for the immune system. Provoking a febrile or inflammatory crisis (see above) would also come into this category.

On these presumptions it is easier to see why a policy of treating inflammatory skin disease, rheumatoid arthritis, inflammatory bowel disease or other autoimmune conditions with remedies working on the gut, mucosal surfaces or other distant sites might be justified.

In further attempting to interpret autoimmune disease the traditional herbalist might intuitively have taken a leaf from Dr Grabar's book. Rather than attempting vainly to crudely disentangle a horrendous immunological knot, the herbalist usually falls back on first principles: the initial health of the tissues involved. A modern practitioner might put it in technical terms: 'What manner of tissue disturbance is it that either overwhelmed the normal (lysosomal) breakdown of intracellular protein thereby necessitating an immune response; allowed viral or other infective organisms to prosper and colonize, thereby damaging or transforming the cells and inviting immune responses; or so diverted or damaged the normal phagocytic surveillance?'

The answer might lie as much in the sphere of herbal treatment as in any conventional immunosuppressive prescription. Identifying 'toxic' factors (see 'The Toxicity Thesis of Disease', on p. 117), earlier assaults on the body ('primary lesions'), and disorders of *circulation*, *assimilation* and *rejection* are strategies that might arise from times when there was little choice, but they should not be ignored for that.

Propositions:

the processes of assimilation and rejection are inseparably intertwined;

the earlier in assimilation an undesirable element can be rejected the more efficient is the process and the fewer complications will arise.

Summary

In summary, the processes of assimilation and rejection include such aspects of cellular and human physiology as:

food searching behaviour
upper digestive functions: secretions, absorption
thirst
reabsorption, especially at the bowel and kidney
macrophage and immune surveillance
fever and inflammation
respiration: the lungs, haemoglobin, gas exchange

Processing

What happens when nourishment reaches the interior is, as expected, mysterious. At a material level the processes involved have been explored within the discipline of biochemistry. Intricate colour diagrams of the chemical changes in the metabolic pathways have decorated the bedrooms of biochemistry undergraduates since the 1960s. Most pieces in the puzzle have been worked out and attention has switched to detail. This detail is fascinating, particularly the role of the essential catalysts of metabolic activity, those proteins called enzymes that can produce, without disturbance, energetic changes otherwise only seen in a bonfire. There is also the marvellous storage of calorific energy in the form of high-energy phosphate bonds, in such molecules as ADP and ATP.

Yet much of this is of little immediate relevance to herbal therapeutics. Such clinical interest is in the gross signs of metabolism, those that can be appreciated subjectively and that might be affected by other gross influences. From this perspective metabolism has three main facets: catabolism, anabolism and heat production.

Catabolism

Catabolism is the breakdown of large molecules into smaller units and, ultimately, with the consumption of oxygen, into carbon dioxide, water, waste products and *the production of energy*.

In the cell this activity is conducted primarily in the mitochondria, fascinating semi-autonomous entities with their own genetic blueprint and legacy. Mitochondria are possibly descendants of bacteria-like organisms which made a momentous symbiotic deal early in evolutionary history: complete security within the newly evolved cell in return for bringing the capacity to utilize what had so far been a poison, oxygen, for the production of energy.

Each major food constituent has its own route to breakdown. *Proteins* are split into their constituent amino-acids and these are then deaminated into keto-acids and nitrogen in the form of ammonia. The latter is highly toxic, so it is converted by liver cells into urea.

The keto-acids join the sugars from *carbohydrates* to form glucose-6-phosphate, the source material for the common glycolytic pathway towards the production of carbon dioxide, water and energy. They are joined at the last step, the Krebs cycle, by acetyl-coenzyme A, the breakdown product of *fatty acids*. Energy is either produced as heat (see below) or saved for cellular functions in the form of high-energy phosphate bonds, mainly in the form of adenosine di- and tri-phosphate (ADP and ATP), a process called oxidative phosphorylation.

Of the various sources of catabolic breakdown and energy supply, carbohydrate is the most immediately available. It is held in store as glycogen by the liver for short-term replenishment of blood-sugar levels between meals. Fat is the most concentrated in terms of eventual ATP production and is thus the most efficient long-term store; its catabolism is increased during starvation and exercise (and decreased in overconsumption and sedentary lifestyle!). Protein is substantially used as an energy source only when other sources are inadequate, although a certain proportion of normal protein turnover is also directed to this end. It may, however, be catabolized in place of fat in an individual who is chronically unused to aerobic exercise.

Catabolism is generally increased in exercise, in a cold environment, in stress and disease, and by high-protein diets. Hormonal stimulants are thyroid hormone, in the long term, and adrenaline and noradrenaline in the shorter term.

Catabolism is marked by negative nitrogen balance, i.e. more nitrogen is excreted, as urea and uric acid, than is consumed. At high levels the urine will be strong and highly coloured.

Closely associated with catabolism are the processes of *detoxification*, performed in the liver, in which fat-soluble waste products from the tissues are converted by various processes, conjugation (to glucuronates or sulphates) or demethylation, oxidation, or reduction, into polar, water-soluble materials suitable for excretion by the kidneys.

Anabolism

Anabolism is the assembly of building blocks to form new complex molecules such as enzymes and other proteins, essential fatty acids, cholesterol, lecithin and other phospholipids, porphyrins (such as haemoglobin), mucopolysaccharides and other structures. It is essentially *energy-consuming* (largely ATP-consuming), and is the basis of tissue growth and repair.

A considerable proportion of the body's anabolism is conducted in the liver, and it is the dominant activity in all those tissues responsible for growth and repair, such as the bone marrow, fibroblasts, chondroblasts and osteoblasts. It is also prominent in early life and in growth spurts, after debilitating illness or injury, and generally speaking at night.

It is marked by a positive nitrogen balance, i.e. more nitrogen is consumed than excreted, less appears in the urine as urea and uric acid.

Anabolism is promoted, in different ways, by the hormones insulin, growth hormone and those steroids from the adrenal cortex and gonads collectively referred to as 'anabolic', notably testosterone.

Heat production

Heat is principally a 'waste product' of catabolism but, ultimately, as Newton reminded us, of all metabolism, as well as of such sources as friction from muscle contraction and fluid flow.

The rate of heat production generally follows the rate of, and is influenced by, the same factors as catabolism, and is actually the unit of measurement for assessing 'metabolic rate'. Adrenaline, however, has a notable heat-generating effect through uncoupling oxidative phosphorylation (reducing the formation of ADP and ATP), so making catabolism less efficient, more 'wasteful' of heat and thus ensuring that more catabolism (and heat) is necessary for the same ATP production.

The latter effect is largely dependent on the amount of a tissue called 'brown fat'. This is a form of fat tissue packed with mitochondria with the specific role of providing heat under the influence of adrenaline (whose production is in turn increased by cold). It is found especially in hibernating mammals in whom it provides sufficient heat for life in the otherwise suspended animation of winter sleep. In humans it is found to any extent only in infants and is likely to be responsible for maintaining their body temperature against adversity. In adults adrenaline-mediated heat production accounts for at most 10 to 15 per cent of the total, and is only evident hours after activation.

The effects of thyroid activity on heat production take even longer to manifest. Acclimatization to cold over several months is accompanied by increased thyroxine levels and eventually thyroid size (Eskimos have very large thyroids). The main short-term rise in heat production is provided by muscular activity, either exercise or, particularly effectively, shivering.

One cannot ignore behavioural and other influences on the balance of heat in the body. Searching for heat, avoiding cold, eating hot food and drink, putting on more clothing, chopping the firewood, are at least as important as physiological factors in the overall balance.

The traditional view of a heat generator in the living body – sited, for example, by Chinese medicine in the right kidney – can only be sustained as a reflection of all the foregoing. Whether the heat arises from metabolic, hormonal or behavioural activity, there is enough evidence to see it all as a broad pattern of interwoven influences.

This is a fascinating subject. The obvious association of heat with life, and of cold with disease and death, referred to later, has given heat generation a powerful place in traditional therapeutics. The idea that vitality can be enhanced in this way is subjectively attractive, just as the warmth of the campfire has been since prehistory. In the sense that increased body temperature means increased circulatory activity (and thus more blood flowing through the tissues), then an antipathogenic effect can be agreed. To what extent it may help otherwise is still tantalizing speculation.

Traditional herbal strategies for generating heat, the acrid remedies like cayenne, ginger and cinnamon on the one hand, and the Chinese *yang* tonics on the other, may have a number of effects on metabolic activity: considerable attention will be given to them later. The verdict throughout history is that they occupy a primary position in medicine. No discussion of herbal therapeutics can minimize their importance.

The liver

The importance of the liver in all metabolic functions can hardly be overstated. It is central to most outlined above, and accomplishes many almost entirely on its own. It is particularly vital for:

> protein synthesis and breakdown and the conversion of ammonia to urea (the latter is the liver's most urgent life-saving task);
>
> the synthesis of 'non-essential' amino-acids (those not necessarily obtained from the diet) from keto-acid precursors;
>
> short-term buffering of glucose levels in the blood through its constantly replenished glycogen store;
>
> synthesis of cholesterol, lecithin and other phospholipids, and lipoproteins;
>
> conversion of sugars like fructose and galactose, as well as amino-acids, to glucose;
>
> the conversion of acetylcoenzyme A to acetoacetic acid so that this particularly concentrated energy source can be exported to other tissues in the body.

The liver has, *inter alia*, many other essential functions, including the storage of many vitamins (notably A, D, B12) and iron (for haemoglobin production), the formation of blood-clotting factors, and the regulation of the immune system.

It is also, as we shall see, a vital part of the body's eliminatory effort (see 'The Bile', on pp. 103–6), detoxifying many waste products as well as new materials like food additives, agricultural chemicals and drugs.

If the body's processing functions are to be sited anywhere, it is in the liver. This lends support to the herbalist's preoccupation with the organ. There are many herbal remedies, *hepatics*, used for varying degrees of liver stimulation. Many work simply by increasing bile production (*cholagogues*, see later), with the traditional view being that this generally improves the liver's ability to look after itself. Others have been shown to increase liver RNA levels and otherwise to show signs of promoting general hepatic activity.

Summary

Processing can be taken to include the following activities:

> the metabolism of carbohydrates, fats and proteins
> cell and tissue repair and growth (e.g., haemopoiesis)
> the processing of vitamins and minerals
> the thyroid and other hormonal determinants of metabolic
>   rate
> the liver functions

Circulation

The cell's view

The conventional approach to circulation is to start with the mechanics of its major components, the heart and the blood vessels, and to consider such clinical phenomena as diseases of the heart and circulation, and high blood pressure. The obvious and justifiable motivation for this orientation is the predominance of deaths arising from these causes.

There is, however, another place to start a review of the subject, one that does not deny the usual preoccupation but puts it in a different context. It might perhaps be described as a phenomenological view: one that looks at what the circulation actually is from the perspective of its only consumer, the cell in its tissues.

A single cell living alone can move through its fluid environment to find areas of nourishment and avoid areas of toxicity. A cell permanently embedded within a mass of other cells in a tissue is entirely dependent on its fluid environment being regulated by other mechanisms (in fact by other cells working in other tissues). It has basic requirements for nourishment and elimination (the theme of this physiology review) that need adequate circulation of nutrient-rich fluid to its surface, and an opportunity in turn to have its discarded wastes flushed away. If these requirements are not met, the cell will become diseased and may die.

It is thus not surprising that to ensure cell and tissue survival, for the good of the whole body at least, there are powerful mechanisms available to each tissue to maintain its own minimum circulation. The central point to make though is that from where the cell sits circulation is the measure of the fluid bathing it. What happens in the heart or the main blood vessels is as immediate to its minute-by-minute experience as the city and motorways are to a country smallholding.

The cell's *experience* is of its own microcirculation rather than the broader macrocirculation, just as a citizen's experience is of his own microeconomics rather than the State's macroeconomics. In the latter case economists argue, with justice, that no man is an island insulated from macroeconomic movements, but the most successful politicians know that, to use a Chinese saying, governing a large state is like cooking a small fish, that what the voter perceives as his own economic state counts more (literally) than what the economist sees.

A similar attitude to the cell's 'vote' would lead the wily physiologist to look first at the world as it affects each cell and then at the global mechanism's role in delivering. If such a perspective were applied clinically, it would give 'circulation' a quite different meaning from that which it has in modern medicine. It is suggested later that the traditional medical view is based on just such a different perspective.

Oceanic currents

The first challenge to convention is in the nature of the circulation itself. The school textbook view, following Harvey's conclusions of 400 years ago, is of freshly aerated blood being pumped through the arterial tree, into the network of capillaries where diffusion into and from the tissues takes place, back into the small veins, through the large veins and back to the heart for dispatch into the lungs.

Close scrutiny of the physiology of the body's tissues produces a different view. The 'stuff' between the cells, 'intercellular matrix', is a colloidal fibrous gel that is actually rather impermeable to fluid flow. There are no gross currents of fluid as suggested in conventional hydraulic theory. Instead, movement of fluid is by bumper-to-bumper diffusion through the gel, with excessive fluid being mopped up by the lymphatic drainage system.

The 'Harveyan' notion of a global flowchart is replaced, as far as the cells are concerned, with a demand-led diversity of supply and flow. The currents are local, determined by a combination of structural factors and ambient influences. They resemble the multiplicity of oceanic currents: some grand and predictable, most infinitely variable and changeable.

At the core is the fact that the circulatory mechanism is set up to provide for the body's tissues and cells and that it is these that are its ultimate determinants. There are a number of powerful chemical mediators of circulation, produced by the tissues, to open up the blood vessels in their vicinity when that is needed. Many are actually metabolites, like adenosine. These substances like bradykinin and kallidin had an almost anarchic connotation when first discovered. They are very active, often short-lived, and not generally produced by central controlling organs or glands. They represent the raw power of the rank-and-file cells, in their billions, to look after their own survival.

Appreciating this de-centralized control of tissue circulation may be useful in following some of the approaches to the circulation developed in the past. However, before returning to such practical applications it will be necessary to review briefly the other main features of circulatory physiology.

Autonomic controls

Without the benefit of modern insights into tissue physiology, early physiologists and theoreticians at the turn of the century established the view that circulation was determined by central diktat, specifically by the autonomic nervous system and by higher nerve centres in the brain. We can now see that in reality circulation services the tissues and is primarily responsive to their demands. The role of the central control mechanisms is to mediate the body's global strategy for survival. Maintaining blood flow against gravity, to stop fainting when getting up suddenly, for example, involves such regulation.

Heat control is another such function: the movement of fluid, as every radiator engineer will confirm, is also the most effective way to move heat, in this case away from or up to the body's surface. Mechanisms have to exist which can respond to changes in internal and ambient temperature and translate such information into gross movements of the body's circulation. There also needs to be a mechanism to channel extra blood into muscles, heart and other tissues involved in emergency activity.

The main central control reflecting the level of activity and mobilization in the body as a whole is the autonomic nervous system.

As far as tissue circulation is concerned, the autonomic nervous system divides very conveniently. While the body is at rest the *parasympathetic* nervous system essentially lets the tissues' metabolic demands set the pace of circulation. When the body is mobilized or active the *sympathetic* nervous system, with its hormonal adjutant, adrenaline, can screw down metabolism and its demands in the short term, and shift vast quantities of surplus blood to zones necessary for the body's immediate survival, the muscles, heart and brain.

A considerable part of modern medicine is concerned with the effects of the sympathetic 'fright, fight, flight' or stress response; this is particularly true of the area concerned with cardiovascular disease. The problem, put simply, is that the response is designed to get the body moving, usually out of trouble, but that in an age when we tend to take our troubles sitting down, it is out of place. It is pointless moving blood to the muscles if they are not used; it is actually counter-productive to distort important metabolic functions so that, for example, blood levels of sugar and cholesterol are increased, or to stimulate heartbeat or increase blood pressure, if none of these can be safely diffused by accompanying physical exertion.

Our forebears were an active lot: the average hunter-nomads, representing humankind for a million years or more, could easily cover 65 km a day on foot. Their lives were possibly even more stressful than ours: but they took it on their feet, their responses were almost always physical. The stress response was in its rightful place, the same place as it is in all other mammals. Our stresses now arrive in the mail, or in the bank manager's office, or in a traffic jam: our stress response has to stew without relief.

If, to this disastrous uncoupling of the stress response and exercise, is added the new coupling of inertia and overconsumption of food, alcohol and tobacco, then much of the catalogue of circulatory problems affecting modern society can be explained. The catalogue might read as follows:

high cholesterol levels (through unrequited stress and overconsumption) lead to fatty infiltration of the artery walls and, in time, to *arteriosclerosis*;

this, with persistent constriction of blood vessels in the sedentary stress response and associated changes in the kidneys' control of the quantity of body fluids, is the most likely cause of *raised blood pressure*;

the extra workload thereby imposed on the heart, along with sympathetic stimulation, makes *arrhythmias* more likely;

arteriosclerosis of the heart's own circulation, the coronary arteries, makes *angina* or *coronary heart attacks* possible;

the change in blood chemistry and in blood-vessel lining due to high cholesterol, the suppressed stress response and arteriosclerosis, increases the chance of spontaneous blood clotting, *thromboses* and *embolisms*;

persistent heart strain, high blood pressure and fluid retention can lead to *heart failure*;

smoking simultaneously increases the stress response, reduces the oxygen-carrying capacity, and thus the efficiency of the bloodstream, provokes pathological deterioration, and probably exacerbates all the above problems.

That much of circulatory physiology is geared towards understanding these phenomena is understandable. The fact, moreover, that they are so obviously linked with modern urban lifestyle means that traditional herbal medicines have not been obviously directed towards them. The considerable lapse of time between cause and effect in circulatory disease has not helped the old empirical techniques either. But none of this means that the traditional techniques have no place. After all, the basis of the most widespread modern treatment for heart disease was the use of foxglove for dropsy, a condition we now know as heart failure.

The heart

The powerhouse of the circulatory system has been a focus of interest from the earliest days of human inquiry. Its obvious life-and-death importance and its hypnotic pulse have guaranteed such attention. Its role at the centre of the blood flow, the apparent source of heat and passion, has given it a strong identity in the collective unconscious (an importance still reflected in the German association of ill health with 'heart weakness': *Herzlosigketry*).

While sharing an intense interest in the organ modern science has discounted much of this. It has dissected the heart to an unparalleled degree. It has shown it to be a pump of remarkable sensitivity, adaptability and robustness. Its components, valves and blood supply, and finally the whole heart itself, have been the subject of routine replacement surgery. A range of powerful drugs, starting with the foxglove glycosides and including the remarkable beta-blockers, as well as a battery of electronic gadgetry, have brought its activity under close control.

Yet even under this intensive scrutiny the heart can still surprise: it is only recently that it has been found to also be a secretory gland, producing small quantities of a polypeptide hormone that increases sodium and water excretion from the kidney and thus reduces blood pressure.[15] It will obviously maintain its fascination for a long time to come.

The traditional medical record in handling heart disturbances has not been good. Although the digitalis glycosides of foxglove, lily-of-the-valley, strophanthus and other plants had been selected and used intuitively for dropsy this was not seen as heart failure: in few other cases were clear clinical strategies developed. Of course, heart disease has always been the hardest to treat intuitively: taking years without symptoms to develop, and then often striking fatally in seconds. Many of the herbs now used for cardiac conditions are modern discoveries. The high ground is still firmly held by technological medicine.

The bloodstream

Intrinsic to the passage of nutrient and oxygen to the tissues is an effective transport mechanism. The bloodstream fulfils this role very well indeed.

It is an effective carrier of dissolved food materials, glucose, amino and fatty acids, vitamins and chelated minerals. It flows round the system at gratifying speed and spreads itself through thousands of kilometres of microscopic capillaries to provide maximal exposure to the tissues.

Most striking is its flexible capacity for carrying oxygen and carbon dioxide. This is dependent on the presence of a complex molecule called *haemoglobin*, packaged up in unusual semi-dormant cells called erythrocytes, or red blood cells. Haemoglobin has the extraordinary ability to grab molecules of oxygen when there are a lot of them and to let them go when there are few, and of doing something similar for carbon dioxide. At the lungs therefore, where there is much, the oxygen-carrying capacity of the blood is vastly increased; at the tissues, where there is little, the haemoglobin yields its oxygen, picking up carbon dioxide instead for its return to the lungs.

The oxygen-transporting property of these molecules has its variations: foetal haemoglobin holds on to its oxygen more than the adult equivalent, so it can grab oxygen from its mother in the placenta; this would be too possessive of its oxygen for tissue demands after birth so a critical phase occurs when foetal haemoglobin is replaced by the adult version in the last months in the womb. Myoglobin, a similar molecule in the muscles, is also able to grab oxygen off haemoglobin and ensure adequate muscle supplies.

Haemoglobin is carried through the blood within the red blood cells. These have an unusual double-concave cross-section, which gives them the highest surface-area-to-volume ratio possible, so maximizing gas exchange. The shape also allows the cells to bend and squeeze through capillaries with diameters smaller than theirs. The result is that concentrated packets of oxygen can be delivered right up to every cell in the body.

The early view

It has long been assumed in traditional systems of medicine that one of the fundamental therapeutic interventions is to help improve the circulation to a disturbed tissue. The simple act of massage, hot and cold water applications, the ancient practice of steaming, or applying hot packs of heating herbal remedies, have all been justified in their own time in terms that can be translated as 'improving vital circulation to aid recovery'.

In addition herbal dispensaries are full of remedies that 'heat', either gently or vigorously, and which are now classified as *vasodilators* or *circulatory stimulants* (see 'The Temperaments of Plant Remedies', on pp. 174–83).

The universality, and thus presumed popularity, of these approaches (and they will certainly feature strongly in this review of herbal therapeutics) means that they were associated with at least some apparent benefit. It is not enough to dismiss the practice because feeling warm so often feels better. Such an observation actually begs the questions: why? and what does feeling better mean in this context?

Nor is it accurate to see the primary aim in dealing with the body's circulation as to increase it only. We shall see that 'cooling' was as valid a strategy as 'heating' in traditional medicine, and oedema was an obvious contra-indication for circulatory stimulants from the beginning. In any case the concern with heating was restricted to illnesses, and not applied to health: it was not seen as a general requirement for life (with the possible and justified exception of using hot spices as a prophylactic against enteric infections – see the chapter 'Remedies').

Nevertheless, it is fair to conclude that in any case of duress the original instinct was to open up the affected tissue to extra heat or circulation. Whatever the explanation proffered through the ages, at its core there always seemed to be a concern for the basic health of these tissues. Heat meant life, as we shall see: by using warmth or circulatory stimulants a diseased or painful tissue could be almost visibly suffused with vitality. If, as so often, this was accompanied by relief and other benefits, the conclusion that diseases might be linked with tissue deprivation was unavoidable.

There is a modern justification for this primitive instinct. It is a basic tenet of medical science that all pathologies start with a relative deficiency of oxygen to the affected tissue (from whatever cause). Finding ways to increase oxygen levels to tissues is an accepted, though otherwise unrealistic, strategy for heading off disease deterioration.

The mechanism for increasing blood flow to the tissues is barely understood. In one case (cayenne) there is evidence of an alkaloid

93 Circulation

with prostaglandin activity (see 'Alkaloids', on pp. 327–31); in many others there are volatile oils present and this suggests an action by these molecules, perhaps directly on the metarterioles that control perfusion through the capillary bed. Some effects are only apparent under certain clinical or individual circumstances: most *diaphoretic* remedies only induce sweating in feverish states and most 'heating' remedies have very variable effects. All this implies a complexity of receptor stimulation.

It is almost certain, however, that any such effects would be at the tissue level: the suggestions made by herbalists in nineteenth-century North America that there might be an effect on the autonomic or other central control system is at best only likely to apply to the diaphoretic phenomenon, and perhaps not even then. It is most likely that explanations for any effect on tissue perfusion will be found in looking at circulation as a local event.

> **Proposition:**
>
> **many herbal remedies benignly increase tissue perfusion: this is accompanied by an appreciable effect against pathologies.**

Summary

The process of circulation can be said to include the following functions:

> interstitial fluid flow and local vasomotor control
> the heart, vascular circulation and systemic vasomotor control
> lymph and the special fluid systems
> temperature regulation, peripheral blood flow and sweating

Removal

Many disparate physiological functions will be discussed together under this heading. That this is so is a further example of the different approach to physiology being pursued here.

There is much sense in seeing the task of eliminating wastes as an overall requirement. The suggestion is that there is an inter-dependence between the several eliminative functions: if, for example, one of them is failing to make the grade, there is a greater load on the others and a risk that they might manifest symptoms of distress as a result. The implications go further in calling into question modern conventional views of the eliminative organs and their output. One example: the herbalist is not so quick to see unusual excretions as a problem, working somewhat on the principle that 'it is better out than in'.

The main channels of removal from the body are the bowel, the kidneys and urinary system, the sweat glands, the biliary system, and the lungs and upper respiratory system. Minor roles are played by various secretory glands around the surface of the body and in its cavities, and in women by the menstrual flow. Overlap with the earlier category of rejection brings in such functions as emesis (vomiting) and coughing.

The Lymphatics and Tissue Drainage

Cleaning the cells

On the principle, established earlier, that the perspective of the cell in the tissue is paramount, then any review of the removal of wastes ought to start there as well.

The immediate channel into which cells cast their metabolic waste products is the intercellular fluid bathing them. This, as has been pointed out, is not a vast volume of fluid but a fast-moving stream of diffusion. It is enough to ensure that the great majority of small molecules and ions excreted by the cells are removed to the venous capillaries.

This is usually a reliable elimination system. It is however not a complete one. Larger molecules, notably proteins, do not pass easily through the walls of the venules. Instead they, as well as any excess fluid, are taken up by the blind end-capillaries of the lymphatic system. The walls of these fine vessels are made up of cells in an overlapping mosaic, with each piece actually welded to neighbouring tissue cells rather than to each other. The result is a very porous membrane indeed, with pores potentially large enough to pass even cellular migrants.

The lymphatic system is quite active in its removal of fluid from the tissues. Rise in intercellular fluid pressure, through muscle contraction or other tissue movement, arterial pulsation or physical pressure in the vicinity, forces fluid through the pores into the lymphatic. Backward flow is prevented by operation of the 'flap' mechanism. As the fluid moves down the lymphatic it passes simple valves, like those in the veins, which further resist flowback. Between each valve smooth muscle rings appear in the lymphatic wall. These contract in sequence down the ducts to act as a 'lymphatic pump'.

At intervals in the system lymph nodes straddle the lymphatic ducts. They effectively concentrate the lymph, by bringing it alongside fluid of higher colloid osmotic pressure. They are also the batteries of lymphocytes and phagocytes, charged with screening the lymph for potential antigenic proteins and micro-organisms.

If they encounter trouble beyond that which they can easily handle, the lymph nodes can inflame and enlarge, manifesting, if they are at the body surface, as 'swollen glands' or lymphadenopathy. These are most often seen in the neck, armpit and groin.

Lymphadenopathy was always a traditional indication for the use of lymphatic herbal remedies. Clinical experience suggests that this is a useful treatment, but probably not for the reasons often given. These remedies were understood to flush the lymphatic system through: to be effectively lymphatic stimulants. However, one experiment has suggested that none of the traditional lymphatics actually stimulated lymph flow as much as simple lager![16] In fact, the best lymphatic stimulation, as suggested earlier, must come from massage and exercise.

Tissue cleansing?

From all this it seems difficult to find any physiological model to justify the traditional herbal idea that it is possible to 'cleanse the tissues', at least if this is taken to be a literal task.

It will be possible, however, to develop the notion that the tissues may be cleansed by improving the function of the major eliminatory channels in the body, those downstream of tissue drainage. It is most likely that those remedies classed as 'blood purifiers', 'depuratives' or 'alteratives' to the extent that they 'cleanse' anything, operate mainly at remote stations discussed below. They may of course have conventional anti-inflammatory action or otherwise change metabolic functions instead (see also 'Alteratives', on pp. 486–504).

Whether or not it is possible to find a pharmacological lever to influence them it is still the case, however, that the lymphatics are an important eliminatory channel in their own right. Although they usually cope with only one tenth of the fluid that is returned to the veins, they are an essential overflow system and their failure is certainly implicated in some types of oedema, a condition in which fluid accumulates in the tissues.

97 Removal

Oedema

The origins of oedema give significant insight into the normal mechanisms for draining the tissues. They fall into five main categories:

1 *obstruction to venous flow*, notably seen in heart failure and accumulating back pressure in the venous system. Oedema in this case is seen in the most gravity-dependent regions first, i.e. in the ankles. A special case of such oedema, known as ascites, is seen in the portal circulation following obstructive liver disease. It leads to fluid accumulation in the abdomen. Localized tissue oedema can form behind occluded or obstructed veins, as seen after venous blood clots and injury.

2 *low levels of plasma protein*. This means that the colloid osmotic pressure in the capillaries, which effectively acts as a brake on fluid movement into the tissues, is reduced. This loss must be extreme and is only seen locally with severe burns, and systemically with terminal kidney disease or near-starvation.

3 *lymphatic obstruction*. This is seen most dramatically in the tropical infection filariasis, in which nematode worm larvae are introduced into the lymphatics following bites from infected mosquitoes. If untreated, the subsequent inflammations can lead to scarring and eventual occlusion of the lymphatics in a region. The consequences have been given the name elephantiasis, such can be the severity of the oedema. A lymphatic oedema can also follow surgical removal of lymphatic tissue in operations to clear cancerous tumours. This is often only temporary.

4 *increased capillary fragility* leading to passage of protein from blood cell to tissue. The dramatic change in the balance of osmotic pressure can lead to tissue oedema. Burns, allergic reactions, and radiation damage can all lead to fluid swelling in the tissues affected through this cause.

5 *kidney failure*. Fluid retention at the kidneys will inevitably lead, if serious, to extensive oedema.

98 Physiology

The obvious point to make is that oedema is not a common condition and that in health there is a considerable safety margin built into tissue hydraulics to ensure that all excess fluid is easily mopped up. The main interest in drawing up this list is that it highlights the many factors influencing tissue drainage and acts as a suitable preface to the review of other eliminatory functions.

The Bowel

How often?

Of the eliminatory routes, clearly far and away the most important is the bowel. The bulk of food residue, various metabolic wastes, and a considerable quantity of dead bowel micro-organisms are voided through this channel. It is also the only normal route for bile products to leave the body.

Opinions vary widely as to the necessity for regular bowel evacuation. Conventional medical opinion has been that it does not matter either way, as long as faecal impaction does not occur. On the other hand it has also been claimed that anything less than daily effective movement will risk toxin accumulation and reabsorption. This latter view is taken to extremes in those who promote the use of colonic irrigation and enemas as ultra-efficient 'detoxification' techniques.

The likely truth, as always, is somewhere between the two views. In natural circumstances all mammals, including humans, will tend to have a daily evacuation. The average diet of our hunter-nomad and pastoral predecessors was sufficiently high in fibre that the stool was bulky, light (floating on water), and generally of low odour. The primitive transit time was also brief, taking 12–18 hours, compared with the 18–36 hours common in inhabitants of affluent societies.

Set against this long-established evolutionary precedence, it is most likely that modern bowel performance falls short of the ideal. Some of the consequences of this have been recognized in medicine: the increased incidence in affluent societies of such bowel diseases as diverticulitis and colon cancer has been firmly linked to lack of fibre, and bran has become the universal panacea of the medical profession since the mid-1970s.

The toxic argument

It is likely that the slower transit time, more compact and costive stool and the odorous evidence of greater fermentation in civilized humans have wider consequences. A transit time double that of the primitive bowel means that there is approximately twice as much opportunity for toxic fermentation and for reabsorption. A notable factor is the fate of bile and the extent of the entero-hepatic circulation. This is the cycle of bile secretion from the liver; bile and other metabolism in the gut; and reabsorption by the liver of both bile and metabolites. Certain drugs, like the morphine alkaloids and the foxglove glycosides, are known to go round and round this cycle, being initially excreted into the bile, and it is certain that other metabolites do likewise. The effect is to increase the time taken to remove them, and, in the case of the affected drugs at least, to raise their average blood levels. The slower the transit of material, the more this retention of wastes. It is, after all, not surprising.

It is however likely that some of the responses to this scenario are misplaced. The use of colonics, originating in middle Europe but most popular among sections of the health movement in the USA, follows the assertion that sluggish bowels are complicated by an insidious adulteration of food in modern times and by the effect of drugs like antibiotics on healthy gut flora, and that only drastic measures, like irrigation, can hope to satisfactorily cleanse the bowel. The considerable mucus that is produced by irrigation is held out as evidence of a valuable 'descaling'. A counter-view might be that the act of irrigation is intrinsically disturbing and that long-term protection and even bowel health might be compromised.

It is even more likely that excessive use of laxatives and even bran itself are harmful. It is generally accepted that the former easily leads to a persistent constipation in later life, possibly as a result of desensitizing the normal triggers for bowel movement.

Bran and fibre

What is less often recognized is that bran can exacerbate existing bowel disease. Its automatic prescription by doctors, even gastro-intestinal specialists, after years when the response to bowel disease was to cut out fibre altogether, can sometimes appear as a cruel irony. Many practitioners report they see more improvements in taking patients off bran than in putting them on it. Bran represents the most insoluble fraction of cereal fibre. The product of cooked cereal, as seen for example in porridge oatmeal, is largely soft and soluble, with mucilaginous properties. Bran is what is left when this is washed away. It can simply be too rough, especially for inflamed or irritable conditions like ulcerative bowel disease, diverticulitis and spastic colon. The overenthusiastic use of other excessively rough foods, like muesli and brown rice, may be similarly inappropriate, especially for those who have grown up on low-fibre diets and who are making a late conversion.

There is evidence too that in these individuals there is less ability to break the formation of insoluble complexes that form between calcium, iron, zinc and other minerals with the phytates present in cereal fibre, thus risking a dietary deficiency as well.

The balanced remedies

The main conclusion to be drawn is that the modern bowel does tend to be less effective than its evolutionary predecessor and that this inadequacy may be compounded by some of the more vigorous attempts to move it along. The ideal solution seems to be to consume a diet as high in *natural fibre* as can be safely tolerated and to increase exercise, which is a powerful stimulus to regular bowel movement. Disturbances of bowel regularity that cannot be helped in this way can be treated by *bulk laxatives*, *visceral relaxants*, liver remedies (especially *cholagogues*), all generally referred to as *aperients*, or the judicious use of *stimulating laxatives*, as will be explained in later parts of this text.

Under normal circumstances the bowel musculature is in a state of variable tension, there being a rhythmic pulsation of gentle contractions throughout the 24 hours. At approximately eight-hour intervals these contractions increase in time and intensity, to climax as major peristaltic contractions and potentially as a 'mass movement' of the contents of the ascending and transverse colons down to the descending colon and rectum (at which point it reaches consciousness as an urge to empty the bowels). In most cases two of the three mass movements each day stop short of completion, though quite often they are all productive. On the other hand, with the modern lifestyle, lack of exercise, sedentary occupations, and a life dictated by the clock, it more often happens that the call to defecate that results from the mass movement will be dulled or ignored. In this case the movement goes into reverse and the chance is lost till the next one, perhaps eight hours later. Repeated often enough, or if the consumption of dietary roughage is too low to fill the bowel, a habitual loss of tone can occur and so-called atonic constipation can set in. One can begin the process of correction by gradually increasing the amount of fibre in the diet, and possibly augmenting this by taking some of the tougher gums and mucilages like psyllium seed (*Plantago psyllium*), flaxseed, or linseed (*Linum usitatissimum*), or the seaweed gums, often available commercially as proprietary 'gels'. However, at some time or other it is usually necessary to apply a discreet touch of the stimulating anthra-quinone laxatives.

A visit to a traditional practitioner in early times would very often lead to the use of a purgative, to rid the body of its toxic load. As will be made clear elsewhere, such a strategy is only suitable for the robust constitution engaged in an acute disorder. Vigorous stimulation of bowel activity, achieved by using cathartics, is an innately debilitating manoeuvre. It fits in with the traditional target of diffusing disturbances arising from acute infectious diseases. In modern clinical conditions it is very rarely justified.

The use of the stimulating laxative is nevertheless sometimes justified. For persistent or acute constipation due to a sluggish bowel tone, either as a short-term treatment in isolation, or as part of a broader prescription, there are undoubted benefits. There are even accounts of small doses of senna (*Cassia* spp.), particularly in mixed prescriptions, being used to help restore normal bowel activity.

There are however considerable problems with excessive or prolonged use of stimulating laxatives which include exacerbating innate bowel laziness and complicating that type of constipation that comes from a spastic or irritable bowel.

Much preferable are the range of bulking laxatives providing a soft, fluid-retentive gel that gently restores natural bowel tone, whether it is initially lax or excessive. Whole cereal fibre, agar-agar, the seaweed gums, psyllium seed and linseed are examples of remedies that are usually benignly supportive to normal bowel function.

The Bile

The bile–bowel axis

The function of the bowel can rarely be dissociated from the secretion of bile and the wider function of the liver. At its simplest the relationship can be expressed in the fact that bile is a natural laxative. This means, for example, that some cases of persistent constipation can be relieved where appropriate by using remedies with primary *cholagogue* (bile-stimulating) effects. On a wider front, it means that the state of bowel function can often be linked to liver health.

Some bile constituents are also metabolized in the gut, particularly by the bowel flora. Some of the metabolites are irritating, providing the main laxative effect on the one hand, but being implicated in the origin of colon cancer and ulcerative bowel disease on the other. That these metabolites may be partly reabsorbed, or further influence the population of the gut flora, simply leads to further complications.

There are other connections. The final elimination route for bile is through the bowel. It is not, however, a direct route. Much bile, intrinsically fat-soluble, is reabsorbed before excretion and returned to the liver, and thus re-enters the cycle. The proportion of bile that has actually been round more than once before is largely dependent on the overall transit time through the bowel (see previous section). In the average near-costive Westerner three-quarters or more of the bile may be recycled. This clearly is significant, if bile is being used by the liver as its own eliminatory channel.

Bile – secretion or excretion?

The conventional view of bile is not principally as an excretion at all. About half its constituents are bile salts, breakdown products of cholesterol, that are important in emulsifying fats in the gut and providing for their absorption. It is pointed out that far from trying to eliminate these bile salts, the body tries to retain them by providing specific pumps for them in the lower small intestine, and that they in turn are the major internal cholagogue in the system, i.e. the amount of bile volume secreted is in direct proportion to the amount of recycling bile salts.

There is a simple point to make here. Bile salts form only a proportion of the whole, and an ionized, non fat-soluble, portion as well. Much of the rest of the bile is fat-soluble and reabsorbs very easily. This is certainly true of the drug and other metabolites that are also found there.

The liver's primary detoxification role is to break up the more fat-soluble metabolites in the bloodstream into less fat-soluble or ionized fragments so that the kidneys can get rid of them. Certain metabolites, including some drugs and food additives, are not so easily broken up, and the liver may have additional troubles in ill health. These fat-soluble materials usually end up in the bile. Their tendency to reabsorb is much less desirable.

Important drugs like the morphine alkaloids and digitalis glycosides are effectively retained in the body, if their excretion in the bile is reduced (and this also means if bowel movements are sluggish).

Bile problems

Bile also contains cholesterol in levels that are reflective partly of dietary levels, partly of innate production by the liver, and partly of the degree of reabsorption of cholesterol from the gut. Apart from dietary reduction, the most effective means of reducing bile cholesterol is by increasing the dietary intake of fibre, notably fruit pectins, and otherwise promoting effective bowel movements.

The cholesterol content of bile can be significant: under certain circumstances the cholesterol can come out of solution and gel into globules that in turn can calcify to form gallstones. If gall-bladder and bile activity is sufficiently vigorous, these may be simply passed as gravel or small stones. If the system is sluggish, small crystals can grow to become large stones that become increasingly difficult to pass. These gallstones can irritate and inflame the gall-bladder, causing considerable pain.

Gallstone problems are most likely in women, in the obese, and are also interestingly associated with constipation (in a syndrome, with hiatus hernia, called 'Saint's triad'). To avert and contain gallstone problems, it makes sense both to reduce dietary fat and cholesterol intake and to increase fibre consumption.

The other frequent problem involving bile is jaundice – the accumulation of bile products in the bloodstream as a result of liver disease or bile-duct blockage.

The consequent yellowing of the complexion was easily recognized in early times and the frequent associated liver inflammation equally obvious.

The herbal approach

Many traditional remedies were directed to the problem of jaundice on the specific grounds that they were re-directing the bile back into its proper channels. So-called *cholagogues* or *choleretics* were thought to increase the production and flow of bile through the bile duct. The vast majority are notable bitter remedies whose effect on bile flow is confirmed. Their actual effect on conditions like hepatitis is less certain and their use in any individual case is largely conjectural. Nevertheless, many are gentle enough and are popular treatments in areas where hepatitis is endemic.

The use of bitter cholagogues may be further justified in the treatment of gallstones on the basis that they could dilute the bile. Again, they provide a popular resort, along with consumption of sour materials like lemon juice, which also are likely to trigger reflex bile secretion by stimulation of taste buds. (There are many cases where the use of large quantities of lemon juice with olive oil by the more robust members of the British populace has been followed by the passage and eventual proud production of gallstones, sometimes of considerable size! The risk of impaction, however, means this is not to be recommended.)

There are a number of other miscellaneous bitter and non-bitter remedies, particularly used for liver and bile disorders, sometimes included under the general title of *hepatics*. They include such herbs as milk thistle seed (*Silybum marianum*), artichoke (*Cynara scolymus*), and dandelion root (*Taraxacum officinale*).[17]

The common view is that biliary problems are widespread: the notion of 'biliousness' to describe nausea, and the two Greek temperaments 'choleric' (emotional, unstable extrovert and literally meaning 'yellow bile') and 'melancholic' (depressive, unstable introvert and literally meaning 'black bile'), are all evidence that bile problems were seen to be central to many disorders. With the advantage of modern insights into liver and bile functions it is easy to dismiss such notions as primitive. Nevertheless, medical science probably errs in the other direction by neglecting the role of the liver and bile in a wide range of normal body functions. The modern herbalist often finds signs that liver and bowel disorders coexist with other syndromes, particularly those which are sometimes referred to as 'toxic': migraine headaches, chronic skin disease, allergies, inflammatory and other bowel disease (and constipation, of course). Following traditional therapeutic principles this herbalist often effectively deals with such conditions by using remedies that have hepatic or cholagogue effects.

The herbalist view is certainly that the full role of bile production in health has not yet been elicited.

The Kidneys

A marvellous mechanism

The kidneys are the precision instruments of elimination. Every day they filter about 120 litres of plasma from the bloodstream. All but a half to one litre of this is reabsorbed straight into the circulation. What is usually left in the urinary tubules is a large portion of the body's circulating wastes.

It is an extraordinary mechanism. It is all accomplished by about two million microscopic kidney tubules or nephrons. At their top end coils of capillaries called glomeruli evaginate into the tubule, separated from its lumen by an extremely fine porous 'basement' membrane. Through this filter passes a considerable proportion of the bloodstream in the glomerulus; the pores are large enough to allow the passage of quite large molecules, up to, but not usually including, proteins.

The filtrate is passed down the tube and is immediately subjected to a series of pumps. The main one claws back sodium ions, and thus water, and all the glucose and amino-acids and other essential components are also retrieved. This reabsorption is matched by further secretion, of positive- and negative-charged ions. The result is that by the time the filtrate leaves the first stage of its journey, through the 'proximal tubules', its contents are already largely selected. Metabolic wastes like urea, oxalates, urates and creatinine have become relatively concentrated.

The filtrate, however, is still actually very dilute. In the next stage, the 'distal tubule', an ingenious concentrating mechanism, is employed to extract the majority of the water. It is also the stage where either potassium ions or hydrogen ions (depending on the concentrations in the blood of the latter) are swapped for sodium ions in the filtrate. This is the major route of excretion in the kidneys for hydrogen ions or acid.

The overall degree of water reabsorption, and thus of the quantity of urine, is largely determined by hormonal control of the reabsorption mechanism. Antidiuretic hormone (ADH), produced by the posterior pituitary gland, effectively opens pores in the tubule and

107   Removal

thus allows more reabsorption of water. It has the major role of overseeing total fluid levels in the body. It is secreted to avoid dehydration and suppressed in over-hydration or after over-drinking (or after even small quantities of alcohol – as is usually obvious!). Other hormones may influence the process, notably adrenal steroids like aldosterone, and the sex hormones, notably progesterone.

Hormonal controls serve another purpose: the control of blood pressure. Small glands located at the glomerulus respond to lowered blood pressure by initiating a hormone cascade, the renin-angiotensin system, that further reduces fluid loss at the distal tubule.

The kidney thus has simultaneous roles in excreting acid or other metabolic wastes, and in regulating overall fluid balance and blood pressure. These linked roles are helpful in understanding the use of diuretics, especially in herbal medicine.

The herbal diuretics

In traditional herbal medicine diuretics have been applied to a wide range of clinical conditions, including fluid retention and high blood pressure, arthritis and other inflammatory conditions, urinary stones, and urinary infections like cystitis. It is possible that all these uses might be justified.

Most plant material has diuretic action: some plants appear to lead to urine production over and above the norm. They all work primarily as 'osmotic diuretics'. Other things being equal, all material successfully excreted by the kidneys, will, to maintain osmotic balance, take water along with it. There are many such constituents in plants including certain types of sugars, volatile oils and many aglycones (constituents forming glycosides with sugars). This is a very gentle and usually not very dramatic diuretic mechanism. It is likely that there are other effects as well: caffeine and other xanthines increase glomerular blood flow, for example, but few plants possess the aggressive diuretic actions of most conventional chemical diuretics. These often directly interfere with the pumps that reabsorb water.

Nevertheless, it is often reported that taking herbal prescriptions does increase urine flow. The impression is that this is a very variable response, the same herbs having very different effects on different individuals. The positive response is reported more frequently by those suffering the conditions mentioned earlier. The conclusion reached is that when appropriate the gentle herbal diuretic action can be quite adequate.

More urine may either be urine containing more water, or urine containing more wastes that in turn bring out more water. There is insufficient evidence in most cases to make a distinction. It is however claimed in herbal tradition that some herbal diuretics are particularly good at increasing waste excretion as well as increasing water loss. These are most often applied in the treatment of arthritic and other inflammatory diseases.

The use of diuretics for fluid retention is an obvious application and is endorsed by conventional pharmacology. It is also appreciated, however, that the cause of the fluid retention has significant bearing on the approach used, and on the outcome of treatment.

The most dramatic form of fluid retention in former times was dropsy. In advanced cases it would lead to gross swelling of the lower limbs and abdomen before death intervened. It was universally considered to be an indication for diuretics, but the effects of such an approach were never dramatic. Some herbalists were nevertheless treating it successfully, and one of the best stories in medicine tells how Dr William Withering in 1785 took the trouble to analyse the prescription of one of them. He found the most active ingredient was not a diuretic at all. It was a foxglove (*Digitalis purpurea*), the poison and heart stimulant.

It was this insight that led to the development of the digitalis glycosides as one of the most effective modern remedies of all, and to a recognition that dropsy was in fact the advanced stage of heart, not kidney, failure. Diuretics are still often necessary, but only as an adjunct to a powerful heart stimulation. As a result the symptoms of heart failure today rarely progress further than puffy ankles (see 'Cardioactive Glycosides', on pp. 310–13).

The role of diuretics as an adjunct to digitalis in heart failure has its own complications. The process of diuresis by definition leads to a net loss of potassium from the body fluids as it is swapped for sodium in the distal tubules. Lowered potassium levels can disastrously upset the effect of the digitalis glycosides. To compensate most conventional diuretic drugs used for the purpose incorporate potassium supplements (often marked by the use of chemical shorthand for potassium, K). It is interesting, therefore, to note that all plants are good sources of potassium. One case widely used as a diuretic in heart failure, dandelion leaf, has so much potassium that it leads to a net increase in blood potassium levels (see 'Dandelion', on pp. 431–4).

Fluid retention may also follow hormonal upset (as seen in premenstrual syndrome in women) or genuine kidney disorder. In many such cases the use of herbal diuretics can be clinically effective. Other sources of oedema (see pp. 98–9) may also be helped with diuretics, but usually require other appropriate treatments as well.

Urinary problems

Herbal diuretics are also applied to urinary troubles. The basic principle is simple. Any dilution of the urine will reduce the concentration of potentially irritating constituents.

The most obvious application is to urinary stones. The urine normally contains substances that are barely soluble in water: calcium phosphate, calcium urate and oxalates are most frequent examples. These are usually carried in a most vulnerable state of solution, the 'supersaturated solution', in which sedimentation is prevented entirely by the glassy smoothness of the urinary tract walls.

School science tells us that if, for example, sugar is dissolved in hot water until the solution is fully saturated and the water cools, it will be carrying more sugar than it can hold in solution (this is because sugar is more soluble in hot than cold water). If, however, this experiment is conducted in a glass beaker, the excess sugar cannot be deposited – the solution is supersaturated. The insertion of a piece of string will provide a seeding surface and a growing sugar crystal will appear almost instantly.

This rather elegant demonstration well illustrates the twin requirements for preventing crystals forming in the urine:

    1 *to keep the urine as dilute as possible*: the essential

recommendation in cases where urinary stones become likely is to drink more fluid. The use of gentle herbal diuretics can almost certainly be justified on the same principle. There is a strong tradition for just that effect, a tradition forged in the days when the excruciating pain of kidney stones might otherwise only be relieved by potentially fatal surgery.

2 *to maintain the glassy smoothness of the urinary tract*: under normal circumstances, the smoothness of the urinary tubules prevents even insoluble salts like calcium oxalate, urate and phosphate from depositing. It is however known from histological examination that any urinary infection will lead to persisting damage to the tubule wall (as well as an increased likelihood of recurrence). There are a number of herbal diuretics used as urinary antiseptics with apparently long-term effect, and others with a reputation for healing damaged urinary mucosa (as evidenced, for example, by bleeding into the urine).

A combination of diuretic, urinary antiseptic and urinary 'astringent' remedies might yet be shown to justify the traditional reputation for herbal remedies in cases of urinary stones.

Eliminating acids

It is a persistent notion that arthritis is an 'acid' condition. It is pointed out, in support of the idea, that acids effectively constitute the majority of cell wastes, being the end-product of most metabolic pathways: carbon dioxide, lactic and uric acids, sulphates and phosphates are notable examples. To these are added the many non-metabolized acids extracted from foods, such as oxalic and tartaric acids. It is concluded that ridding the body of these acids must be a prime requirement of the eliminatory machinery. The lungs clearly remove much in the form of carbon dioxide, but the kidneys are charged with getting rid of much of the rest.

The early unravelling of the pathogenesis of gout, caused by the accumulation of uric acid crystals in the joints, probably cemented the notion of acid accumulation as a general factor in arthritis in nineteenth-century Europe. It is moreover a stubbornly popular explanation. The idea of 'acid' as a toxin is especially common in

Britain. Arthritis is widely thought to be an indication for the reduction in the consumption of 'acid foods'.

In naturopathic traditions foods have been divided into those that yield acidic and those that yield alkaline residues (a classification originally based on the analysis of the ash left after combustion). Protein- and starch-rich foods were shown to be the most acidic; vegetables and fruit the most alkaline. (This latter causes endless popular confusion! In fact, most fruit acids readily metabolize to alkaline bicarbonates.) A reduction in the consumption of animal protein and refined carbohydrates has for long been widely recommended on these principles.

There is some support for the suggestion that vegetarians have less likelihood of arthritic disease.[18] As in most such things, of course, the protection is probably more true for some individuals than for others. It is nevertheless with a similar explanation that diuretic remedies like celery (*Apium graveolens*) and parsley (*Carum petroselinum*) seed, wild carrot (*Daucus carota*), birch (*Betula* spp.) and nettle (*Urtica dioica*) have been applied to arthritic conditions.

We now know that arthritis is far more complex a disorder than these ideas suggest. There are in fact no references to acid metabolites in conventional explanations. It must be noted, however, that as yet little is known of the disease: it is difficult at this stage to dismiss herbal claims that relief may be had by improving elimination of wastes through the kidneys.

The Sweat Glands

Is sweat an excretion?

To the modern physiologist the sweat gland is essentially a cooling mechanism that can also be invoked in the sympathetic 'fright, fight, flight' response.

There is no doubt that sweating can be very effective in getting rid of heat under maximal conditions. The effect of evaporating sweat from the body surface can be to remove ten times the amount of heat generated by the body's metabolism.

It is also the primary mechanism for cooling in fever. In ways discussed elsewhere sweating usually marks a turning point in the course of fever, a point where heat needs to be lost rather than gained. Again its effect on reducing body temperature cannot be in doubt.

In the process, however, a lot of body fluid can be lost. In hot climates more water can be lost through perspiration than all other routes of elimination put together.

The question of relevance to this discussion is whether the sweat glands excrete anything other than water and the normal ionic constituents of the body fluids. There is no doubt as to the answer.

The sweat gland extracts a filtrate from the plasma, from a network of capillaries opened up by action of sympathetic nerve fibres. This filtrate is not as rich as that passing through the pores of the basement membrane in the kidney glomerulus, but small metabolites like urea, metabolic acids and creatinine pass easily enough. There is a degree of reabsorption as the filtrate passes along the tubule, but this largely affects the amount of sodium and water left in the eventual secretion. The quantity of metabolites passed in any sweating is thus largely independent of the total amount of perspiration.

The overall result is that *even small quantities of sweat can lead to the excretion of a significant proportion of the body's wastes*. This can sometimes be noted in the odour of the body's perspiration or even in secondary irritation of the skin. It is perhaps not surprising that such waste excretion is especially obvious in kidney failure or disease.

It is difficult to avoid the conclusion that the functions of sweat glands and kidneys overlap. In hot weather, and after prolonged perspiration from other causes, the kidneys excrete very much less urine. In cases of kidney failure the sweat glands pass more wastes. Anatomically and physiologically there are similarities in the two processes.

Clearing fevers

In traditional medicine sweat was seen primarily as an excretion, most notably in fevers where it was seen as flushing out the poisons

113   Removal

that brought on the problem. As will be seen traditional thera-peutics put the promotion of perspiration as the first step in treating ancient clinical disorders, with the implication that fever was the first indication that the body was hitting trouble and that helping the natural perspiration not only helped in managing the fever but most quickly and obviously eliminated the external intruder.

It is probably accurate to say that the sweat glands were only seen to be clinically significant as eliminating channels during fever. This reflects the way treatments influenced sweat production. There are a number of herbal remedies, the *diaphoretics*, with minimal impact on sweat production under normal circumstances, that in the febrile state provoke quite considerable perspiration.

We might smile benevolently at such archaic ideas. Who today could take seriously the thought that sweating flushed out the poisons that caused fever?

Yet, there is likely to be elimination involved after all. Physi-ologists need not go primitive to see a value for it, if they accept that there are overall requirements in the body for the removal of wastes.

The Respiratory System

The trouble with air

In creating the lungs the Maker faced several intriguing engineering problems. Exchanging oxygen and carbon dioxide in a fluid environ-ment, initially by simple diffusion through cell walls, and then through specialized gill structures, is a relatively uncomplicated business. Air breathing is much harder. Because gas exchange is less efficient between air and fluid, a relatively much larger surface area of body fluids has to be exposed for aeration. A way of passing large quantities of air over these fluids has also to be devised.

The resulting design is the lungs, vast networks of fine blood capillaries surrounded by air whose movement is powered by an efficient bellows unit, the diaphragm. It works extremely well!

However, there remains a problem. Air is likely to be contaminated with dust, smoke and other pollutants. Sucking all this into a closed moist sponge inevitably means that a lot of rubbish will get trapped inside. There needs to be an effective cleaning system.

Cleaning the lung

The solution is elegant. As the air is inhaled the anatomy of the airways sets it spiralling in a vortex down the bronchial tubes. Centrifugal forces thus ensure that most particles in the air get thrown to the bronchial walls. Here a sticky mucus secretion traps the particles like flypaper. This film is supported on a bed of cilia, contractile filaments projecting from the surface of the epithelium. They are involved in a phased series of contractions, always upwards, to give the effect of repeated waves rising up the airways, carrying the impregnated mucus with them. This emerges at the top, at the throat, as phlegm or sputum usually to be swallowed unconsciously, to be destroyed in the sterilizing vat of the stomach. The whole upward elimination is attractively referred to as the 'mucociliary escalator'.

As a result of this escalator, the air reaching the fine alveoli in the lungs, where it meets the capillaries, is very largely cleansed. It is just as well: there are no cilia or mucus secretions at this level. Those impurities that are either too fine or too copious to be trapped higher up can then only be removed by wandering phagocytes, or possibly by powerful upheavals of the diaphragm, exercise or coughing. As every medical student dissecting and discovering the tar deposits in a smoker's lung knows, however, this last resort can easily be overburdened.

The cough is the back-up to the mucociliary escalator. It is clearly an attempt at removal. The traditional view, unfortunately not always shared in modern times, is that coughing is better helped than suppressed. Only when a cough can be seen to be pointless, as in nervous coughing or in conditions like tumours or other injury, are cough suppressants or antitussives used.

115 Removal

Respiratory problems

All this is very relevant to understanding various respiratory disorders. The mucociliary escalator can fail in two main ways: there may be an insufficient, tacky mucus, or there may be too much.

In the first case, seen for example in allergic and asthmatic conditions and in dry, irritating coughs, the mucus is too tacky to flow adequately. If the problem is prolonged, congestion may occur and a secondary bronchitis can result. Traditional medicine classified such problems as 'hot and dry' and prescribed 'cooling, moistening' herbs, *relaxing expectorants*, most known nowadays to be rich in mucilages. Mucilages, as will be seen, act, possibly by reflex from the upper gut, to increase the fluidity of tacky mucus and may also reduce accompanying bronchial muscle spasm.

The second case is more common in the cold and damp climate of Britain, an obvious connection in traditional medicine. Excessive mucus, otherwise known as catarrh, can overload the ciliary mechanism and a primary congestion can occur. Opportunistic infection can easily supervene and bronchitis and other lung infections are the common result. In these circumstances traditional prescriptions included *warming expectorants* like cinnamon, ginger or garlic, or *stimulating expectorants*, often low-dose emetics, that appear, again by reflex from the upper gut, to provoke a more productive cough.

Catarrh

The production of excess mucus in the lung just referred to leads on to a general consideration of the nature of catarrh. It is still largely a mystery. Many factors are likely to be involved in provoking excessive activity in the mucus cells. Increased blood flow to the epithelium is definitely one; pathogenic or other toxic irritation can be another. There does however remain a considerable internal influence, metabolic and possibly systemic inflammatory activity, that is even less understood.

Again the early viewpoint was that catarrh was an extraordinary elimination, or at least a sign that ordinary eliminatory channels were inadequate. Thus the traditional treatment of catarrh involved the use of eliminative remedies and 'cleansing' diets (usually rich in fruit and raw vegetables). The European naturopathic tradition was that respiratory infections followed catarrhal states as much as they provoked them, but that even in the latter case they were signalling the need for, and actually delivering, an increased eliminatory effort.

The Toxicity Thesis of Disease

In the foregoing sections it is possible to discern the development of a common theme: that in earlier traditions many illnesses were linked with a failure in the co-ordinated functions of elimination.

The illnesses concerned are, almost by definition, of the more chronic variety. They also happen to include a large group of particularly difficult chronic inflammatory disorders: catarrhal problems, skin and bowel disease, arthritis and autoimmune diseases.

Modern medicine has done little more than provide symptomatic relief, late surgical or other drastic intervention for these conditions. It is not in a position to dismiss another therapeutic option that has been a popular choice for millennia. It does, however, justifiably ask that any such approach subject itself to adequate scrutiny.

Traditional herbal medicine will need to show it can make a significant impression on chronic inflammatory conditions. It may also need to elaborate further, with rational physiological and psychological explanations, its view that improving eliminations from the body is a valid strategy. Such a search might have at least one benefit: providing new insight into the causes of some particularly distressing modern illnesses. The following might usefully encapsulate the matter:

Propositions:

the process of removing waste materials from the body is essential to health;

several eliminatory functions share the task: failure in or suppression of one will lead to extra burdens and possible signs of distress in others, and will have potentially widespread implications for general health.

The Control Processes

Inner harmony

In surveying the body's functions, interest soon focuses on those that are responsible for the regulation, integration and control that is manifested as *homoeostasis*.

These functions appear to be at a different supervisory level from the primary functions described so far, acting to connect them with each other and with the wider survival imperative. There is no doubt that at this level they fascinate many for whom other physiological subjects are too mundane.

Yet this view of control as being some higher function is not necessarily the best one, nor is it always helpful in understanding disturbances in homoeostasis. The fact that the nervous system is prominent in control functions is a reminder of the Cartesian split between mind and body. Such a hierarchical view of the human being has had some benefits but, as discussed elsewhere, its wisdom is not accepted in traditional medicine.

In the framework discussed here the *control functions will be seen to arise from that which is controlled*, rather than being superimposed upon it. It is a view that accords well with modern physiological and ecological research.

In the diagram illustrating this review (see Fig. 1, on p. 28), the control processes are envisaged as arranged concentrically, with each level encompassing the processes at its core. There are three such levels:

> 1 at the centre is the primal oscillation of the life form; to the extent that an actual physiological function can be articulated, it is the management and control of these vital pulses;

2 at a second level of control are the functions that balance activity and rest at all stages beyond the cellular;

3 the third level is in two related parts: overall homoeostatic integration on the one hand, the reproductive functions on the other. Linking these two may appear puzzling at first, not least because reproduction might not seem an integrative function at all. It will be seen, however, that there are very close functional overlaps at this level and the association will be shown to have therapeutic value as well.

All the control functions are inseparable from that which they control. Their influence is intrinsic to all vital manifestation. It is difficult to envisage any function that is not also directly involved in control. It may actually be concluded that biological control arises out of the relationship between vital functions.

These are the themes that will be elaborated in what follows.

The Vital Pulse

To explore the nature of the vital motor is to go into very deep water indeed. It will be necessary to detour briefly through more philosophical currents in order to develop any workable model at all.

Mechanism vs. vitalism

As the biological and biophysical intricacies of cell function have been elaborated over the last 150 years or so, it has been tempting to develop the thesis that the living cell is no more than a very complicated mechanism, responding to external forces in ways that, although mysterious, are potentially decipherable.

From the outset this new scientific attitude was countered by those who saw life as essentially miraculous, beyond reason, in which the material was subservient to and powered by a purposive intangible 'Vital Force'. This 'ghost in the machine' was also undefinable, and vitalism declined as an influence in the biological sciences in the face of the explosion of mechanistic discoveries.

Vitalism was revived briefly in the early part of this century by the embryologist Driesch,[19] who, with the benefits of further advances in science, was still able to predict, for example, that no mechanism would ever emulate a living being in being able to regenerate missing components (as the embryo, notably, can do) without help from outside.

Generally speaking, however, the vitalist-mechanistic debate, active in the last century, has not been productive. The lack of any criterion even to define a vital causal force has meant that vitalism itself has taken retreat into the bunker of modern religion.

Organicism

What may provide a more promising scenario is a philosophical view that derives initially from the work of the German mathematician and philosopher, G. W. Leibniz (1646–1716). In seeking to define the entities ('monads') that made up the universe he was drawn to conceive of them possessing an internal 'blue-print', a pre-established pattern of development. Following this, A. N. Whitehead (1861–1947) developed the 'philosophy of Organism', a full-blown metaphysical version of Leibniz's ideas, specifically including physical as well as biological phenomena.[20] In Whitehead's view, 'atoms do not blindly run' as the mechanistic view holds, nor are they directly guided by Divine intervention, as the vitalist view usually presumes, but rather all entities at all levels behave in accordance with their position in the greater pattern ('organisms') of which they are parts.[21]

The idea of a pattern determining the parts has of course been adopted as a feature of modern ecological thought and the holistic health movement. It has led to the idea of morphogenic fields as the determining factor in biological structure and function. The innovative text by D'arcy Thompson,[22] at the time much beloved of biologists with an artistic bent, was an early development of the view. A more recent review, with interesting propositions for the future of the biological sciences, has been provided by Rupert Sheldrake.[23]

The essential difference between the organismic view of life and that of the vitalists is that the former does not insist on a separate 'ghost in the machine'. Rather, it presumes that the behaviour of an organism is *a combination of the intrinsic qualities of its constituents, and the influences bearing in on it from outside.*

It is interesting to note that after initially postulating the *Gaia* hypothesis as a manifestation of some inner, almost vital, homoeostatic force governing the Earth and its atmosphere Professor James Lovelock has modified his views (supported by his model ecosystem of black daisies and white daisies with herbivores to graze upon them) to a balance comprised of the interaction of the intrinsic properties of the Earth's constituents combined with the influence of outside forces, i.e. the Sun.[24]

An organismic view does not in itself preclude further theological or spiritual reflection. The prospect of a divine presence is not reduced by such a scheme. Compared with the previous vitalist-mechanist argument, moreover, it provides a better model for any contemplation of an immanent God. The only view it does challenge is of a Creator as a separated entity.

The choreography in the cell

We may now tentatively apply these concepts to the phenomenon of vital activity within the cell.

It is certainly true that the contents of the cell are in continuous movement. The protoplasm that makes up the intracellular matrix exists in various interchangeable states of relative viscosity with continual movement from one state to the other, especially if a cell itself is moving. There are also internal currents within the cell, that seem to be linked to the fine inner structure of microtubules and to the activity of the fine cell skeleton, the microfilaments. Even the major organelles, notably the endoplasmic reticulum, microsomes and Golgi bodies, are in a state of continual movement, in a way that extends beyond the simple Brownian movement of molecules in solution.[25]

The constant movement within a cell is clearly contiguous with the constant changes in the tissues at large. Throughout biological systems there is a tendency for such changes to be rhythmic in nature. In an exciting new text,[26] Leon Glass and Michael Mackey from Montreal survey, with the aid of mathematical analysis, current knowledge about the nature of rhythmic physiological activity. A tendency for activity in living systems to oscillate, via a number of mechanisms, is confirmed in many case-studies. They however forbear from speculating too far about mechanisms involved in the generation of such oscillations.[27]

While we are not seeking recourse to the 'ghost in the machine' it is obvious that myriad cyclic movements are a central manifestation of biological life. This was often the account of literature. When pressed to ascribe qualities to the Life Force, writers in the past have repeatedly used the analogy of a vibration, a pulse, a sound, a breath. We will see how such ideas inspired at least some views of herbal therapeutics later.

What Glass and Mackey confirm is that, whatever the source of such biological impulses, they are immediately involved in a mesh of interactions and perturbations and in the discipline imposed by the integral steady-state normally reached by physiological functions. The collective patterning that all this implies could be classed as the process of 'maintaining vital rhythms'.

Balancing Activity and Rest

'Alternate labor and rest'

The basic vital pulse is transformed at the level of the tissues and beyond into waves of activity (the 'alternate labor and rest' of W. H. Cook – pp. 159–60).

The heart contracts and relaxes, the alimentary tract has its slow peristaltic pulse, and the bronchial tube its mucociliary escalator. Beyond these are the directed rhythms. They include the central nervous oscillations such as those that drive the diaphragm and ribcage muscles in respiration, the vasomotor tone of the circulatory system and the cerebellar and basal nuclear control of the skeletal musculature that allows upright posture.

Superimposed on such pulses are other tidal cycles. Most obvious are the diurnal rhythms, the phases of activity from day to night.

Day-time sees a general increase in activity, the catabolic 'combustion' of food and the function of the adrenal stress response. Night-time is when the body slows down and the balance of activity switches to repair, growth and healing.

These daily shifts are linked with changes in the levels of a wide range of physiological markers (see Fig. 18, 'Circadian Rhythms', on p. 631).

In the early morning the pituitary ACTH reaches its peak levels. This is followed as expected by a peak in the activity of the adrenal cortex and in the level of stress hormones, the better to balance the simultaneous peak in noradrenaline and to influence its conversion to adrenaline. A similar peak is seen in the level of sex hormones (FSH, testosterone, progesterone), and in the amount of haemoglobin to carry oxygen to the active tissues.

During the day various markers follow the increase in metabolic rate: body temperature, pulse rate, blood protein (followed by blood urea), and average levels of blood glucose, lipids, serotonin and cyclic AMP.

Many other variables, generally associated with parasympathetic activity and repair and growth, peak at night: thyroid, growth hormone, insulin, prolactin, renin (along with diastolic blood pressure), average blood flow to the skin, immunological activity and gastric secretion.

There is obviously much more. Most such changes are clearly set by the external *Zeitgeist* of dark and light and daily activities, but as night-shift workers and international airline passengers will know, the body retains its own tidal rhythms as well. How these are all controlled is still barely understood. There is, however, one effector mechanism that is involved: the autonomic nervous system, the network of fibres and chemical transmitters that regulates many internal functions.

The autonomic nervous system

There are two branches of the autonomic nervous system. The *sympathetic nervous system* is linked with the secretion and effects

123   The Control Processes

of adrenaline and noradrenaline. Its primary role is to stimulate those functions that will be most useful for the 'fright, fight, flight' response. It mobilizes the body for overt action. Blood supply to the muscles, heart and brain is increased, that to the digestive and other vegetative functions is decreased. Activity in the internal viscera is generally reduced. The airways and pupils are dilated; sweating is increased (though blood flow to the skin is decreased – hence the cold sweat) and the hairs rise in gooseflesh; blood glucose levels and metabolic rate also rise.

The *parasympathetic nervous system* reduces the heart rate and bronchial capacity; it increases blood supply to the internal viscera, digestive activity and glandular secretions.

The sympathetic system is set up like a blunderbuss. Central stimulation leads to widespread mobilization. The parasympathetic system is more discreet, subtle, decentralized. It is the complex pluralistic state versus the militaristic one-directional solution.

Exercise and rest

The role of the sympathetic system is prominent in the mobilization of the body in exercise. The aerobic economy that results from vigorous exercise – a high oxygen consumption, a switch to the combustion of fats rather than carbohydrates, and all the other metabolic and physiological shifts one would expect – contrasts markedly with the resting metabolism of sedentary life.

This must have considerable health implications. Early *Homo sapiens*, tramping upwards of 65 km a day through millions of years of hunter-nomad existence, evolved into the human being we are today literally on his feet. Our forebears spent most of their waking hours under the influence of the sympathetic nervous system and of noradrenaline healthily channelled through exercise. The usual day for the modern affluent middle-class citizen of parasympathetic-dominated waking, or even worse, stressful sympathetic dominance without the exercise to diffuse it, must mean that the balance of functions is simply different, and probably less healthy.

The effects of sympathetic activity, adrenaline and noradrenaline when there is no actual exercise are to exacerbate all the problems now referred to as 'stress diseases': e.g. high blood pressure and cholesterol levels, heart disease, thromboses and duodenal ulcers.

If regular daily exercise has any value at all, it must initially be in re-establishing the body's original fluctuation between parasympathetic dominance at night and active sympathetic dominance during the day, with all the benefits accruing from that.

Plant drugs on the autonomic system

Pharmacological interest in the autonomic nervous system revolves around the effects of certain drugs on the chemical receptors found at different synapses in sympathetic and parasympathetic systems. Both systems use nicotine-sensitive acetylcholine receptors at their first stages and thus nicotine has the effect of increasing general autonomic activity. The parasympathetic system is mediated at its target sites by acetylcholine receptors that are stimulated by the poisonous alkaloid muscarine, from the fly-agaric toadstool, but is blocked by the atropine alkaloids from solanaceous plants like deadly nightshade (*Atropa belladonna*), henbane (*Hyoscyamus niger*) and datura (*Datura stramonium*). Caffeine, among its many hormonal effects, extends the action of noradrenaline, the final neurotransmitter of the sympathetic system.

The fact that these influences originate from the plant world is a result of the widespread use of these powerful herbs. The bronchospasm of asthma could be blocked by inhaling fumes of datura or henbane; the original *belladonna* was one of many Spanish ladies who used deadly nightshade in eye-drops to dilate their pupils, a technique at once inducing desirability and myopia! Coffee, tea and tobacco are well-used stimulants and hunger suppressants; magic toadstools and mushrooms, datura, nightshades and other such plant material are used rather more selectively as hallucinogens.

Other mechanisms

There are other components to the regulation of the on-off pulse of body rhythms usually linked to autonomic functions. There is the vast endocrine orchestra and its connections to the diurnal, lunar and seasonal cycles touched on later. There is the fascinating role of the brain centres linked through the reticular activating system, a network of fibres in the brain stem, in determining the level of arousal, relaxation or sleep, and in helping to set the cycles of appetite, thirst, sexual activity and other passions.

It would be convenient if the view of Cook and the physiomedicalists (see 'The post-Thomsonians', on pp. 158–60) were to be borne out and herbal medicines had a pivotal role in improving such regulatory activities. It is however difficult to share their confidence. The herbs just mentioned are special cases, only marginally used in clinical practice. The interest nowadays has shifted to other control functions.

Integration

An awesome physiology

The regulation of levels of activity within the body is just part of a broader array of integrating functions. As organisms scale up in complexity, so do their organizational processes. This is the main reason for the approach adopted here: the traditional view, having appreciated integration as the highest manifestation of vitality, is to leave it well alone. There is little sign of any attempt to tinker with the details: rather, there is an air of reverence and awe. The actual strategies adopted are discussed later, but they tend to be non-specific.

The evidence for integration can be seen everywhere. The following examples illustrate the breadth of the regulatory functions:

> In health, cells in the body's tissues only reproduce to fill gaps caused by damage, disease or in the process of organic growth; a failure in this regulation leads to tumour growth, a relatively rare event given the billions of cells involved.
>
> The levels of fluids and electrolytes in the body, of glucose in

the bloodstream, of blood pressure and of body temperature remain remarkably constant, both within an individual and among all human beings.

The propensity of the blood to clot is on a razor balance. If it is too sensitive, thromboses form; if not sensitive enough, haemorrhage occurs.

The relationship of the body's hormones is a choreography of dazzling complexity and finesse. The most powerful substances in the bloodstream are held in an astonishing symptomless balance even in many states of ill health.

There are several agents of integration identified. They must, however, not be seen as working in isolation. The whole is what determines the parts:

The central nervous axis connecting the limbic system, the hypothalamus and the pituitary is primarily responsible for integrating nervous and hormonal activities with the individual's sense of place in the world.

The same collective central integration unit also modulates activities in the immune system to influence the body's physical relationship with the environment.

The liver provides an essential integration at the somatic level, controlling most metabolic reactions and exerting its own powerful influence on hormonal and immunological functions.

The adrenal cortex, through its production of glucocorticoids and aldosterone, acts as the primary instrument of the hypothalamus-pituitary in maintaining many of the body's constants, notably fluid and electrolyte levels, blood-sugar and amino-acid levels, and blood-cell counts, and in maintaining overall balance after trauma, infection, intense heat and cold, disease and other stresses.

All cells throughout the body, but especially the nerve fibres and cells from the gut, endocrine glands, lymphatic and immune systems, kidney, heart and skin secrete a vast assortment of chemical messengers, neurotransmitter hormones, neurohormones, neuropeptides and immunohumours, that together determine the activity of all the body's other cells.

127   The Control Processes

The broader frame

It is an obvious conclusion that many disturbances of an individual's integrative functions directly reflect that individual's relationships to the outside world. The family and the social, sexual, economic, political and, above all, spiritual fabric in which an individual is enmeshed are the major determinants of health or ill health at this level.

Traditional society usually provided a very different context for human growth and development. Family, social ties and obligations were overwhelmingly strong; the experience of life as a story with a meaning was all-pervasive; the place or prospect of individual self-aggrandizement was minimal. Many strongly traditional societies surviving today, like those in the Far Eastern or Islamic countries, have found it difficult to address the notion of neurosis, anxiety, stress-induced illness and the common malaises of a post-industrial society. They even sometimes deny that such problems exist.

These modern disturbances are now known to cause illness specifically through their effect on the body's integrative functions. 'Holistic' medical practitioners work on the principle that much modern ill health is best tackled by reference to psychological, emotional and spiritual stresses. They might see the mundane preoccupations of the traditional herbalist as rather limited.

The herbalist's approach

In one sense their instincts are correct. Modern illnesses merit modern solutions. Nevertheless, the herbal tradition can inspire a most creative approach to them. The first message lies in the attitude herbalists have had to the whole subject.

In facing the phenomenon of integration the traditional practitioner was drawn to awe at the robust elegance of it all rather than to any aspiration to tinker with the controls. With one notable exception there are no traditional strategies that directly address disturbances of integration as such, and even this, the use of *tonics* in general and of the Oriental *adaptogenic* remedies in particular, is applied in an attitude of reverence for the body's own recuperative abilities rather than with any intention of running the show.

This is not a statement of failure. The living body is an ecosystem. Herbalists are not among those who believe that one can direct ecosystems to short-term gain without repercussions. In another context they would instinctively prefer to prevent drought by preventing deforestation and overgrazing rather than divert rivers or seed clouds. The sense of the whole being more than the sum of its parts is no more dominant than in looking at the internal integration of the whole human being.

In any case practitioners have no doubt that applied with such sensitivity herbal remedies can encourage the body to considerable efforts at this wider level. Some of the adaptogenic and tonic remedies used are discussed in detail in Part II.

The second message is in the herbalist's 'enlightened materialism', the view, expressed in different ways, that a somatic intervention is also likely to manifest in psychological, emotional and even spiritual effects. It is a viewpoint of the well-grounded, the natural consequence of an experience based in ancient rhythms, yet it can speak to modern humans particularly well. There is a risk in modern therapeutic practice that somatic defects can be overlooked. The herbalist's approach to such disturbances can be a useful complement to psychotherapeutic and psychosocial treatment, and can even reach beyond the material world to influence it. Much has been discovered in the last two decades about the role of hormones, neuropeptides and other chemicals in determining emotion, behaviour, mental functions and the immune system. The link between soma and psyche has never been stronger.

Modern endocrinologists are known to express concern that psychiatrists and psychotherapists can underestimate the physiological component in their work.[28] Traditional medicine, notably from China, has proceeded on the assumption that all such levels are borderless and that change at one will lead to consequences at all others. If herbal remedies can be applied in full recognition of their place in the wider scheme of things, then they could be very useful.

Reproduction

An aspect of integration

The evolution of sexual reproduction – as opposed to the asexual cloning of simple organisms – depends on the anatomical development of male and female generative structures. This, and the extraordinary social and sexual behaviour linked to reproduction among all creatures (including sexual displays, territorial behaviour, male competitiveness and libidinous instincts), suggests that all this should be separate from discussion of mundane vegetative functions!

Yet in looking at the process internally, the conditions necessary for the production of male and female germ cells, and particularly for the development of the embryo in the womb, then it is clear that these are specifically linked to the integrative functions discussed earlier:

> The primary hormones of reproduction, oestrogen, progesterone and testosterone, secreted by the ovaries and testes, are also produced by the adrenal cortex and are of the same steroidal type as its own integrative secretions, the glucocorticoids and mineralocorticoids. Embryologically speaking, the ovaries, testes and adrenal cortex arise from the same tissue, the germ-cell layer (a tempting anatomical analogue for the Chinese concept of *Kidney*).

> Increasingly, the activity of the other hormones and chemical mediators within the body are known to interact with the sexual functions, and the sex hormones themselves are known to have effects far beyond their immediate area.

> Two important cycles of physiological activity, the lunar month and the life cycle of puberty, maturation and senescence, are tied directly to sexual function in both sexes. The lunar cycle is particularly directed by reproductive rhythms in the female; it is specifically suppressed in the male by a burst of testosterone at a crucial stage of embryonic development. The female menstrual cycle is a dramatic example of the hormonal

choreography mentioned earlier – even reproductive anatomy is affected by it.

The conception and development of the embryo in the mother's womb put unusual demands on the immune and other physiological functions that can only be met by a fundamental overhaul of all the integrative machinery, this being accomplished primarily by hormonal change, incidentally mostly through foetal direction.

The affective functions, one's state of mind, the way one feels about oneself and others, one's degree of self-confidence, aggression, drive, vanity or passion are directly tied to reproductive hormonal activity. Sex and passion may be one part of love, but much of the rest is associated with other reproductive 'peripherals': parents, children and other family bonds.

Little of this may seem immediately relevant to herbal therapeutics as such. It does however help to set the framework within which this medicine has been applied; and, of course, interest in reproduction was as great in traditional society as today.

The 'wise woman' was very much a midwife and gynaecologist, and there are many useful herbal remedies passed down to us from her times. Herbal medicine has many qualities which make it still a particularly promising therapy for women to use among themselves. On the other hand the male obsession with potency has yielded several interesting androgenic stimulants.

There is also one intriguing piece of pharmacological speculation to add to all this. Several saponin-rich herbs traditionally used in gynaecological problems seem to have the same balancing effect, on the menstrual cycle, for example, as other saponin-rich adaptogens are claimed to have on the adrenal cortex.[29] It seems likely that future investigations will reveal interesting interactions between such herbs and the functions of steroid hormones in general. Further reference to all of these points will be made when saponins are discussed in the chapter 'Traditional Pharmacology' and in the description of the tonic and reproductive herbs themselves.

3 Traditional Pathology

External Ills

Only the dreamer or scholar is interested in physiology. For most people matters of health only impinge in their absence. One might even define health as a time when one doesn't have to think about it.

Illness, on the other hand, is important. It intrudes on one's consciousness and distracts from the business in hand; it affects one's ability to cope, survival itself. It is unpleasant, often painful. It is a time when one feels vulnerable. Illness has always been a major preoccupation: the earliest known texts include comments on illness and ways to treat it.

It is interesting to see how humanity has viewed this malevolent influence, particularly so when it is realized that most cultures seem to have agreed on the fundamental points.

The agreement follows the universal view of early humans that they were microcosms of the world at large, subject to the same laws as the rest of creation. Until rationalism and technology had borne fruit there was simply not enough evidence to support the illusion that *Homo sapiens* was different from or better than anything else in nature.

So, like sailors at sea, our forebears survived by weathering what the world threw at them. If something went wrong, it was because they did not weather it well enough.

Initially most, though not all, disease was seen as arising from without. The obvious metaphors for, in fact incarnations of, illness of external origin were extremes of weather.[1] Cold, heat, dryness, damp and wind were potentially overwhelming influences in the days before central heating and air-conditioning. Diseases and disruptions in the food supply obviously followed in their wake, and everyone could agree on what such weather *felt* like. In older animist times weather extremes were actually incarnate as malevolent demons whose sole aim was to invade and destroy. Correct living and proper atonement to the benevolent beings in nature would help against harm.

The view that climatic extremes are reflected in illness has survived to modern times, even to late-twentieth-century suburban London.[2] The very power of the imagery should impress, even more so when a scrutiny of the principles involved reveals considerable good sense. Many otherwise puzzling modern pathologies begin to take on a new meaning when viewed in this context.

The following is a brief summary of the symptomatology of climatic diseases, as distilled from several traditions,[3] and in terms of the physiological principles outlined earlier in this text. For those working with herbal remedies this view of illness will still prove useful in the clinical context and reference will also be made to herbal therapeutics, as discussed later. Patients who consult with modern medical diagnoses often find the connections here making particular sense to them, and a practitioner versed in these stories will often find them helpful in introducing patients to their disorders.

Cold

Illnesses associated with:

unusual sensitivity to cold, with chills
needing hot or warm influences recently, either topically or
    generally
lack of thirst or desire only for hot drinks
subdued response to illness
intense sharp pain

and/or associated with the following constitutional signs:

tendency to feel cold easily
craving for heat and hot weather
poor circulation
subdued temperament
fatigue
low libido and sexual performance
bladder irritability

Other signs:

symptoms worsening in cold and improving with heat
tendency for catarrh to be fluid and copious
urinary frequency

Clinical findings:

wet, white-coated pale tongue
copious pale urine
pale complexion
pulse slow

Clinical presentations:

pre- and sub-febrile infections
acute or chronic immunosuppression
low adrenocortical/thyroid/adrenergic activity

Processes primarily affected:

distribution (reduced peripheral circulation)
integration (including reduced capacity to accommodate to
   stress)

Herbal treatment:

warm and hot herbs
yang tonics
echinacea (*Echinacea angustifolia*)
garlic (*Allium sativum*)

Heat

Illnesses associated with:

unusual sensitivity to heat
favouring cool and cold applications
thirst, particularly for cold drinks
irritability and sensitive reactions to symptoms
burning, throbbing pain

and/or associated with the following constitutional signs:

tendency to feel heat easily
craving for refreshing and cool weather
excitable, nervous or anxious temperament often driven,
    energetic and passionate

Other signs:

symptoms worsening in heat and improving with cold
    applications
tendency for catarrh to be viscous

Clinical findings:

dry, dark-coated red, rough tongue
scanty dark urine
ruddy complexion and especially nail beds
pulse: rapid, flooding, or agitated[4]

Clinical presentations:

overactive inflammatory response
histamine and other vasoactive overactivity
hyperpyrexia/violent fever
hypersensitive immune responses/allergies
visceral and neuromuscular hyperactivity
raised metabolic rate/hyperthyroidism

Processes primarily affected:

distribution (increased circulation)
assimilation and rejection (reduced gastric activity)
maintaining vital rhythms (tendency to excitability)

perception and response (tendency to exaggerated reflex
responses)

Herbal treatment:

relaxants and sedatives (bitters)
analgesics
yin tonics

Dampness

Best divided into cold-dampness and damp-heat, each looked at
separately. Both, however, have in common that they are essentially
toxic conditions, with a traditional external manifestation as fungal
and similar infections (a possible early observation might have
been the effect of damp in buildings and household articles).

They also both affect digestive and processing functions in the
first place and eliminative functions in the second. Individuals
suffering dampness, as in nature, tend to have a greater sensitivity
to both hot and cold weather, though one more than the other
depending on which end of the spectrum they lie.

COLD-DAMPNESS

Illnesses associated with:

unusual sensitivity to cold and damp
liking for dryness and heat
general copious mucus or catarrh
other qualities of cold conditions

and/or associated with the following constitutional signs:

long-term damp and cold environment
starchy, stodgy diet
'phlegmatic' temperament
sluggish metabolism

Other signs:

white or clear catarrh and discharges (e.g. from vagina)
fungal infections, especially *Candida*
tendency to bloating, congestive dyspepsia, constipation and
   retention
liability to chronic low-grade infections

Clinical findings:

depressed eliminatory activity – constipation and/or oliguria
hydration of the tissues and oedema
low gastric/intestinal secretory activity
mucous congestion on mucosal surfaces
pale, wet tongue with greasy white coating
pulse: slow, slippery, languid, frail or thin

Clinical presentations:

chronic inflammatory diseases
excessive mucosal secretions leading to secondary infections

Processes primarily affected:

assimilation
processing
circulation
elimination

Herbal treatment:

aromatic digestives
warming eliminative herbs (including *Urtica*, *Scrophularia*,
   Echinacea)
diuretics

DAMP-HEAT

Illnesses associated with:

unusual sensitivity to humid conditions
liking for cool and dry conditions
other qualities of hot conditions

139   External Ills

and/or associated with the following constitutional signs:

abhorring humid conditions
long-term fatty, rich and high-alcohol diet, and recreational
and medicinal drug use

Other signs:

malodorous body secretions and excretions
thick, coloured catarrhal or mucosal secretions
difficulty in digesting fats and alcohol
possible jaundice
fevers, generalized inflammations (e.g. peritonitis, pancreatitis)

Clinical findings:

dark, wet tongue with yellow greasy coating
biliary and/or bilirubin disturbances
hyperlipidaemia/hypercholesterolaemia
intestinal infections (including appendicitis)
pulse: rapid, slippery

Clinical presentations:

liver and biliary disturbances
difficulty in metabolizing fats and alcohol; cholesterol and
blood-lipid disorders
associated inflammatory (prostaglandin?) disturbances, e.g.
migraine
intestinal infections and disturbed intestinal flora
disturbances in immunosurveillance: e.g. classic food allergies
and Type 1 hypersensitivities

Processes primarily affected:

assimilation
processing (of nutrient)
rejection (especially liver-related)

Herbal treatment:

bitters and cholagogues

Dryness

Illnesses associated with:

vulnerability to mucosal irritation
dehydration and thirst

and/or associated with the following constitutional signs:

weakness in the body's superficial defences, especially the
    respiratory system, mucosa and skin
tendency to atopic conditions (dry eczema, asthma and allergic
    rhinitis)
difficulty in breathing in dry atmosphere
dry skin

Other signs:

dry unproductive cough
wheezing and breathlessness
allergic rhinitis and conjunctivitis
dry allergic eczema
in extreme cases, haemoptysis (coughing blood)

Clinical findings:

atopy (raised IgE levels, eosinophilia, tendency to allergies)
viscid sputum, dry mucosal secretions elsewhere
dry or even fissured skin

Clinical presentations:

drying of mucosal secretions, especially in respiratory system,
    and other barrier protections, such as the skin
secondary infections and/or hypersensitivities
dehydration leading to pyrexia

Processes primarily affected:

assimilation
rejection

Herbal treatment:

mucilages and mucilaginous applications
yin tonics
inhalations

Wind

In Chinese terms windy weather can induce its own range of symptoms and is sometimes linked with, though not always causative of, 'internal wind' arising from turbulence in the body's distributive functions (i.e. the *Liver*). This in turn is very likely to arise out of a wider debility (*Kidney* deficiency), equivalent to the exhaustion phase in Selye's 'General Adaption Syndrome' (see 'Stress', on p. 210) and most associated with adrenocortical fatigue.

Illnesses associated with:

sudden sensitivity or exposure to draughts
fluctuating symptoms with sudden onsets and remissions
itching
neuromuscular spasms
intermittent fevers

and/or associated with the following constitutional signs:

volatile vaso- and immunoregulation, e.g. migraine
variable food intolerances
rheumatic tendencies or inheritance

Other signs:

arthropathies and muscle spasms
rapid changes in body temperature

Clinical findings:

quivering tongue
arthro-, myo- or neuropathies often with negative clinical
  findings
cerebrovascular disturbances and hypertension and strokes
pulse: taut and wiry

Clinical presentations:

fluctuating and erratic inflammatory conditions
rheumatoid conditions

Processes primarily affected:

maintaining vital rhythms (erratic regulatory cycles)
perception and response (exaggerated reflexes)
integration (disturbed balance)

Herbal treatment:

local heating
'sour' and other specific Chinese remedies
Kidney tonics
peripheral vasodilators

Other Ills

Not all diseases were seen to arise through climatic changes. There were other malign influences as well. Each culture characterized the causes in its own way and the result is that there appears little agreement on details.[5] Nevertheless, it is possible to extract a few further simple elements from traditional medicine.

Accidents, fighting (with men or beasts), and other causes of injury were always present, and often the most frequent reason for seeking herbal treatment.

The quality of food was obviously important. Insufficient food clearly led to disease, and dietary imbalance could do it as well. Like everything else food was classified as relatively warming or cooling. Too much meat might exacerbate or provoke a hot disease, too much fish might cool the digestion unduly.

Other causes were associated with communal illness. Contagions and pestilences were clearly the result of other human ailments and human contacts.

Internal causes of illness tended to be perceived in terms of codes of morality and social conduct. Right living, family loyalty, sexual prudence, cleanliness, good neighbourliness were qualities that were linked with good health; transgressions of such codes carried their own punishment as illness.

There were also the myriad illnesses of the emotional and spiritual world, linked with dreams, portents and the malign influences of the gods and their agents, working either through the individual or the whole community. Magic, shamanism, trance states, communal rituals and sorcery were variously invoked to deal with such disturbances. With increasing social order such disturbances were channelled into the work of the priest caste and eventually into organized religion. With the growth of a communal faith and spiritual order it became more difficult to express personal anxieties and crises, so that these in turn became new illnesses.

There is no doubt that the last categories of disease causation are of less relevance to the prescribing of herbal remedies. Plants have of course been used for their psychoactive properties, and also as talismanic emblems in shamanism, but this is peripheral to the great proportion of herbalism, which has been concerned primarily with correcting physical forces of harm.

4 Therapeutics

The Herbalist's Approach to Health and Disease

The Rural Tradition

Before the beginning

There can be little doubt that plants were the first source of medicines. Even animals are observed to use them intuitively for more than simple nourishment. They were, and remain, easily accessible to everyone, and among plants in any habitat, even deserts and inner cities, there are always some with established pharmacological or other medicinal effect.

So, given the native intelligence of the human being, it is not surprising to find that all but the most technological of societies have an immense wealth of knowledge about the plants in their vicinity. There is often anthropological evidence of an extraordinary insight into the botanical and pharmacological character of plants in pastoral and hunter-nomad communities.[1] All this was originally acquired, transmitted and understood entirely within the limits of personal experience and the oral language and symbolism appropriate to that experience.

In recent times herbal medicine has fared badly. The modern preoccupation is with constructing a tidy well-behaved world as a protection against the insecurities of raw nature: crude plant drugs are too unpredictable, messy and anyway have a gut-wrenching taste! They lack the cool efficiency of the modern breed of man-made drugs, working with broad strokes rather than precision cuts. Matters are not helped by the fact that the essence of traditional herbal practice has hardly ever been recorded: traditional practitioners worked with pre-rational concepts and were almost never interested in scholarship, whilst scholars themselves seem to have reciprocated in kind: *it is after all just an old country craft.*

If, in spite of this dubious prospect, the modern citizen is interested in learning more, then it makes sense to try to understand how and why herbal remedies were applied. So far, much modern use of herbs has been very superficial, with the remedies being used mainly as soft-option substitutes for conventional drugs. Regulatory authorities, like Britain's Department of Health and the USA's Food and Drug Administration, confirm this attitude by applying the bureaucratic standards that have been evolved to judge the efficacy and safety of new drugs. It would be almost impossible for them to do otherwise. To expect them to develop an entirely different mechanism for monitoring medicines, without the support of an established body of knowledge and expert advice and a level of consensus at all stages, is frankly absurd.

It is thus incumbent on those who would claim a different model for herbal medicine to set out their case clearly. An attempt has already been made here to put forward an appropriate framework of medical science. We must now attempt to explore the use of herbs in their rural heartland.

Shamanism and the craft tradition

In every rural community since prehistory there were likely to be individuals, most often women ('wise women'), regarded as specialists in the art of using the healing plants. They would satisfy the demands of basic health care, treating injuries and illness, and usually acting as midwives as well.

They were usually not the shamans, witch-doctors or priests, practitioners of a distinct calling, who specialized in treating wider, peculiarly human malaises of a spiritual or emotional nature. These individuals, often men, would be asked to come to the aid of the community as much as of the individual; they might use only a few plants, and these more often as talismanic emblems in a therapy based on dreams and trance. The shamans provided a uniquely holistic service for their times, and even an example of personal commitment to the inner life of their patients that we could respect. However, many were also becoming a power in the community, a process that ultimately diverged from the quiet and even effective health care actually prevailing where women, children and men went about their daily business.

Although there were doubtless many individuals who were both shamans and herbalists, it is important not to confuse these two traditions. The modern medical herbalist does not claim descent from the shaman (and is also not particularly amused by jokes about witches' brews). Herbalism is seen as a craft tradition. It is, of course, always the case that the therapist powerfully influences the therapy, but as in other crafts it is the nature of the material, the character of the remedies, that is the determining factor.

Rural herbalism and the classical medical traditions

Like most crafts too, rural herbalism has never been adequately articulated. Yet the tradition inspired the medical concepts of early civilizations. With the move away from the rural community to the city states, plants remained the only significant source of medicines and so were transferred to the new circumstances. The importance of plant remedies is evident in every civilization for which we have records. In looking at these written accounts and at their transmission through succeeding cultures, it is surprising to note how much of the substance of therapeutics is common to them all. It really does appear that there are fundamental principles in using plants as remedies that all humans have had to discover and to which most have adhered.

In ancient Greece the Hippocratic and in Rome the Galenic schools elaborated concepts that were to underlie Western thought for 1,500 years, and that inspired the Islamic civilization which has survived till the present day. Farther east the approaches formulated over 2,000 years ago in India and China are still developed to this day. In the latter case they provide the most subtle and elaborate exposition of traditional medicine available. There are also substantial surviving traditions in Tibet, Japan, Laos, Vietnam, Cambodia and Thailand, among many others.

If the insights of Graeco-Roman and Chinese medicine are

compared, for example, one finds expressed views of the human being in health and illness, and a therapeutic approach to the latter, that have much more in common with each other than with modern views of medicine.

It will be valuable to try to rediscover these principles and to articulate them into modern terms.

In this review the Chinese view of herbal therapeutics will provide the major source of information, but this will be titrated with insights from the European traditions. The story will start, however, where the last major attempt to formalize traditional wisdom for the West left off: in North America prior to this century.

The white Indian doctors

During the eighteenth and nineteenth centuries a largely dispossessed European population moved into the large tracts of North America for a new life in the 'New World'. They were often remote from anything that resembled civilization, and usually a long way away from anything like a satisfactory medical service. Being on the whole of rural stock themselves, they generally found it easy to fall back on traditional practices, and to this end imported many familiar medicinal plants with them. (The wild flora of North America, especially around the eastern seaboard, has a great deal in common with Europe to this day.)

However, these settlers could barely ignore the vast native botanical wealth around them, and there were opportunities to discover that the indigenous population of 'Indians' were adept at using these plants as medicines. There were many stories of trappers and other explorers falling ill and being taken in by friendly native tribes to be treated; there were also many contacts at trading posts and between settler and native subsistence farmers (neither of whom tended to be of fighting stock). In the eastern states particularly there was considerable grassroots contact between the two peoples, jointly facing an often hostile climate and environment.

It became quite common for settlers to use Indian lore in formulating their home remedies. There were specialists, both women and men, who became well known for their ability to use the herbs. As this was already an enterprise society, several of them took to the road, moving from one homestead or town to another, often peddling dubious nostrums, and setting up their 'travelling medicine shows'. Several were actually quite proficient, but all were disparagingly lumped together as 'white Indian doctors', obviously implying that they had gone native.

One 'white Indian doctor' stood out from the crowd: Samuel Thomson (1769–1843), brought up on a farm in New Hampshire and introduced to herbs as a shepherd boy by a 'wise woman', Mrs Benton, who was versed in Indian lore. So impressed was he by the value of the remedies compared with the performance of 'Regular physic' at the time, that not only did he take up herbal medicine as a career but he resolved to learn to read and write, the better to figure out this different but solely oral tradition.

It was this that marked Thomson out. Accounts of herbal practice from the inside, as it were, have always been extremely rare. Thomson set out a principle that at once encapsulated this tradition and fired the public imagination. The book in which he propagated his views[2] was a runaway publishing success, and at the time it was calculated that over half the population of Ohio were adherents of Thomsonism.

Thomson's language was simple, even simplistic; his audience was made up mainly of the untutored God-fearing farming families of the Midwest, many of whom probably owned only one other book, the Bible. He was also, as we shall see, lucky in selecting a message that fitted the times. Yet it was almost as though he had plumbed a secret code. He seems to have touched a gut instinct, one that the 'Regular' physicians had missed: that life and health are positive virtues, to be protected or recovered through personal self-sufficiency using the medicinal aids provided by the Maker.

The combined factors of a sturdy, self-sufficient population and a desire to shape out a life different from the often oppressive Europe many had been fleeing, meant that this was a fertile climate for innovation. North America had already an enterprising climate. In the nineteenth century it saw the formation of two of the major complementary medical systems of modern times, the manipulative therapies osteopathy and chiropractic.

Thomsonism was to develop in the second half of the nineteenth century to inspire both eclecticism and physiomedicalism, at the same time as osteopathy and chiropractic emerged. Unlike the latter however, the medicinal therapies did not fare well. The main colleges of physiomedicalism and eclecticism, along with those of homoeopathy, were 'invited' to come within the umbrella of established medical training in talks held with the American Medical Association at the turn of the century. They never emerged.

The National Institute of Medical Herbalists, UK

Physiomedicalism, with its Thomsonian roots, survived only by virtue of the fact that a few of its proponents had already travelled to Britain, where their message was eagerly adopted by a newly urbanized herbal profession in the industrial cities of the Midlands and North.

It was a fascinating situation. Britain was also facing an unusual new environment in public health care. The Industrial Revolution, affecting Britain more than any other nation, had seen a massive depopulation of the countryside and the creation of new proletarian cities like Nottingham, Halifax, Leeds and Manchester. These newly urbanized country folk, living in their back-to-back houses and working in the 'dark Satanic mills', nevertheless maintained many of their old rural habits. They grew vegetables in their 'allotments', kept pigeons and ferrets, and stayed faithful to their old remedies. The herbalists who provided for them, by now mostly male, in looking for a new role in the city, literally 'set up shop'.

Herbalists still survive in these working-class cities as shopkeepers. Today there are very few. In the last century they were on every block and prospering. In times when there were no welfare payments and little sentiment, working men patronized herbalists instead of doctors because they got them back to work faster. For minor acute and chronic complaints like coughs, dyspepsia or headaches, they would simply go into the shop and get a product 'over the counter'. If they had a more complex or serious condition, the counter flap would be lifted and they would pass into a back room for a more considered treatment. This might be quite alarming: there are records of minor amputations, and blistering and emetics would have been commonplace.

These practitioner-retailers were often very successful and there are accounts that many regularly had queues forming out in the street. This clearly presented a visible political threat to the new British Medical Association, and herbalists were forced, possibly for the first time in history, to associate. Several regional associations were set up, finally coalescing in 1864 as the National Association of Medical Herbalists, with Jesse Boot of Nottingham, sire of the multimillion-pound empire Boots the Chemists, as one founder member. It still survives as the leading professional association of herbal practitioners in Britain, the National Institute of Medical Herbalists.

It was quite obvious that these new urban herbalists had no philosophical foundation they could articulate. With an infinitely complex heritage of purely oral traditions there were no clear principles that they could use to establish what made them different from 'Regular' physicians. They clearly needed something written down that they could all agree on. So when a Thomsonian, Albert Coffin, arrived with *Botanic Guide to Health*, his own successful version of Thomson's book,* to form his own movement in 1847 ('Coffinism': a gift to the satirists!) he found an appreciative audience. As further developments in North America also filtered over physiomedicalism was eventually adopted as the founding philosophy of the NAMH.[3]

Right up to the late 1970s the training for herbalists in Britain was based on physiomedical principles and almost half the remedies taught were American. Without this fortunate reverse colonialism the whole Thomsonian experiment might have been buried in the specialist history books. As it was we are now able to look fairly well at the first opportunity for modern Europeans to attempt to articulate the practices of their rural forebears.

Thomson and the four elements

The prevailing medical problem for all urban or semi-urban cultures up to the mid-twentieth century was the killer febrile diseases. The allopathic tradition developed in medieval Europe

---

*In Britain his book sold 40,000 copies and ran to 44 editions by 1884.

required that remedies be used that as effectively as possible stifled the disease symptoms. With the discovery of the selective toxicity of the mineral ores like the salts of arsenic, mercury, antimony and lead, a new medical profession developed to provide training in the application of the appropriate dosage necessary to suppress the symptoms without killing the patient suffering them (see also 'Fever', on pp. 63–7).

Although allopathy was to have its day with the discovery of antibiotics and the new drugs, these early physicians were not successful. They were powerful in the community, possibly because their treatments were more dramatic, but contemporary accounts of their work sound horrific to the modern ear. Fatal or near-fatal doses of poisons with nightmarish side-effects were interspersed with blood-letting and leeches. It is very unlikely that they provided much net contribution to the health of society.

Thomson was among those appalled by all this. He was convinced that the techniques of the country folk were more promising. He himself had saved the lives of several patients whose suffering of an infectious disease had been compounded by 'Regular' attempts at healing. He learnt to read and began to look for the language to express his basic conviction that the role of remedies was to support the body in its illness, not threaten it. The following is perhaps the cornerstone of his efforts:

I found that all animal bodies were formed of four elements. The Earth and Water constitute the solid; and the Air and Fire (or heat) are the cause of life and motion; that the cold, or the lessening of the power of heat, is the cause of all disease; that to restore heat to its natural state was the only way health could be produced, and that, after restoring the natural heat, by clearing the system of all obstruction and causing a natural perspiration, the stomach would digest the food taken into it, and the heat (or nature) be enabled to hold her supremacy.

A brief introduction to ancient views of the world is appropriate here. In Europe and the Near East all creation was seen to emerge from the action of four fundamentals, or 'elements'. Earth was the solid and Water the fluid principle. Their mixture, referred to in the book of Genesis as 'clay', was the stuff of which creation was constructed, each material being a unique blend of the dry and the wet.

155   The Herbalist's Approach

Air was not as we now know it. The still air of an enclosed room was barely known in the days before windows. If anything this would have been 'ether', or nothingness. Air to the ancient was what he felt on his cheeks most of the time. We might call it 'wind'. Wind has always been the metaphor for movement, the result of approximating hot and cold air. Air was the principle of motion.

A ball rolling down the hill is a blend of Earth, Water and Air. When it rolls to a stop it loses most of its Air and is largely Earth and Water again. These were the ways phenomena were understood.

There was clearly a special element needed to explain the phenomenon of something that not only rolled down the hill (under the influence of gravity), but was able to pick itself up and walk back up. Life, with its capacity for transcending physical laws like gravity, with its transforming presence, with its self-perpetuation, needed a uniquely powerful metaphor. The symbol was clearly Fire, or heat: rising against gravity, self-perpetuating and transforming everything in its path, and uniquely attractive to all life forms. Just as life breathes something transcendent into the body (how *do* we manage to stand upright?) so is heat a life-giving force (life requires a minimum temperature, cold-blooded creatures can only move when warmed to a certain point). The ancients must have watched a large bird soaring up propelled by no more than rising warm air, or indeed marvelled at the rise of smoke, or the agitation induced in water by boiling.

Above all else, nothing would have convinced the early observer of the equation of life and heat but the feel of a corpse. It was this that Thomson picked upon. Heat was not only life but also health. Cold was the cause of all disease, and ultimately of death itself. If one could only maintain vital heat then the body would be able to fend off illness – *it would be able to look after itself*. It was an old and very simple notion, but it suited him very well.

As referred to earlier, the major clinical condition facing Thomson and his contemporaries was infectious diseases, marked of course by fever. The 'Regular' approach then, as it is now, was to see the high body temperature and other unpleasant symptoms of fever as a potentially very serious threat, something to be removed as efficiently as possible. By contrast, Thomson was pointing out, the ancient vitalist herbal tradition was to see fever as *extraordinary vital activity*, as the desperate generation by the body of extra vital heat to fend off the invasion of cold disease.

Thomson followed the Indian technique of actually heating the body further in support of these efforts. He was well aware of the 'sweat lodge', a tent erected over fire-heated stones on which water was dropped; sufferers would sit there sweating out their toxins. He advocated another Indian technique, the administering of cayenne pepper (*Capsicum minimum*), which has a direct effect in increasing body temperature. He would use this if he judged that the body's efforts in repelling the invasion were flagging (as they often and sometimes fatally did in serious infective diseases). At earlier and more robust phases of fever his primary concern was to manage the process, to stop it getting out of hand. His most famous remedy here was lobelia (*Lobelia inflata*), originally used as an emetic ('Indian pukeweed') but in lower doses a notable relaxing remedy, which he found considerably reduced the spasms, convulsions and pains of many fevers and was incidentally an effective expectorant in bronchial infections. He also advocated the use of bayberry (*Myrica cerifera*) for its relaxing effect on the bowels, reducing – but not suppressing – the potentially debilitating eliminations of diarrhoea. Both these remedies were also incidentally warming.

His secondary concern was to help clear the body of toxins. In this he was pursuing firm herbal principles of detoxification using cleansing herbs referred to repeatedly in this text. It is noted from the quotation above that he saw the healthy (hot) body being quite able to cope with digestion and clear obstructions on its own. Like other herbalists before him he saw the vomiting, coughing, diarrhoea and sweating of fevers as another extraordinary attempt at self-help. These eliminations were not to be suppressed unduly but again were to be managed, so as to reduce their debilitating effects.

Thomson's message was almost absurdly simplistic, being applicable to a narrow albeit common range of illnesses. Yet the radicalism of his position was not lost on his audience. In seeing the maintenance of body heat and vitality as the primary duty of the practitioner he was directly accusing the regular physicians of criminal neglect. He clearly stated that the usual mineral suppression of symptoms was adding more 'cold' to an already threatening situation, running entirely against the interests of the body. He ranked these physicians with the diseases that they were being charged to eliminate.

Thomson's popularity and his outspoken attacks on the medical profession earned him their unbridled wrath. He was hounded through the courts, accused of manslaughter and murder (without success, except for one charge of assault when in a loss of temper he actually attacked one of his more persistent tormentors with a scythe!).

The central point, of course, was that Thomson had articulated, with popular success, an essential feature of the herbal tradition: that the primary task was to support the body's own recuperative efforts; everything else was secondary. He also sounded the essential difference between that tradition and what had already become conventional medicine. The fact that his relationship with the medical establishment was almost entirely acrimonious only served to reinforce his position as a fundamentalist.

Some of his followers were less keen on absolute simplicities. Much to the old man's disgust several started developing variations on his teachings, recognizing, for example, that there were conditions that could be diagnosed as excessive heat. There were different emphases on the need to control heat (in fact, circulation) and variations in the mechanisms for keeping the blood 'clean'.

The post-Thomsonians

Wooster Beach of the 'reformed' or eclectic school, borrowing some principles from European naturopathy, paid particular attention to the subtle adjustment of the circulation, bringing in an integrated nervous mechanism for the first time and even countenancing 'cooling' at times. He was most insistent that the body fluids be kept alkaline, as a metabolic metaphor for reducing accumulated waste products.

Two years before Thomson's death, one of his followers, Alva Curtis of Cincinnati, founded the physiomedical movement, attempting to elaborate Thomsonian simplicities while retaining their robust effectiveness. At its peak in the latter part of the century it produced a number of accomplished individuals well versed in current medical advances who provided thorough reviews of the theoretical basis of herbal medicine.

Three figures particularly stand out. T. J. Lyle produced a particularly thorough materia medica,[4] concentrating on the observed influence of each remedy on the human being rather than listing its symptomatic indications.

J. M. Thurston provided definitive statements on the nature of the Vital Force, health and disease, on the distinctions between functional symptoms and those arising from organic ('trophic') origins, and on the need to use only such remedies as supported vitality. He also, rather prematurely, sought to classify remedies in terms of the newly discovered autonomic nervous system, reasoning that in its vasomotor activity control could be exerted on local circulation and thus on all tissue functions, including digestion, elimination, and hormonal and nervous activity.[5]

Of the physiomedical theorists W. H. Cook might be considered to have made the most lasting contribution. Like the others, Cook attempted to link the rapid new discoveries of medical science to traditional approaches. Like Thurston, he was tempted into blind alleys and most of his conclusions about the detailed effect of herbal remedies on various parts of the body do not bear close examination today. However, in the following and other passages he seemed to have grasped a useful principle:

Regularity in periods of alternate labor and rest is characteristic of all vital action . . . the earliest departure of the tissues from under the full control of the vital force will be in the lack of ability either to relax or to contract some of the tissues as readily as in the healthy state.[6]

Cook was writing as scientific investigations were opening up internal body functions to a remarkable degree, and in particular as the first implications of the discovery of the autonomic nervous system were beginning to sink in.

Here was the first scientific model that could underpin that mysterious balance of life, that balance for which W. B. Cannon was later to coin the term 'homoeostasis'. The self-righting fluctuations and rhythms in activity of the heart, gut, nervous system and other functions from hour to hour and through day and night could at last be explained. Here was a whole network of nerve fibres that variously increased or slowed down these many activities.

159   The Herbalist's Approach

Immersed as medical science is now in the myriad interweaving control systems it is difficult to see the force of Dr Cook's vision. If health depended on each function tuning its activity to wider needs, and it could be shown that there was an integral network apparently controlling these functions, then it seemed obvious that illness would start with trouble at this level, probably long before disease was evident.

There were also implications for medical intervention. If herbal remedies were to be used principally for improving recuperative faculties, then this implied that they were to have a *benign, non-manipulative influence on normal body functions*. This is an important theoretical point. It requires the development of fundamental new principles of pharmacology.

A vitalist pharmacology

Conventional pharmacology is an entirely pragmatic, unprincipled science. Suppressing inflammation, killing pathogens, blocking pathological deteriorations and potentially damaging physiological responses: these are specific tasks requiring specific investigations, with little regard for normal body functions (or even the wider implications of the treatment). A therapy that seeks specifically to improve normal functions needs an over-arching schema of pharmacological theory. How do such remedies actually achieve their influence?

What is needed is a view of normal human physiology that provides a space for the effect of herbal remedies. Cook asked his readers to assume that a feature of health was *a regularity of vital rhythms*: that an early (the earliest?) move from health would be to a state either of relative tension or relative flaccidity. A constipated bowel might have started in a state of atony or of spasm; blood-sugar levels could drop from excess insulin or insufficient glucocorticoid secretions; migraine might follow either vasoconstriction or vasodilation; peptic ulcers could follow either excess acid production or inadequate mucus secretion.

Cook reckoned that by a gentle nudge it might be possible to help the body restore normal balance. Remedies could thus either *contract* or *relax* depending on the direction in which they nudged a particular disturbed function.

It was always assumed that any such nudging remained within the bounds of normal vital activity. The physiomedicalists avoided any remedy that they felt had an adverse effect on normal functions. *They sought only remedies that worked to improve normal body functions.* The remedy should always have a net enhancing effect.

It is pertinent that physiomedicalism was born in an atmosphere of religious fervour: the Bible was the fundamental source of wisdom. There was a sense of absolutism and even damnation in their view of therapeutic compromise. Regular physicians were castigated for reasons that went further than professional rivalry.

Few would apply today strictures that included a repudiation of sedatives and analgesics in favour of remedies that helped the body tackle the pain or distress at source. Nevertheless, the core of the physiomedical message sets a high standard and might still be transferred to more venial climates.

Cook was attempting to set out a new basis for understanding remedies, one quite different from the one that had developed by default for 'Regular' medicines. We might now create a schema to illustrate the position he had reached.

A first step would be to illustrate the central vital force. Taking the metaphor of heat rising upwards from Thomson, we could have it as a vertical line pointing up.

Following Cook we can add a horizontal axis showing levels of activity, from no activity to the right, to maximum practical activity on the left. Taking his point further we could add an oscillating sine-wave to indicate that in life there is a rhythm between activity and inactivity at all levels (see Fig. 2).

It is then possible to superimpose upon this diagram a second version (Fig. 3) to illustrate the basis of herbal therapeutics as conceived by Cook and the other physiomedicalists. A positive health-giving remedy was seen to be either relatively relaxing or contracting, to provide the appropriate counter to whatever deviation existed. Above all, however, the remedy had to exert an enhancing influence upwards in the direction of the vital force; in other words its line of action had to fall within the hemisphere illustrated, and preferably as vertical in direction as possible. The alternative was seen to go down the road of 'Regular' physic and actually to depress vitality.

Cook, like the other physiomedicalists, began to classify remedies

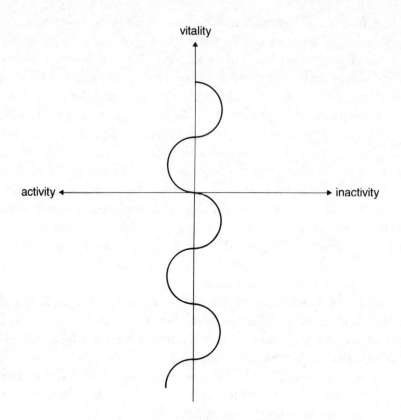

Fig. 2 The pulse of life (after W. H. Cook)

according to whether they relaxed or contracted various organs or functions. The categories quickly became unhelpfully complex, but this was a feature of their times rather than a substantial failure in the approach. It is quite feasible to envisage a new version of such a schema being developed in the light of modern insights.

It was also an unfortunate but irresistible conclusion for Cook that the autonomic nervous system was the mechanism on which herbs primarily acted. This was clearly a mistake, a lesson in the value of controlling one's enthusiasm for a good idea. Some herbs do work on the autonomic nervous system (see 'Plant drugs on the autonomic system', on p. 125), but they are in a minority.

Cook's other residual contribution was in drawing attention to the importance of body functions as constant activities. He presaged

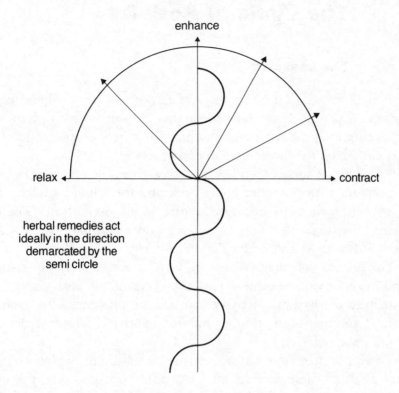

enhance

relax

contract

herbal remedies act
ideally in the direction
demarcated by the
semi circle

Fig. 3 The effects of herbal remedies on vital functions (after Cook)

the modern enthusiasm for biological rhythms and provided the germ of a therapeutic basis for handling their disturbances. Unlike those holding the modern view, who saw cyclical activity as something extra to be tacked on to the main core, however, he was claiming that *if herbal medicine meant anything at all in physiological terms it was as a medicine that corrected disturbances of functional activities from the start.*

If we are to agree with this approach, it will be helpful to move on from Cook's position and look more closely at human experience of biological activity. It happens that there is a widespread agreement through history on the meaning of cyclic change and the way in which herbs might influence it in the body.

163 The Herbalist's Approach

The Cycle of Activity

The seasons

If herbal remedies are to be understood as primarily affecting normal rhythmic body functions, then it will be helpful to look more closely at the nature of rhythmic activities as such, and at the ways in which they were seen in earlier times.

So far Fig. 2 shows 'activity' and 'inactivity' as opposite poles of a spectrum with the pulse going back and forth like a shuttle. This is of course not an accurate depiction of oscillation. There is instead a rising and falling, a waxing and a waning: rather than a straight line there should be a circle, a *cycle*.

The primary elements of nature's cycle were widely understood. The most obvious example was the cycle of the seasons and the principles of rhythmic activity can best be illustrated by reference to it. If summer is the time of maximal activity, winter is the time of minimal activity.

There are then two seasons, spring and autumn, which are half-way phases. These contain the two points in the cycle, the equinoxes, when activity and inactivity are exactly matched. Although they are of identical value there is, of course, a fundamental difference between them. In the one case there is movement towards more activity, in the other a movement towards less. These phases may thus be designated as 'potential activity' and 'potential inactivity' respectively. The four poles of this cycle equate exactly with the 'four phases' recognized in many cultures, which substitute for the Graeco-Roman four elements discussed earlier.

In Eastern cultures activity was translated as *yang* and inactivity was equated with the inert or 'structive' principle *yin* (from the Latin *struere*: to form concretely, as in 'structure'). Maximum *yang* was the literal meaning of Fire and maximum *yin* the literal meaning of Water (originally ice). The imagery is fairly obvious: in Anglo-Saxon Britain the poles were represented as Fire and Frost.[7]

Potential *yang* was the ideogram that became Wood, while potential *yin* became Metal. The wider correspondences for all these phases will be introduced in the Chapter 'A Traditional Physiology',

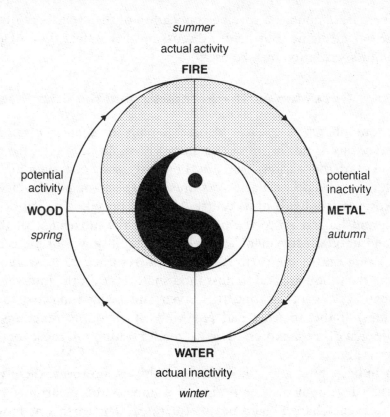

summer

actual activity

FIRE

potential
activity

WOOD

spring

potential
inactivity

METAL

autumn

WATER

actual inactivity

winter

Fig. 4 The four-phase cycle

in the Appendixes section. (See also Fig. 4.)

Although Chinese imagery is used here, there were similar alignments in other cultures. In most, attempts would have been made to pursue the correspondences through all human activity so that these phases could underlie and characterize all phenomena, including diseases and the remedies used to treat them. It is difficult to overemphasize the extent to which early humans thought of their world as cyclic. As Mircea Eliade has so impressively explained,[8] even their view of history and destiny was cyclic rather than linear. Every event was on the point of a wheel, endlessly turning. Only in the mystical tradition was there considered any opportunity to stand apart from the wheel of destiny and other mundane rhythms. Otherwise their hold on experience was complete.

There is, of course, a specific application of the cyclic perspective to herbal medicine. But before discussing this a final dose of picturesque speculation may be useful.

Out of the earth – herbalists and the fifth phase

The four phases of cyclical change actually presume a fifth. The observer needs to be fitted in somewhere. In the cycle of the heavens, of the seasons, there is implicitly someone standing on earth to experience it. Earth was thus recognized as a fifth stage in the cosmos, originally at its centre.† Human beings came out of the earth and looked up to the heavens to see the movement of their life and nature. Movement was celestial, stability was of the earth. One came out of the earth (mother) and returned to it, womb to tomb ('dust thou art and to dust thou shalt return'); the intervening lifespan was spent aspiring to heaven and being subjected to its rhythms. If the ancients had any view of rhythmic functions, it would have been expressed as a manifestation of those of the heavens above.

In India, China and other Eastern cultures, however, there was another development. The notion of a universe only partially subject to cyclic change could not be tolerated. The earth was moved out to join the four phases in the cycle. How such a step was taken, and why the earth was placed where it was can only be speculation, but one metaphor from nature is revealing.

The simple movement of the seasons appears to be very familiar. Winter is seen as the time of minimal botanical activity when seeds and subterranean stores are held in reserve; spring is seen as the time when all that was latent becomes apparent, life springs forth, plants emerge and begin to grow profusely; summer is the maximum fulfilment of this potential; autumn is the beginning of retrenchment for the winter. There is the familiar cycle of death, rebirth, life and decay.

However, this is not the exact state of affairs at all. Closer

†As Needham has noted, quoting Granet (*Science and Civilisation in China* [1956], vol. 2, p. 288, Cambridge University Press) in Chinese science space itself was divided 'into regions, south, north, east, west, and centre'.

examination of the botanical cycle reveals that there is a period before the decay of autumn when the next year's spring growth is actually being laid down. Seeds are formed, and buds appear. On microscopic examination the latter are seen to contain in miniature the embryo shoots ready for emergence after the winter (and as 'Lammas growth' in any unusually extended warm period in autumn). Thus spring is not the season when new life begins. It is *late summer*. The same is true for other organisms: the larger mammals, for example, conceive then so as to give birth in the spring; it is a time of notable abundance, a time for laying down reserves for the privations of winter.

As the metaphor for the origin of life and for the supply of nourishment (the 'earth mother'), it is thus only appropriate that in the grand cycle Earth is fitted between the Fire phase (e.g. summer) and the Metal phase (e.g. autumn). It also fits in with the metaphorical generative cycle in which each phase generates the one following: as simultaneously ash and ore, Earth is an appropriate stage between Fire and Metal.‡

Putting Earth out into orbit created a very interesting new dynamic. Earth ceased to be a fixed concrete dependency. Instead it assumed the quality of an ideal boat, steady in a swell, able to transcend the disruptions of life by maintaining a stable balance. Some movement is essential in all things: in Earth it is movement around a point of balance. Earth is manifested in the living body as homoeostasis, as poise, steadiness, balance.

It is as if the sailor had said to the non-sailor: 'You can never know earth until you leave it, and have to recreate it yourself, and especially within yourself.' Only in not taking its stability at our feet for granted can we see that Earth has movement like everything else.

A cycle divided by four poles is intrinsically inert. It easily divides up into static entities with neat relationships between each. It is

‡The full generative cycle is as follows: Water is the basis of Wood, which is the fuel for Fire, which leads to Earth (ash); Earth (ore) gives rise to Metal and (a useful divinatory tip this), Metal plates left out at night sometimes generate Water (dew!). Each phase, as befits all ecological systems, also checks the second phase along, so as to provide necessary balance. Thus Wood (spade) controls Earth; Earth (dam, irrigation channel) contains Water; Water quenches Fire; Fire melts Metal; Metal chops Wood.

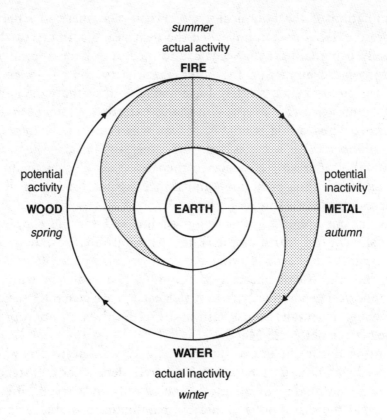

Fig. 5 The Earth and the four phases

reminiscent of the four elements of Graeco-Roman tradition, where movement is not an issue. Introducing a fifth pole to the cycle brings an exciting instability: the cycle cannot be drily dissected into equal, balanced portions. Movement is implicit in the relationship between the five phases.

In Chinese philosophy there are almost thirty formal relationships recognized between the five phases, and that does not exhaust the possibilities. The five-phase basis for Chinese medicine gives it a powerful vibrancy and subtlety. Yet for herbal medicine the perspective seems to have remained Earth-centred, the universe is still *geocentric*. This is a subtle point, and it is easy to overstate it, but the following comments might be made.

Plants are, of course, 'out of the earth'; the prevailing impression

168   Therapeutics

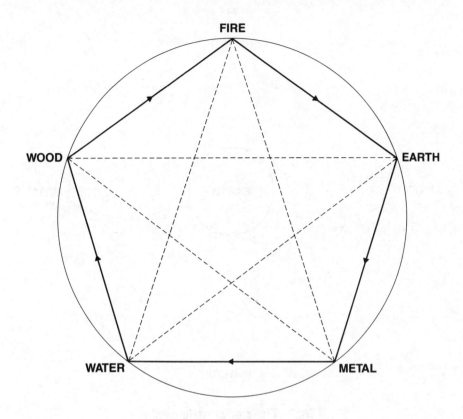

Fig. 6 The five-phase cycle

about traditional herbalists is that they are rather parochial (to the extent that a village wise woman may not recognize a plant, even of a familiar species, if it was collected from a distant location). Like the plants at her feet she would quite possibly die in the same region as she was born: even her mineral intake would be the same as theirs, determined by the soil they both shared. Although this is an extreme example, herbalists as a group do seem to have stayed close to the earth.

There is more. The functions of the body, in Chinese terms, corresponding to the Earth phase are the *Spleen* and *Stomach* (those concerned with digestion and metabolism – see Appendix). Herbal medicines enter the body and have many of their effects through these functions. We shall also see that the Chinese five-

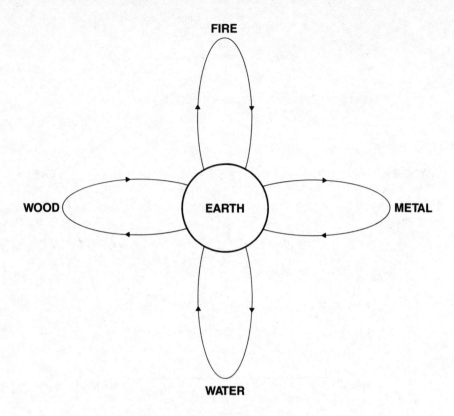

Fig. 7 The geocentric cycle

phase interpretation of pharmacology, the so-called 'five *Tastes*', can only be understood within an older geocentric framework.

As late as the Sung dynasty in China there emerged a major theoretician Li Tung-Yuan who, in his 'strengthening the Earth' school of medicine, effectively reinstated the original position of the Earth phase, in particular insisting that the harmonious function of the *Spleen* and *Stomach*, of digestion and metabolism, was literally central to any medical treatment. He championed a variation on the relationship between the five phases in which the Earth phase resonated independently with each of the other phases.

Li Tung-Yuan's position is extremely close to that held intuitively by the herbalist.

Plant Cycles

Understanding plant remedies

It is now possible to return to the early human view of plants and their effects on the body in terms of the primary four-phase cycle. We will see that the physiomedical view that plants could be classified in terms of the direction in which they nudge a disturbed rhythm (by 'contracting' or 'relaxing') receives strong endorsement and elaboration. Here is the beginning of a traditional herbal therapeutics.

Understanding the character of plants was of course an essential requirement for the herbal practitioner. There was, in fact, a dual task: to acquire insights into the nature of health and illness in the human being, and to recognize those qualities in the remedies that might best correct such disturbances. The latter called for the skills of the craftsman: an ability to appreciate and work with the qualities of the material at hand. Like all crafts it was not something that could be learnt through books. Long apprenticeship and daily handling of the material were the obvious training.

In the second part of this text a modern appraisal of the action of plant remedies will be offered. It contains a considerable portion of book knowledge. No amount of that, however, would produce a good practitioner. Learning to use herbs wisely takes a great deal of simple hands-on experience. The following are the tenets that might provide the foundation for such an instruction.

Looking at plants as cyclic phenomena assumes that they are moving. The characteristics drawn from such a view must therefore be dynamic, not only changing themselves (to the next point on the cycle) *but exerting an influence on their environment as well*. This effect is as much felt by the body as rationalized by the mind.

There is no modern terminology to express the stages in the plant cycle so the following headings are the author's suggestions. Because the associated characteristics are apparent in the effects they exert, and because they are not absolutes, we will refer to them as 'tendencies'.

THE FOUR TENDENCIES

The four tendencies can be termed 'rising', 'floating', 'condensing' and 'sinking'.

The plant was seen in terms of both its parts and the current state of its life cycle. On no account must the conclusions drawn be applied too literally. It is always necessary to take all circumstances into account before making a balanced judgement of the probable predominant tendency. Even then each conclusion should be seen as approximate and subject to many exceptions: a starting point only.

Rising is associated with emergence and maturation, with the plant in spring, in the early morning and at the waxing moon, with rapidly growing tissues, the leaves, green tips, and other parts when green. (In Chinese it is the Wood phase, or 'minor *yang*'.)

Floating is associated with fulfilment and transcendence, with the plant in midsummer, at noon and at the full moon, with the mature parts of the plant, the flowers, fruit, and associated structures. (In Chinese it is the Fire phase – passing into Earth, perhaps – and 'major *yang*'.)

Condensing is associated with retrenchment and withdrawal, with the plant in autumn, in late afternoon and during the waning moon, with drying plant tissues, stalks, fallen leaves, parts of the plant that have lost their full colour, the rhizomes and tubers that condense nourishment for the following year. (In Chinese it is the Metal phase, and 'minor *yin*'.)

Sinking is associated with dormancy, latency, hidden potency, with the plant in winter, at night and at the new moon, with quiescent tissues, especially seeds, buds, and rootstocks. (In Chinese it is the Water phase, and 'major *yin*'.)

As these classifications represent dynamic qualities of the plant they are subject to alteration during handling and preparation.

All harvesting is a condensing influence and all storage a sinking one, so one can assume that using dried herbs is providing a more condensing influence than using fresh ones. This is more so, of course, if the plant is harvested late in the day, in the autumn or even during a waning moon, and less so for collection at rising times of the day, month or year. Reference to the phases of the moon in traditional medicine usually provokes a wry smile today. However, a force that can make an ocean surge up to its high tide level twice a day is not one to be dismissed lightly: it is certain to exert an equivalent pull on all masses of fluid everywhere, including those in humans, animals and plants.

Methods of preparation will also affect the direction of influence of the remedy in different ways, as will the presence of other herbs in a mixture.

The point of all this is to estimate the effect of any plant remedy after ingestion. This was predicted in wholly consistent ways.

The effect of rising and floating remedies (collectively referred to as rising) is to emphasize upward and outward movements in the body; there is an increase in heat, of superficial defences against external pathogens, of activities in the head and thorax. One would use such remedies to disperse cold, to assist superficial defences against both cold and heat, and to counteract symptoms of excessive sinking in the body (such as prolapse, diarrhoea, excessive menstruation), or excessive penetration (i.e. disease conditions moving past primary defences to establish themselves as chronic pathologies).

Rising remedies might include emetics and expectorants, the astringents, the peripheral vasodilators and heating remedies (all discussed later).

The effect of the condensing and sinking remedies (collectively referred to as condensing) is to emphasize downward and inward movements in the body; there is a reduction in heat, and a general increase in the activities of the lower regions of the body, and in those with nourishing and eliminatory functions; one would use such remedies to counteract symptoms of excessive rising in the body, such as vomiting, coughing, headaches, convulsions, spastic conditions such as asthma and nervous dyspepsia, and neuro-muscular tensions.

Sinking remedies might include the antispasmodics, sedatives, bitters, antitussives, purgatives and diuretics (all discussed later).

For those brought up in the modern medical tradition these broad sweeps of the brush will seem laughable – the work of a simpleton. How can all the diverse and complex clinical conditions that humans are prey to be lumped into just two categories of illness?

These are, however, very broad sweeps. No practitioner would underestimate the difficulty of dealing with real illnesses. These categories are for orientation purposes only: they are rarely binding. Nevertheless, as will be apparent in the rest of this text, there are indeed strong themes touched on here that will re-emerge again and again in discussing herbal remedies. It is already known that plant sap rises and falls as suggested here, that alkaloidal and volatile oil principles (definitely candidates for rising influences) are more concentrated in the morning and that bitters and anthraquinone laxatives with clear sinking properties are found more in roots and in the later part of the year.

We can now turn to a slightly more specific and much more powerful variation on this same theme.

THE TEMPERAMENTS OF PLANT REMEDIES

In highlighting the link between vitality and heat Thomson was picking up a theme that has been almost universal among traditional herbal practitioners. Heat was life, cold was disease or death: it was the obvious conclusion, only cast into doubt by the invention of the clinical thermometer, which showed that what we feel is not always reflected in measurable changes.

Of all the qualities of herbal remedies that have been used, their ability to affect the apparent degree of body heat has been the most widely applied. The categories were completely tied to the framework just discussed, so that rising energies were seen to be warming, floating hot, condensing cooling and sinking cold.

The Graeco-Roman physician Galen picked on this apparent property of medicinal agents to provide the basis of one of his most notable classifications. His empirical methods might have been faulted but his theoretical framework would have been recognized all over the world. We can quote from Culpeper's translation:

All medicines considered in themselves are either hot, cold, moist, dry or temperate.

The qualities of medicines are considered in respect of man, not of themselves; for those simples are called hot which heat our bodies; for those cold which cool them; and those temperate which work no change at all . . .

Such as are hot in the first degree, are of equal heat with our bodies, and they only add a natural heat to them, if it be cooled by nature or by accident thereby cherishing the natural heat when weak, and restoring it when wanting. Their use is 1. To make the offending humours thin, that they may be expelled by sweat or perspiration; 2. By outward application to abate inflammations and fevers by opening the pores of the skin.

Such as are hot in the second degree, as much exceed the first as our natural heat exceeds a temperature. Their use is to open the pores, and take away obstructions, by relaxing tough humours and by their essential force and strength, when nature cannot do it.

Such as are hot in the third degree, are more powerful in heating, because they tend to inflame and cause fevers. Their use is to promote perspiration extremely, and soften tough humours, and therefore all of them resist poison.

Such as are hot in the fourth degree, burn the body, if outwardly applied. Their use is to cause inflammation, raise blisters, and corrode the skin.

Such as are cold in the first degree, fall as much on the one side of temperate as doth hot on the other. Their use is, 1. To qualify the heat of the stomach and cause digestion; 2. To abate the heat in fevers; and 3. To refresh the spirits being almost suffocated.

Such as are cold in the third degree, are such as have a repercussive force. Their use is 1. To drive back the matter, and stop defluctions; 2. To make the humours thick; and 3. To limit the violence of choler, repress perspiration, and keep the spirits from fainting.

Such as are cold in the fourth degree, are such as to stupefy the senses. They are used, 1. In violent pains; and 2. In extreme watchings, and the like cases, where life is despaired of.

The themes introduced here are so important in understanding traditional therapeutics that they will repay clause-by-clause interpretation.

All medicines considered in themselves are either hot, cold, moist, dry or temperate.

Galen was referring here to all four elemental influences. Other sections of the passage refer to moistening and drying but have been left out for this discussion (they are however referred to in the chapter 'Traditional Pathology'). In this context 'temperate' means a neutral influence.

The qualities of medicines are considered in respect of man, not of themselves; for those simples are called hot which heat our bodies; for those cold which cool them; and those temperate which work no change at all . . .

A reiteration of a recurrent principle: what follows is how things feel when these remedies are applied. The language used is often very apt for observations of personal experience.

Such as are hot in the first degree, are of equal heat with our bodies, and they only add a natural heat to them, if it be cooled by nature or by accident thereby cherishing the natural heat when weak and restoring it when wanting. Their use is 1. To make the offending humours thin, that they may be expelled by sweat or perspiration; 2. By outward application to abate inflammations and fevers by opening the pores of the skin.

The first degree of heat is that which appears to support normal body temperature. Blood heat is something that most can appreciate. (The common assessment of the best temperature for a baby's drink by dropping it on one's wrist is a familiar application.) Remedies 'hot in the first degree' induce such a level of heat in the body: they gently warm it when chilled, maintain ('cherish') it if threatened.

This is a property almost always applied to febrile conditions in which such remedies tend to have a stabilizing effect on body temperature and on the course of the fever. What is also implied in fact is that when the body temperature is too high these remedies will actually *lower* it.

Heating the body fluids thins 'offending humours'. Referring back to the Thomsonian position again, cold was seen as the noxious influence. Its effect on body fluids was possibly taken from seeing meat stock congeal when cooled. To clear congealed matter one simply brings the stock back to body temperature again!

As with Thomson, fever was seen as the usual vital response to cold – the body's own attempts to thin the congealed matter. In this context it is not surprising that the pores or sweat glands were seen to be the immediate route of elimination, and the sweating, after the fever's crisis, a sign that clearing out was under way (see also 'The Sweat Glands' on pp. 112–14). The remedies 'hot in the first degree', like yarrow and elderflower, are *diaphoretic*, that is they increase sweating but, interestingly, only when the body is in a febrile state.

In brief, therefore, these remedies are applied for either of the following reasons:

> in the pre- or sub-febrile state, to move it nearer to the point where a flush-out through the sweat glands can occur;
>
> to get the body to a more healthy vital temperature;
>
> to temper a fever already under way.

This latter point is made in the final sentence: there is little modern experience of using external applications of these remedies, but lukewarm bathing in general is a well-known method for containing the high temperatures of fever, and Galen would have classified such a manoeuvre as a remedy of this class.

Such as are hot in the second degree, as much exceed the first as our natural heat exceeds a temperature. Their use is to open the pores, and take away obstructions, by relaxing tough humours and by their essential force and strength, when nature cannot do it.

This first sentence is easier to understand if 'a temperature' is read as 'room temperature'. These remedies are clearly more heating and we are asked to imagine about doubly so. The point is well made that they are definitely more dynamic than the previous category, being used to take over from 'nature' rather than simply allowing it to take its course. Remedies such as cinnamon, angelica, fresh ginger and raw garlic would fit this category: they are used where firm heating is indicated, but at a level that is not too powerful. The first three especially, sometimes referred to as *aromatic digestives*, make a sound foundation for a heating prescription.

Such as are hot in the third degree, are more powerful in heating, because they tend to inflame and cause fevers. Their use is to promote perspiration extremely, and soften tough humours, and therefore all of them resist poison.

Remedies 'hot in the third degree' are powerfully heating. They will literally raise body temperature, whatever its initial situation. They will induce sweating under any circumstances and so they could be expected to be particularly effective in 'softening tough humours'. The last phrase is especially revealing: poisons in Galenic medicine are clearly equated with cold. It is a point that Thomson would have endorsed. His favourite remedy, cayenne, along with the other hot spices, dried ginger, the peppers, chillies, mustards (*Sinapsis* spp.), and horseradish (*Cochlearia armoracia*) are all of this category. Their effect is well known and as *circulatory stimulants* or *rubefacients* will be discussed further.

Such as are hot in the fourth degree, burn the body, if outwardly applied. Their use is to cause inflammation, raise blisters, and corrode the skin.

The final category of heating is too strong for internal application. It includes the blistering agents croton oil, and formic acid nettle stings. These were dramatic remedies for local inflammations, especially arthritic joints.

The technique, sometimes known as 'counter-irritation', was almost certainly quite effective, albeit for a short time, and was a favourite way of getting sufferers back to work quickly in the working-class herbal practices of northern England. The theory was that a therapeutic inflammation could provide a relatively pain-free boost to the body's painful and crippling histamine-mediated inflammatory process, i.e. bring massive increased blood supply to the affected region. If a blister could be cultivated and then punctured, it had the added and apparently obvious benefits of directly drawing out the local toxins. It was a fitting extreme to the spectrum of heating remedies.

To understand the action of cooling remedies better we shall start by looking at the penultimate two categories, and then backtrack to look at those 'cold in the first degree'.

It is important to remember that cooling was essentially anti-vital, and that too much cooling produced a corpse! The use of cooling remedies was therefore less on the side of the angels, so to speak, than supporting vitality with heating remedies. Nevertheless, there were conditions that were marked by excessive heat, and the cooling remedies were appropriate to correct this, *but only as far as necessary*. The points are well made in the following paragraph:

Such as are cold in the third degree, are such as have a repercussive force. Their use is 1. To drive back the matter, and stop defluctions; 2. To make the humours thick; and 3. To limit the violence of choler, repress perspiration, and keep the spirits from fainting.

To put it simply, 'repercussive force' is what it feels like to be hit on the head by a brick! The first point to make about remedies of this type is that they tend to be sedative, to be depressive of vital functions. They are used where the vital reactions to illness get out of hand and begin to lead to more problems than solutions.

'Matter' is what is often thrown out of the body in the throes of serious illness; 'defluctions' is an earlier term for discharges. In other words the cold remedies suppress some of the more alarming manifestations of old-fashioned infectious diseases: vomiting, diarrhoea, purulent discharges, and weeping skin inflammations. Although all these might be seen as eliminations, they were also debilitating and in extreme cases at least would merit careful control.

The 'violence of choler' refers to the complex of convulsions, spasm, delirium and other excessive activities that often accompanied infectious diseases and fevers. The call for *sedatives* and *antispasmodics* might sometimes be urgent: such remedies would fit into this category.

Repressing perspiration was also a possible requirement. Excessively violent fever was often fatal: fever suppressants might sometimes save a life, and even give the body a chance to recoup its energies.

Keeping 'the spirits from fainting' sums up the indications for all remedies of this group: old diseases were usually very alarming and debilitating. While a weakened body would be more likely to succumb to the onslaught and would require heating remedies in its support, a robust body, in the violence of its reaction to the intrusion, might bring about its own downfall. Holding it in check might be for its own good.

Such as are cold in the fourth degree, are such as to stupefy the senses.

They are used, 1. In violent pains; and 2. In extreme watchings, and the like cases, where life is despaired of.

The qualities of cold remedies are dramatically extended here. 'Stupefying the senses' is plain enough: Galen was talking about strong sedatives or *hypnotics*. Their use in violent pains is also easy to follow: we would call such remedies *analgesics*. In fact, there was one remedy above all others described here: opium still provides modern medicine with many drugs of this category.

The final phrase is in some ways the most fascinating. 'Extreme watchings' is a potent image for the last hours before death, when it is impossible to leave the patient. There is a dramatic clinical technique, requiring the knack of an experienced practitioner, that can be used here. At a time when the violence of an illness is at its most extreme and terminal, one gives a massive sedation. The result is a blanket shutdown of all activity, vital and pathogenic. This may either lead to a hastened (though probably less painful) death, or, just possibly, freeing the patient from the burden of the fight, it may provide a last chance for the spark of vitality to rekindle and life to be grasped from the very jaws of death.

There is a final, important point to make about these last two categories. *If Galen had been presented with the contents of the modern doctor's medicine cabinet, he would most probably have classified almost all of them as cold.* They are all primarily concerned with relieving what would have earlier been thought of as vital signs: fever, inflammation, pain, diarrhoea, vomiting, coughing, stress responses, visceral tension and so on. If pushed to justify this strategy, the modern physician might suggest that relieving the body of the burden of the fight not only provides direct relief, but also might, just might, allow it the opportunity to recoup and fight better another day. This is a variation on the extreme thought introduced by Galen at the end.

It is an argument, but not a new one. And Galen and his successors through the ages were surprisingly well aware of its limitations.

Having seen where this type of remedy is heading, it is now time to consider the less extreme categories.

Such as are cold in the first degree, fall as much on the one side of temperate as doth hot on the other. Their use is, 1. To qualify the heat of the stomach and cause digestion; 2. To abate the heat in fevers; and 3. To refresh the spirits being almost suffocated.

It may have been noticed that there is no category of remedies 'cold in the second degree'. This is possibly due to minimal requirements for mild sedatives in the more robust days of old. It may also reflect a view that there was a substantial gap between remedies 'cold in the first degree' and the rest of the group.

The key to the identity of this class lies in the first use provided. These are the *bitter digestives*, about which a great deal will be said in this text. All traditional cultures are unanimous in characterizing the bitters as cooling. In the case of fevers they do indeed lead to a reduction in apparent body temperature ('abate the heat in fevers').

As will be seen later, however, the primary effect of the bitters is to increase overall activity in the upper digestive system, to 'cause digestion'. A possible scenario is that this may lead to greater circulatory investment in the digestive process, and, in a way reminiscent of the advice against swimming after a meal, draw blood (and thus heat) away from the rest of the body.

Whatever the mechanism, bitters were credited with a unique feat of medicinal alchemy. They were seen not to cool excess heat so much as to *convert it into improved nourishment*. This means that, alone among the cooling influences, the bitters do not intrinsically depress vitality, and can apparently have a useful enhancing effect. In general they are indicated for hot (inflammatory) disorders where the competence of the upper digestive system and especially of the liver is suspect, or where there is other evidence of poor assimilation.

Bringing blood to the digestive system does not contradict the description 'to qualify the heat of the stomach'. This refers to fevers of enteric origin, and notably hepatitis, both conditions for which bitters are strongly indicated.

The bitters then clearly occupy a privileged position in the spectrum of heating and cooling. Their net effect is gentle, falling 'as much on the one side of [room temperature] as doth [blood heat] on the other'. Finally in a lucid passage they are likened to a splash of water on a stifling hot day 'to refresh the spirits being almost suffocated'.

In modern times when syndromes of anxiety, neurosis, visceral tension and spasmodic conditions are perhaps more widespread than they were in the past, we might be tempted to slip another category into the list. Perhaps remedies 'cold in the second degree' might include the gentle *relaxants*, less than sedative and unlikely to depress. The mirror images of warming yarrow (and containing similar constituents), the cooling chamomiles (*Chamomilla recutita* and *Anthemis nobilis*), as well as lemon balm (*Melissa officinalis*), peppermint (*Mentha x piperita*), scullcap (*Scutellaria* spp.) and even valerian (*Valeriana officinalis*) and passionflower (*Passiflora incarnata*), are widely used today to ease troublesome tensions in even the very young. They contain a blend of other constituents, warming volatile oils and cooling bitters for example, that reassure as to the gentleness of their calming (i.e. cooling) action.

THE THERAPEUTIC CHOICE

Just as everyone knows the difference between heat and cold, so the temperaments are the most universally understood qualities of herbal remedies. They are also surprisingly useful in developing prescriptions even today. We will return to the diagnostic criteria used for determining how to apply this approach in a following section (see 'Traditional Herbal Therapeutics', on pp. 196–228). In essence, though, the herbalist can still ask a primary question: whether the prescription should be predominantly warming or cooling. All other diagnostic questions follow. *A prescription with the wrong temperament can rarely be corrected by subsequent tinkering.*

In modern physiological terms the choice can be translated as follows:

Heating implies increasing blood flow and/or metabolic rate. Blood is the main vehicle for transferring heat around the body; generally speaking increased blood flow increases the temperature of the tissues. Conversely, any apparent increase in tissue warmth usually signals an increase in the amount of blood flowing through it, the amount of oxygen and nutrients supplied, and the amount of carbon dioxide and waste products removed. The apparent benefits accruing to heating remedies may well be a reflection of improved perfusion of the body's tissues (see also 'Circulation', on pp. 86–94).

Increasing metabolic rate is a less certain pharmacological effect of the heating herbs. It is just possible that some, particularly the stronger heating remedies, might have such an effect, either locally or generally. But the position remains unclear.

Cooling, as we have seen, involves either an increase in digestive activities and assimilation, or sedation. The first is a positive increment in the body's fortunes. The other is at best a palliative, a way of relieving an intolerable and otherwise untreatable condition; at worst it can be a dangerous suppression of inconvenient manifestations of vitality.

Chinese Pharmacology§

Whereas cooling and heating are universally applied properties of herbal remedies, most cultures have developed their own approaches as well. One of the most interesting for our purposes is that developed in China.[9] Here was an attempt to order medicinal properties in five-phase terms, as the five *Tastes*.

There is always an element of artificiality in such systems of classification,[10] but the Chinese do seem to have spotted a number of important pharmacological principles. They also cast an interesting light on our previous exploration of the traditional cyclic view of natural phenomena.

Many of the interpretations for the action of the five *Tastes* are explicable only in terms of Chinese physiology (see Appendix) but these will be translated as well as possible in what follows.

§To those unfamiliar with concepts of Chinese medicine the following will make much better sense after referring to the introduction to Chinese concepts of physiology in the Appendix.

THE FIVE TASTES

The choice of taste as the means of herbal classification is an interesting one. In days before laboratory investigations, taste was obviously a major arbiter of a plant's quality. It is easy to see how a taste would come to be associated with particular types of pharmacological activity and would readily be seen *to be that quality itself*, and then become a remedial force in its own right.||

The five *Tastes* are considered to arise from the mingling of the four tendencies with the energies of Earth (the temperaments by contrast are seen to involve celestial energies). The *Tastes* are thus specifically tied to the Earth and its manifestations. In some accounts there is reference to a sixth *Taste*: mild, neutral or no-taste: as this also has interesting qualities we shall include it in our discussion, referring to it as *bland*.

Two of the *Tastes* are primarily *yang* and tend to disperse upwards in the body. They are the *acrid* and *sweet Tastes* (the latter is usually yoked with the *bland Taste*).

Three *Tastes* are primarily *yin* and tend to flow downwards in the body. They are the *sour*, *bitter* and *salty Tastes*.

As is the way in Chinese thought, the *Tastes* were soon assigned to the five phases and their functional manifestations in the body (see 'A Traditional Physiology', on pp. 595–609). In turn this came to mean that the normal role of each *Function* included being a vehicle for the activity of its own *Taste* and depended on acquiring a quantum, primarily from food, but if necessary from medicine. Thus:

||Manfred Porkert, in *The Theoretical Foundations of Chinese Medicine*, MIT Press, Massachusetts, p. 113 (paperback edition 1978), and elsewhere, has drawn attention to the semantic inaccuracy of using the word 'taste' to translate the Chinese word *wei*, considering that this attribute of a substance is strictly a quality defined by taste. He uses the word 'sapor', derived from the Latin, to denote this quality and to reduce confusions that might arise. It is unfortunately true, however, that the use of the word 'taste' is widespread so we shall use it in the same way as other authors, but using the first capital letter.

Taste	Phase	Function
Sour	Wood	Liver/Gall-bladder
Bitter	Fire	Heart/Pericardium/Small Intestine/Triple Heater
Sweet	Earth	Spleen/Stomach
Acrid	Metal	Lungs/Large Intestine
Salty	Water	Kidneys/Bladder

While a moderate amount of each *Taste* is necessary for its corresponding *Function* there are also wider effects deriving from its consumption. Fig. 8 (see p. 186) illustrates the main relationships.

It will become clear that while this starts out as a basic five-phase cycle the need to accommodate asymmetries and irregularities has produced a considerable variation on the previous cyclic theme. It will be obvious that sourness is not a rising or warming influence, and as we have seen bitterness is certainly not. The cycle only begins to make sense when all the relationships of the *Tastes* and *Functions* are filled in. In particular the central position of the Earth phase needs to be understood.

The *Tastes* were seen to be properties refined from foods and medicine by the *Spleen*, the body's Earth *Function*, and which in modern terms would be understood as the metabolic processes of the body. The *Spleen* then distributes the *Tastes* to the other *Functions*, sourness to the *Liver*, bitterness to the *Heart*, and so on. Having distributed four of the *Tastes*, *it keeps the sweet Taste for itself* (and in some accounts the *bland Taste* by default, it being without sufficient character to be moved at all!). As would be expected from such a central position, the relationship of the *Spleen* to the *Tastes* is unusual. The interesting point, referred to earlier, is that in matters pertaining to herbal medicine, the Chinese have in essence referred back to the old Earth-centred, geocentric view. Using this perspective it is much easier to understand what would otherwise be a puzzling list of correspondences.

185   The Herbalist's Approach

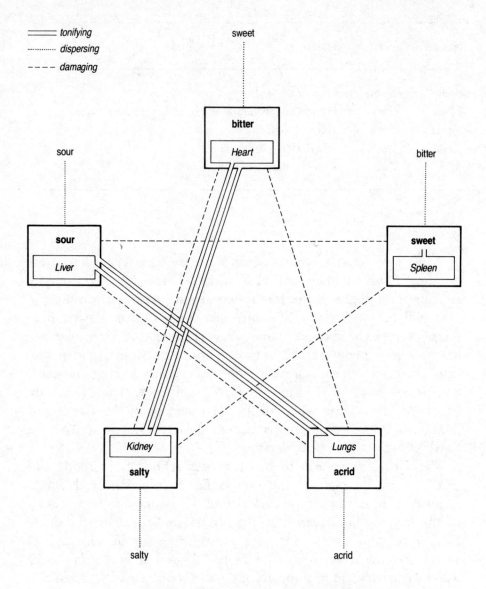

Fig. 8 The five *Tastes* and their relationships

Tonification

As well as being associated with one *Function* each *Taste* is also seen to tonify another *Function* in the body. That means that at moderate levels it positively supports that *Function*. Looking at Fig.

8 it will be seen that the *sour Taste* tonifies the *Lungs*, the *bitter* tonifies the *Kidneys*, the *acrid* the *Liver* and the *salty* the *Heart*. The *Spleen*, however, as well as expressing the qualities of *sweet* as its own *Taste*, is also tonified by it. All this will be elaborated later.

Dispersion

The general principle is that selectively giving extra amounts of each *Taste* disperses excessive activity in the *Function* with which it is linked. The rationale seems to be that mediating the action of a *Taste* in the body involves and exercises the linked *Function*, like any exercise draining off excessive energy. Thus excess tension or activity in the *Liver* can be dissipated by keeping it well fuelled with the *sour Taste*, and likewise for the *acrid* and *salty Tastes* and the *Lungs* and *Kidneys* respectively.

There is, however, a problem to resolve. While the *Spleen* might manage to extract two roles from the *sweet Taste*, it could not manage three. It appears then as though it arranges a swap with the *Heart*, so that the *sweet Taste* disperses excess activity in the *Heart* and the *bitter* disperses excess activity in the *Spleen*.

Damage

The effects of taking excessive amounts of any particular *Taste* follow a conventional five-phase relationship, in fact the *ko* cycle. Thus, excessive salt will damage the *Heart*, sourness the *Spleen*, bitterness the *Lungs*, sweetness the *Kidneys*, and too many hot spices will harm the functions of the *Liver*.

THE PHARMACOLOGY OF TASTE

All this might seem to be the sort of cosmic tinkering that cultures like the Chinese have a reputation for, except that in this case at least valuable and unusual insights into the pharmacological properties of foods and medicines seem to have been drawn. Some of these can now be elaborated. (Text set in small type below provides commentaries on the conclusions drawn from Chinese traditions.)

Salty

It is the taste of common salt and seafood, physiologically the result of the presence in the mouth of substantial quantities of ionized molecules, these particles acting to stimulate the salt receptors on the tongue and palate. The salty *Taste* is not well represented in the herbal materia medica, though seaweeds are occasionally used in maritime cultures (e.g. bladderwrack in the British Isles), and particularly so in Japan. It is possible to classify the occasional remedy like celery seed in this category. In China the main group of drugs classified as salty includes animal remains and tissues, and the minerals.

The salty *Taste* is directed by the *Spleen* to the *Kidneys*. It is *yin* and tends to flow downwards in the body, and it moves particularly to the most *yin* tissue in the body, a manifestation of *Kidneys*, the bones.

It is interesting to note that sea-salt was possibly the world's original currency, so vital was it in hot climates: its association with *Kidney* may thus have other connotations.

It is said to 'moisten' and 'soften'.

Salty remedies are used for 'dry, hard' pathologies, such as tumours, fibroses (e.g. liver cirrhosis), constipation and other abdominal swellings. Some of these conditions are more likely to respond to treatment than others!

It disperses excess activity in the *Kidneys*.

This has little to do with urine production, and is in any case a rare disturbance.

In moderation it tonifies the *Heart*.

In the sense that the *Heart* is, like its Western counterpart, responsible for maintaining the movement of the circulation the ancients would probably have noticed the increased fluid and improved heart stroke that results from taking salty foods, particularly in hot weather and where salt has become deficient. Salt has always been seen as essential to life: its association with Water and the *Kidneys* is a recognition of that here. At a more speculative level, one might now note the primacy of the sodium/potassium pump in the regulation of all fluid movement, and in fact for the life of the cell itself.

In excess it damages the *Heart*.

The pathological consequences for the circulation of a high-salt diet have been recognized, rather belatedly, in modern medicine.

Sour

This is the result of the stimulation of the sour taste buds by acid, or to be precise hydrogen, ions (H^+). It is the taste of fruit acids, vinegar, and tannins (apparent in a cup of over-steeped tea). In herbal medicine it is the latter that are of most interest and they are covered in some depth in the chapter 'Traditional Pharmacology'. The properties of fruit acids including ascorbic acid (vitamin C) are also of interest in this context.

The sour *Taste* is directed by the *Spleen* to the *Liver*; it is *yin* and tends to move downwards in the body. It moves particularly to the muscle fibres (or 'sinews').

It is said to 'absorb' and 'bind'.

It is applied to discharges, excessive diuresis, incontinence, perspiration and premature ejaculation (a preoccupation in China at least as much as in the West!). Some of these indications recur in the discussion of the effect of tannins later.

It disperses excess activity in the *Liver*.

This would manifest at least in part as disturbances in the flow of body fluids.

It tonifies the *Lungs*.

Among other roles, the *Lungs* are concerned with the maintenance of the body's defences against external pathogens. The role of fruit as a protection, particularly against respiratory infections, was certainly not a new discovery.

In excess it damages the *Spleen*.

Excessive consumption of tannins at least is known to interfere with assimilation of foods. On the other hand it is now known that stimulation of the sour receptors leads to reflex increase in the flow of salivary juices and bile: the effect of excessive stimulation is not known.

Bitter

This taste is mediated by bitter taste buds in the mouth which are stimulated by a number of chemical structures. Many plant constituents can evoke the taste, including alkaloids, terpenoid derivatives (such as many volatile oils), and phenol derivatives (see the chapter 'Traditional Pharmacology'). It is thus a quality recognized by the Chinese, and others, as intrinsic to herbal remedies.

The bitter *Taste* is directed by the *Spleen* to the *Heart*; it is *yin* and tends to flow downwards in the body. It moves particularly to *xue* ('blood').

The association of bitterness and *xue* is interesting. As the most dense of the circulating energies in the body (see Appendix), *xue* is in effect the speculative force behind the more somatic events in the body. Compared to acupuncture, which is seen to primarily affect *qi*, the more rarefied circulating energy, the archetypal bitterness of herbal remedies is strongly associated with treating more substantial deep-seated clinical problems. In some accounts there is actually a geographical stratification: acupuncture needling from the surface, initially affecting the most *yang*, superficial level of *qi*, *wei qi*, then successively penetrating to the more *yin*, deeper layers of *qi*, with ever more potent effects. *Xue* is too deep for needling (in practice it would be the level that actually leads to bleeding), so herbs were seen to be the technique to affect that layer, from the inside.

It is said to 'sedate', to 'dry', and to 'harden'.

The first can be loosely approximated as we have seen to bitter's cool temperament; 'drying' refers to bitter's use in 'damp-heat' conditions (see the chapter 'Traditional Pathology'); 'hardening' may be better understood in energetic terms, if translated by the term 'consolidating' and used to express the effect of improving assimilation and nourishment.

It disperses excess in the *Spleen*.

One modern manifestation of such a condition is the excessive consumption of sweet foods with the disruptions in blood-sugar levels (reactive hypoglycaemia and/or late-onset diabetes) that often result. There is impressive clinical evidence of the benefits of bitter herbs in stabilizing such disruptions and in other ways counteracting the effects of excessive sugar.

It tonifies the *Kidneys*.

As these are the repositories of one's constitutional reserves, any influence that can claim to tonify the *Kidneys* is clearly very impressive indeed. Above all other features, even its association with the Fire phase, this claim for bitterness establishes its position at the top of the pharmacological hierarchy. Such reverence is found in other traditions as well, with the bitter herbs often claimed as the prime tonics in the materia medica.

In excess it damages the *Lungs*.

Bitters are cooling; excessive cooling suppresses vital defences; the *Lungs* are the *Function* responsible for harnessing vitality to both its defensive and metabolic roles.

Sweet

The sweet *Taste* needs some interpretation. In a time when sugar was almost unknown, sweetness was a far more delicate taste, and was used to refer to the intrinsic sweetness of the basic foodstuffs of a peasant's diet. Many of those have a clear, if subtle sweetness; for example, the basic cereals, peas, cooked root vegetables, and those fruits suitable for drying and storing as winter food: apricots, figs, prunes, sultanas (all of which are marked by an acid-free sweetness in their fresh state). In days when even honey was an occasional luxury, the taste of extracted sugar would have been considered intrinsically excessive. In herbal remedies the sweet *Taste* is exhibited particularly by the saponins, a fascinating group often with balancing pharmacological effects (see the chapter 'Traditional Pharmacology').

The *Spleen* keeps the sweet *Taste* to itself; it is *yang* and tends to move upwards in the body; it moves to the soft tissues.

Sweetness must really be equated with nourishment: it is the quality of a simple agrarian diet, and has its most potent metaphor in mother's milk.

There can be no other fate for it than to remain with the *Function* most concerned with assimilation and nourishment. It is also not surprising that it should manifest in the soft tissues, and thus in overall body shape. (It is worth noting that the Chinese ideal build was that usually credited to the Buddha – his is thus the shape of a healthy *Spleen*!)

It is said to 'tonify' and to 'balance'.

As archetypal nourishment, sweetness can do little else but tonify and restore. It is however also interesting to see a reflection of the other (moving) Earth quality: the capacity to stay in balance in a turbulent world. The Chinese were in effect saying that a good stable agrarian diet is the most effective way to maintain homoeostasis; it is also a point that many saponins (e.g. those of ginseng (*Panax ginseng*) and liquorice (*Glycyrrhiza glabra*)) have a similar clinical reputation.

It disperses excess in the *Heart*.

Many symptoms of anxiety and nervous tension were attributed to various excess syndromes affecting the *Heart*. This property thus follows closely the preceding comments.

In excess it damages the *Kidneys*.

This is a more or less terminal effect in Chinese medicine, resulting in premature ageing. In other words they would have predicted an enfeeblement of general vitality through the sugar-consuming habits of modern affluent society. We may live longer, but are they wrong? This was incidentally another reason for recommending bitter as an antidote to the problems of excess sweet.

Acrid

Sometimes also called 'pungent', this is the taste of the hot spices, cayenne (*Capsicum minimum*), ginger (*Zingiber officinale*), mustard, the peppers, horseradish (*Cochlearia armoracia*), and raw onions (*Allium cepa*) and garlic (*Allium sativum*) (both the latter become sweet when cooked), and more subtly of all the 'heating' herbal remedies. Unlike the other four *Tastes* the acrid *Taste* is not linked to any special taste bud, but simply follows direct irritation of any exposed tissues and sensory nerve fibres. The association with the Metal phase may have followed inhaling the fumes given off from any smelting plant.

The acrid *Taste* is directed by the *Spleen* to the *Lungs*; it is *yang* and tends to move upwards; it moves particularly to *qi*.

The heating properties of the acrid *Taste* are always its dominant feature. Reference back through this text will provide many resonances with this and following points.

It is said to 'move *qi*', 'disperse', 'activate the body fluids', 'cause expulsion from the *Lungs*' and 'open the pores'.

It tends to be used therefore for superficial, external disease conditions, to counteract external pathogenic influences, especially 'wind' and 'cold', and to mobilize stagnant body energies. Again reference to the traditional role of heating remedies and to the *Lungs* will show how consistent these attributes are.

It disperses excess in the *Lungs*.

Notably that manifested by congested bronchial inflammations.

It tonifies the *Liver*.

The *Liver* is charged with ensuring a balanced dispersal of all the body's energies and activities.

In excess it damages the *Liver*.

As one might expect: fire burns out as well as providing heat.

Bland

A substance classified as bland is one which is literally seen as having no character, as being neutral, without dynamic action in the body.

It is not therefore a typical *Taste*, and is not recognized in all accounts. Where it is, it is said to slip through the body without hindrance or interaction. It moves straight through from the *Spleen* to the *Bladder*, i.e. the urinary system, and thus out of the body.

Its only effect therefore is that it is a *diuretic*. Many of the diuretics used in herbal medicine have a characteristic blandness of taste: in modern assessment they would be seen to operate on osmotic principles, the result of excreting simple carbohydrate or mucilaginous constituents.

In modern practice, the mucilaginous remedies that would fit into the 'bland' category are also used as *relaxing expectorants*, as detailed in the chapters 'Physiology' and 'Traditional Pharmacology'.

The Doctrine of Signatures

The Doctrine of Signatures is one of the features of medical history that in modern eyes most confirms herbalism as a humorous relic from the past. To suggest that a plant with a kidney-shaped leaf should be used for urinary diseases, or one that was speckled for lung disease is patently laughable.

In such a form it would deserve relegation to history: even the explanation that God left signs ('signatures') as to the purpose of His creation does not ring true outside fundamentalist circles today.

If, however, these simplicities are put back into their true perspective, then they make more sense. If, as we have seen, the early view of life was as a uniform whole, with each manifestation, each living thing a microcosm of the whole, and subject to the same natural laws, then it is indeed the case that natural phenomena should match, one with the other. We have seen how rising and sinking, heating and cooling, moistening and drying were qualities of plants met upon the human consuming them. We have also seen how in at least one tradition these qualities came to be assessed by their taste.

It is not surprising then that in a desperate attempt to make sense of the healing potential of the natural world, early humans would have looked for any clues possible to read the appropriate qualities of the medicines.

It is certain that the 'professional' version of these signs, some of which were transmitted in the rare written texts on the practice of medicine still available from other early cultures, were suitably complex and subtle. The popular view, the basis for the oral transmission of folk medicine, was more simple. Like many caricatures the simple image has been the more lasting.

Traditional Herbal Therapeutics

Having sketched out the traditional perspectives in the previous sections, it may now be possible to construct, as a synopsis, an interim approach to the use of herbal remedies that keeps faith with the experience of the past. This will also act as a simple groundplan upon which to set the more specific (and fragmentary) material in Part II and will be a suggested basis for effective clinical application. An assumption is made that these remedies actually work as claimed: a more searching review of efficacy will be made later.

Real clinical practice will never be as easy as what follows. *Nor will these simple principles replace the rigorous study of clinical medicine that any practitioner in a developed society must now undergo.* They may however help to set the application of herbal medicine into a context different from conventional practice. They may also be helpful for those who wish simply to use herbs a bit more productively for themselves or their family.

This approach will be based both on historical precedent and on current practice among herbal practitioners around the world.[11] It will be presented systematically, perhaps more so than in reality, as a hierarchy of questions illustrated as follows:

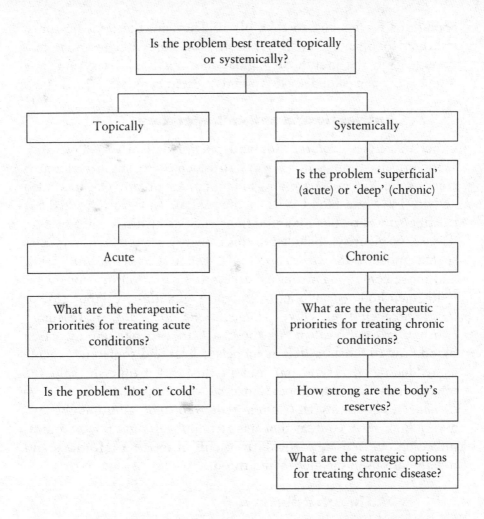

| Is the problem best treated topically or systemically? |

| Topically | | Systemically |

| Is the problem 'superficial' (acute) or 'deep' (chronic) |

| Acute | | Chronic |

| What are the therapeutic priorities for treating acute conditions? | | What are the therapeutic priorities for treating chronic conditions? |

| Is the problem 'hot' or 'cold' | | How strong are the body's reserves? |

| What are the strategic options for treating chronic disease? |

Is the Problem Best Treated Topically or Systemically?

Healing

A very large proportion of herbal remedies are eminently suitable for topical treatments. This is because many contain appreciable quantities of *mucilage* and *tannins*. These exert a soothing, protecting and binding influence on any exposed tissues and so provide the optimum conditions for healing to take place. They are the remedies most indicated for open wounds, ulcerations, abrasions, mucous inflammations (e.g. in the mouth or vagina), haemorrhoids, fissuring, and weeping eczema (skin disease is mainly treated by systemic medicine).

Antiseptic and anti-inflammatory

Other principles (*volatile oils* and *phenol* derivatives) have antiseptic effects, though not always so much as to sterilize the area completely. Yet more are anti-inflammatory or provoke increased activity by white blood cells in the region, and are indicated for treating subcutaneous inflammations such as arthritis, chronic skin disease, or pleurisy. Included in this category are the *acrid* remedies such as mustard (*Sinapsis* spp.) and cayenne (*Capsicum minimum*), and those containing strong volatile oils such as oil of peppermint (with menthol), eucalyptus (*Eucalyptus globulus*), cajaput (*Melaleuca leucadendron*), cloves (*Eugenia caryophyllata*) or rosemary (*Rosmarinus officinalis*): all these act to provoke an increased blood flow to the area (felt as increased heat and sometimes visible as reddening, or erythema) and in this way painlessly help the inflammatory process along. Tinctures of marigold (*Calendula officinalis*) and gum myrrh (*Commiphora mol-mol*) additionally have a very high *resin* content that has strong local antiseptic and anti-inflammatory action, particularly useful in treating infections and inflammations in the mouth and throat.

The internal surface

Reference to the chapter 'Traditional Pharmacology', will provide more details of these actions and will also reveal that they do not stop at the exterior of the body. One of the central themes of any herbal treatment is that the digestive system is in the front line of any internal application and that the lining of the gut is as accessible to the topical actions of the remedies as any external surface. Moreover, the incredible complexity and sensitivity of the whole alimentary apparatus mean that any influences on its surfaces have potentially profound reflex implications elsewhere in the body. Such treatment can barely be considered topical in the conventional sense, but it underlines an important point: most topical herbal remedies, if swallowed, carry their effects through to the interior, with expectorant, diuretic, laxative, emetic and anti-emetic, carminative, and a diverse range of other actions. Again elaboration of this point will be found in the chapter 'Traditional Pharmacology'.

Topical treatments for the interior

Topical treatment can be entirely external or partly systemic. It is, in fact, often difficult to make the distinction, or to choose between applications. It is frequently the case that a problem is best dealt with in both ways. There are traditions which favour external treatments for almost all conditions, relying on the beneficial principles of the plants diffusing through the skin. The French herbalist, Maurice Messegué,[12] is a prominent advocate of this approach.

There are other more specific routes of administration where the boundaries are also blurred. Vaginal and rectal treatments have pronounced systemic effects, as do mouthwashes, gargles and inhalations. The techniques for applying all these preparations may be found in 'Pharmacy', on pp. 365–87.

It is a significant point that material absorbed into the body elsewhere than at the gut is not subjected to the effects of digestion and particularly the 'first-pass effect' of liver metabolism. The systemic effects of topical applications are thus likely to be different from those resulting from oral administration.

If it is concluded that topical treatments are not appropriate or sufficient, then the practitioner will look to the next question.

Is the Problem 'Superficial' (Acute) or 'Deep' (Chronic)?

The penetration of illness

The nature of any treatment depends considerably on the extent to which the problem has 'penetrated' the system. A passing cough, cold, headache or dyspepsia can be treated very simply and usually safely with home remedies, such as might be discussed at a symptomatic level in the average herb book; these treatments often combine reasonable efficacy with a lack of interference in vital processes. Most such problems are self-limiting anyway: they would pass on whether they were treated or not.

However, a condition that has involved the system over a long period of time, either persistently or recurrently, is seen in traditional thought to have penetrated superficial defence measures. It will require increasingly substantial and carefully directed treatments, and a greater practical expertise as well. There will be greater involvement of the body's tissues and structures, and increased likelihood of the appearance of conventional, tangible pathologies.

It is thus necessary to assess the degree of penetration of any condition and its suitability for any particular treatment.

The vital resistance

Generally it may be said that at the early, acute or superficial stages of disease the body can be expected to defend its integrity stoutly. *This defence is often uncomfortable or distressing and is often thought of as the illness itself.* Symptoms include vomiting and diarrhoea, coughing, fever, inflammations and skin eruptions. These are all mechanisms the body can call on to rid itself of some noxious presence within its boundaries. If such symptoms have occurred recently, then it is unwise to suppress them unduly.

One can reduce the ferocity of the symptoms, make a cough more productive, manage a fever (so as to help the body maintain a temperature of around 38.5–39°C (101–102°F) for example, while perhaps stimulating perspiration and digestive activity, see 'Fever', on pp. 63–7), reduce the inflammation by stimulating extra blood flow to the area, and so on. But the priority should be *management* rather than suppression, and the need to see such symptoms as signs of healthy resistance to attack rather than as illness.

The subdued resistance

If, however, such symptoms are recurrent, have been persisting for too long, or seem to have arisen out of another more substantial problem, then they should not be treated in quite the same way. An important point here is that in modern affluent societies most apparently acute conditions are in fact *sub-acute*, that is they are recurrent attacks from essentially a chronic condition. Repeated bouts of bronchitis, sore throats, or rheumatic pains, even if these happen only every year or so, are more likely to be deep-seated than superficial problems.

This raises some interesting questions about the average state of health in modern times. There is no doubt that advances have been made on some fronts, but the whole weight of modern medicine has been directed to reducing the symptoms of short-term vital defence measures: it might be expected that these vigorous encounters occur rather less frequently than of old. If the purpose of the vigorous encounter is to hit a problem hard before it has an opportunity to get established, then it might also be not too surprising to see more insidious, less tangible illnesses develop instead. This is certainly a current impression.

Other symptoms

Apart from the question of time and persistence, there are other ways to help ascertain the degree of penetration of an illness.

The pulse is a helpful sign: in acute conditions it is much more 'superficial', i.e. easy to feel on the surface; in chronic or deep-seated conditions it tends to be 'deep', i.e. only palpable on pressure.

In chronic conditions there is a tendency for other vital signs to be subdued, for eliminatory functions like those of the bowels and urinary system to be diminished. Respiratory passages tend to dryness and sensitivity rather than the initial production of profuse catarrh.

If an assessment of the problem has thus been made, it may then be possible to review the different therapeutic options to be taken.

What are the Therapeutic Priorities for Treating Acute Conditions?

FOUR STRATEGIES

If it is determined that the problem is short-term or acute, then treatment divides into four main strategies:

1   to maintain and if necessary increase eliminations from the body, in order to fulfil the minimum requirements for preventing the condition proceeding any deeper;

2   to make such functional adjustments as may seem indicated to reduce distress and improve the body's capacity to manage the problem, while always avoiding undue suppression;

3   to balance up the final prescription so that its temperament best counters the temperament of the illness;

4   to ensure that there is adequate time planned after the illness for full convalescence and recovery.

1 Eliminations

Improving eliminations means using remedies that induce perspiration (*diaphoretics*), remove material from the airways (*expectorants*), the stomach (*emetics*), the bowel (*laxatives* or *aperients*), the urinary system and kidneys (*diuretics*), and the liver (*cholagogues*), as well as non-specifically 'cleansing' the tissues and bloodstream (*alteratives* or *depurients*), or specifically the lymphatic system (*lymphatics*). These may be selected either for obvious reasons or as part of a broader strategy.

It is difficult to overstate how important this stage is in herbal tradition: a majority of remedies have some effect on eliminatory pathways and in former times, when acute diseases were the norm, the use of eliminatives might have been the only treatment used.

2 Functional adjustments

Making other functional adjustments in this context could be described as fine tuning. Nevertheless, they may be necessary. There might be a need for visceral or nervous relaxants to reduce the risk of spasms and convulsions, either generally or selectively, for bowel, stomach, bronchial muscle or elsewhere. A flagging circulation may need support, or excessive gastric activity need to be reduced. It is often necessary to augment natural defences either locally (at the mouth, throat, or near a lesion) or generally.

There is, of course, the particular task of managing the vital defence mechanisms themselves. Undue vomiting, excessive diarrhoea, coughing or discharges can, at least in the hands of experienced practitioners, usually be gently contained with herbal remedies, without having to have recourse to conventional suppressants.

3 Temperament

For all those planning to use herbs, whether the novice in day-to-day ailments or more experienced practitioners, there remains an important practical question to ask and answer before deciding which remedies to use. It refers back to earlier discussion about the traditional classification of both herbs and illnesses.

Is the problem 'hot' or 'cold'?
This could also be rephrased: 'How actively is the body responding to the problem?' If, as Galen claimed, remedies are allocated temperaments according to the effect they have when taken, then their application will be determined by the temperament of the body at that moment.

A 'cold' illness is one in which the body's responses are subdued: it is usually brought on by a 'cold' pathogenic influence but may also reflect a constitutional sluggishness. It will generally call for a prescription with overall 'heating' properties (for more on these concepts see the chapter ' Traditional Pathology').

A 'hot' illness is one in which the body's responses are excessive: it is usually brought on by a 'hot' pathogenic influence but may also reflect a constitutional vigour. It will generally call for a prescription that is 'cooling'.

The diagnostic signs that will help determine whether heating or cooling remedies are indicated are listed in the chapter 'Traditional Pathology'.

The temperament of the prescription is a matter that also concerns the treatment of chronic conditions, but other factors may also then intervene, as will be shown in the next section.

The most frequently used remedies usually exhibit their own blend of actions here. A good example is the combination of bitter digestive stimulant and visceral relaxant seen in the chamomiles (*Chamomilla recutita* and *Anthemis nobilis*), peppermint (*Mentha x piperita*) and hops (*Humulus lupulus*), or the warming (circulatory stimulant) and carminative effects of ginger (*Zingiber officinale*), fennel (*Foeniculum vulgare*), and the other warming spices. As the remedies become familiar many such combinations of action will be apparent.

4 Restoration

The need for adequate time for recovery after an acute illness is barely accepted in modern medical care. The power of antibiotics and other treatments has distracted health professionals from the continuing need of the body to recuperate; the manic economic imperative has made those taking time off work feel like social pariahs. Yet it is most likely that the earlier view still holds, that an acute illness needs to be treated with respect, that several days' or a week's recovery time should be accepted as the true cost of an average feverish illness, several weeks for a more severe or debilitating case like glandular fever (infectious mononucleosis). The prominence of post-viral fatigue syndromes in modern times would most likely be much reduced if adequate convalescence time was allowed at the time.

The principles of convalescence and restorative regimes are important and are elaborated in full in the following pages.

PRESCRIBING

It is advisable in drawing up a prescription to see the management of eliminations as the primary task and to select such herbs as are appropriate; then, given that most will have a blend of activity, to see what other remedies are necessary to balance out the treatment; and last, but certainly not least, to get the temperament right. It might then only be necessary to have one, two, or three individual herbs in a mixture. This will usually make it easier to keep on top of the prescription and its subsequent alterations.

There are two further important points to make about treating superficial conditions:

> the condition changes very rapidly: any one prescription will often need to be taken only for a day or two, sometimes much less;

> the dosage of the herbs used can be relatively large.

Short sharp adjustments are the order for acute conditions. The dosages found in popular herb books are usually derived from old texts that were referring to primarily acute disorders; they are sometimes called 'heroic' dosages and are acceptable, *but only if a robust vital reaction is under way.*

Fortunately most of the herbs available for popular consumption in the shops are relatively gentle. They may, with a little practice, be used at near-heroic levels, for the common aches and pains, with the prospect of almost instant effect.

Even the experienced practitioner will rarely if ever prescribe emetics or violent cathartics as was done in the past: the tempo of modern life does not permit such unpleasantness and in any case it is now rare to encounter the indications for such treatment outside the hospital casualty department!

For this is the final point: traditional herbal medicine was all there used to be for almost everyone. It had to find ways of coping with conditions that we would immediately refer for emergency medical treatment with drugs or surgery. If traditional herbal medicine is to adapt to modern health-care needs, it will only be by recognizing that some of its received principles were geared to the high ground of medical emergencies.

What are the Therapeutic Priorities for Treating Chronic Conditions?

Taking care

If the problem has been of such ferocity that it has penetrated the peripheral defences, or (as is now more likely) if the body's reserves have been weakened by many unresolved disturbances, repeated suppression of vital resistance, other accumulated stresses and fatigue, inadequate nutrition, or simple neglect, then the therapeutic measures outlined above will not be appropriate and *may even be counter-productive.*

With repeated or excessive assaults on its integrity the body begins to lose bounce: it becomes less and less able to mount a vigorous defence against disruptive influences (especially if this has been repeatedly suppressed). It becomes slow on its toes, punch-drunk. It falls back increasingly on to secondary and tertiary defences, like the phagocytes and the immune system; its internal regulatory machinery becomes more vulnerable to long-term imbalance; *chronic patterns of disturbance* and *diminished adaptability to stresses* are the most likely consequences.

Chronic diseases

These take myriad forms such as the following:

> a persistently oversecreting mucous membrane (as in chronic sinusitis or bronchitis);
>
> an excessive production of stomach acid (peptic ulcers);
>
> a progressive accumulation of auto-inflammatory or immunological assaults (arthritis, rheumatism, psoriasis, eczema, diabetes, thyroid disease, Crohn's disease, etc.);
>
> a capricious production of violently inflammatory agents within the body (migraines, Raynaud's disease, asthma);
>
> an unresolvable infection with 'slow' pathogens, especially viruses (herpes, chronic hepatitis, pelvic inflammatory disease,

post-viral syndrome, thyroid disease, Crohn's disease, etc.);

progressive pathological deteriorations of the tissues (arteriosclerosis, cirrhosis, fibroids);

a gross failure in the body's surveillance against malignant cells (cancer);

immunodeficiency (post-viral syndrome, Epstein-Barr infection, myalgic encephalomyelitis (ME), Candidiasis, Aids).

The list is almost beyond measure. All these conditions are extremely complex; in fact, almost all still remain largely impenetrable to medical science, and all involve the following:

more than one type of pathology at once;

to varying degrees, deep-seated disturbances of both tissue function and structure, *with an increasing tendency to structural damage as the condition deteriorates*;

a general lack of the sort of vital reaction described for acute conditions.

The modern epidemic?

There is a disturbing trend towards chronic illness in modern times. It is a matter rarely identified in discussions about health care. Most would in any case be too grateful not to have to cope with the epidemics of acute infectious diseases to worry about the implications. However, from the viewpoint of traditional medicine, the consequence of having squeezed out the opportunities to do vigorous battle with adversity is that the adversity will be more insidious: the body will find it harder to clear itself out; the illness will become long-standing, chronic.

Most herbal practitioners in developed countries now deal mainly with chronic disease. They will tend to see acute diseases mostly in children, in a very few still living a robust physical lifestyle, and in recent arrivals from developing countries! Yet even with children it may be too late: the first colds or sore throats or coughs might have already been treated with antibiotics or other quick-fixes and have become persistent catarrh, eczema, or recurrent infections instead.

A different herbalism

This trend towards chronic illness means that the modern herbalist has to practise a therapy quite different from that practised in the past. *It also means that it is inappropriate to use any system of herbal medicine that has not been adapted for modern needs.* The indications, applications and dosages used in Chinese herbal medicine, for example, recently popular in the West, are largely aimed at dealing with the mostly acute case-load of traditional life. Without readjustment, they may be inappropriate for a modern practice.

Fortunately, European traditional herbal medicine has had a century or more to adapt to the changing face of health care. The dosages of remedies, and even their applications, have shifted in that time. Above all, the principles of treatment have had to change.

In traditional terms, chronic conditions are a sign of reduced vitality. It is no good using heroic measures to nudge the system into correcting disturbances more efficiently if that system has shown it cannot rise to the challenge: this may actually harm it.

Before all else the treatment of chronic conditions must be *supportive* of the system. Remedies must first be used that are restorative, tonic or even nourishing. In terms of Cook's scenario (see Fig. 3, on p. 163), the direction of action of the remedies used in chronic disease must be evermore 'vertical', moving more in the direction of enhancement, rather than trying too ambitiously to move the system one way or the other. In terms of the five phases of the cycle, the emphasis should be on 'supporting the Earth', improving nourishment, assimilation, tone.

It is difficult to make this point too strongly. The modern herbalist dealing with a predominantly chronic case-load has to avoid heroic strategies and look to measures that are gentle and supportive instead. These will have the following implications:

> dosages will be smaller than in the past, even a quarter or less of the old quantities;
>
> treatment will take longer (a simple guideline might be that for every year of trouble, treatment might be expected to take a

month – it ought to be noted here that by the time arthritis, for example, has appeared there is likely to have already been five to fifteen years of insidious decline);

there will be considerably more emphasis on augmenting herbal treatment with changes in diet, and particularly with recommendations of rest and convalescence.

The modern reputation that herbal medicine has of being slow and gentle follows only from the problems it is now asked to treat. In the past a patient visiting a traditional herbalist with an acute disease would almost always experience unpleasantly drastic treatment with often very rapid effects. Nowadays it is only because practitioners are often being asked to make up for years of ill health that their prospects for real progress are gradual.

None of this is to say that herbal treatment for chronic conditions is likely to be uneventful. A good practitioner will pursue a strategy that will aim to provide plenty of evidence that work is being done: this might even include reducing the symptoms!

There is no set procedure for tackling these problems. Different practitioners will have different approaches and, in any case, the vast variations in disease will dictate a pragmatic and empirical attitude. There are, however, several general approaches that might be adopted. What they will be will also depend on the answer to another question, which should be tackled first.

How Strong are the Body's Reserves?

This is another clinical question that is not usually asked in a conventional consultation. Even in conditions that are manifestly fatigue syndromes, like myalgic encephalomyelitis (ME) or Epstein-Barr infection, the argument is much more about the virulence or even existence of a virus than about the obvious exhaustion. The state of patient vitality seems to count for little in a medical approach so obsessively preoccupied with germs and the finer mechanisms of pathology.

Stress

The most notable exception to this rule was the man who developed the stress thesis for disease causation. Hans Selye[13] saw the capacity of the body to handle stress as a finite entity, and as much more important than the actual stress itself. In developing the notion of 'General Adaptation Syndrome', he saw a *first stage*, the initial encounter with stresses (which could be physical as well as mental), as being stimulating to the system, as it rose to the challenge; then typically if any stress was prolonged, there would be a *second stage* of acclimatization to it by the body, during which time it would be barely noticed. This stage, however, would involve considerable expenditure of adaptive energies, notably in the function of the adrenal cortex, and, inevitably, at a point determined by many other factors, a *third stage*, one of exhaustion, would set in. Beyond this point *the same stressor* which originally stimulated, or was accommodated to, becomes progressively, and irreversibly, debilitating. The body's capacity to adapt is diminished, not just to that stressor, but in general.

Vital reserves

The implications of this scenario were not lost on Selye. His speculations about the nature of this capacity led him to describe it in terms very similar to the description of the energy of the *Kidneys*, especially *jing*, in Chinese medicine. Here were convergent theses of a finite vital capacity, something that tended to be strong in early life and weakened to varying degrees with age. In fact, Selye, like the Chinese, was drawn to conclude that ageing itself was a measure of the decrease in such capacity: those staying fit and active in old age being the most successful in preserving their adrenal-based adaptability.

In any explanation of illness as an interaction between pathogenic forces and the body's powers of self-recuperation some concept of vital capacity is needed. Selye's is almost certainly not all-embracing but it does provide a good modern model.

The immediate diagnostic question is how to assess the general state of the body's reserves. There are a number of criteria that are drawn from clinical practice and from a number of therapeutic traditions. A patient could be said to have depleted vital capacity if more than one of the following apply:

> there is undue and prolonged fatigue, listlessness and possibly muscle weakness, especially if combined with tension and irritability;
>
> there is a tendency for sleep to be broken in the early hours of the morning;
>
> there is night sweating (seen by the Chinese as the body losing control of its fluids when asleep!);
>
> there are chronically raised lymph glands;
>
> the digestive and assimilative functions are weak, with possibly vague, persistent nausea and abdominal discomforts, low appetite or escalating food intolerances;
>
> the pulse is weak, either deep and frail, or superficial and hollow;
>
> the tongue is smooth.

It is important to note that these are not the same signs as someone suffering a 'cold' problem. It is quite possible (and very confusing) for a person with weakened reserves to react to a condition with considerable 'heat'. Such reactions are usually particularly dangerous because, like a paper fire, the degree of activity may be in direct proportion to the lack of substance underlying it. The state of the reserves is always the most critical factor: thus the complexion can be ruddy, the tongue dark, the pulse superficial, the manner excited, but if these signs coexist with some of those above they should be re-evaluated.

Fatigue

There are several new syndromes that overwhelmingly manifest as exhaustion of the vital reserves. Their symptoms are astonishingly similar and encompass many of the above. The following list might also be offered, including many diagnoses that are not universally agreed:

> post-viral syndrome
> Epstein-Barr infection
> myalgic encephalomyelitis
> Candidiasis
> multiple food allergies
> reactive hypoglycaemia
> hyperventilation syndrome

One approach to such diagnoses-in-search-of-a-cause is to start out seeing them all as manifestations of severely depleted vital capacity and, in fact, of profound fatigue, with an overwhelming need for the restorative measures outlined below. Individual symptoms in any patient may then be handled secondarily. It is likely that any individual sufferer will have persistent slow viral infections, excessive *Candida albicans* in the bowel, food intolerances, volatile blood sugar, and diaphragmatic tension, *all at once*. In other words these 'diagnoses' are almost statements of the obvious, and their populist adherents are mistaking one facet for the whole syndrome.

Fortunately these extreme syndromes of debility are not the inevitable lot of those with diminished adaptive capacity. The assessment can be made for far less obvious conditions. It has very important implications for treatment.

What are the Strategic Options for Treating Chronic Disease?

The first point in deciding tactics is the one just made. *The more debilitated the patient, the less scope there is for active remedies, the greater the emphasis on restorative measures.*

ACTIVE STRATEGIES

Gentle provocation

For most cases of chronic disease there are no serious debilities to worry about and, at a milder level, it is possible to use similar tactics to those used for acute conditions. One can for example gently heat, or gently cool. In the first instance it is helpful to use remedies, the aromatic digestives, like angelica, cinnamon, fennel and ginger, that are also likely to help with one of the more pressing problems in long-term illness, poor assimilation and digestion. This is also a reason why, in choosing cooling remedies, one should opt for bitters as much as possible. Sedatives are increasingly contra-indicated the more debilitated the condition. (It is difficult to conceive of a strategy more likely to further depress than to use conventional antidepressants – actually sedatives – for treating depression.)

The more debilitated the patient the more likely heating or cooling remedies are to over-heat or over-cool, with further exhausting effects.

Gentle clearing out

The main task in the active aspect of a prescription for chronic disease is to resuscitate the eliminatory processes. It will be recalled that the traditional hypothesis for the conversion of an acute to a chronic condition is the failure of the body's eliminatory functions and that this failure is one of the telling features of chronic symptomatology. Thus the prime traditional strategy is to gently stir up a clear out.

Powerful eliminatives are ruled out. Instead mild aperients (often dietary) might be used to ensure the bowels move effectively; mild diuretics might help move fluid and acid-waste accumulations; gentle cholagogues (like dandelion and yellow dock (*Rumex crispus*)) can massage the liver into improving detoxification; and expectorants might be used to help clear congestions in the airways.

Diaphoretics are generally inappropriate, unless the body can be provoked into a healthy, even therapeutic, fever. This can be a powerful tactic in some cases. A lingering catarrhal or lymphatic infection can be cleared very quickly if there is still a febrile fight left in the system: in expert hands a passing cold can be whipped up, by short-term application of moderate or strong heating remedies, into a therapeutic fever. Provided this is managed well, with bedrest and diaphoretic remedies, it can achieve dramatic breakthroughs in an otherwise stubborn condition.

Other eliminative remedies are so gentle they do not have a dominant channel of elimination and are often particularly indicated for chronic disease. The so-called 'alteratives', 'blood cleansers', or 'depuratives', like cleavers (*Galium aparine*), nettle (*Urtica dioica*), red clover (*Trifolium repens*), burdock (*Arctium lappa*), sweet violet (*Viola odorata*) and fumitory (*Fumitoria officinalis*), seem to nudge eliminations into whatever channel is appropriate at the time. Each may variously increase bowel activity, diuresis, or tissue blood flow, or reduce lymphatic engorgement, depending on the circumstances.

Skin disease, catarrhal conditions, arthritis and persistent lymphatic infections are the obvious indications for eliminatives, but any chronic condition could profit. The aim, once again, is to go no faster than the body can stand. The axiom must be: if in doubt, back off!

Remote toxicity

Recent insights into the potential benefits of this traditional approach have been gained in relation to some notorious chronic inflammatory diseases. A persistent association between rheumatoid arthritis and a history of serious or chronic lung infections has been confirmed, and more recently there has been evidence of an immunological cross-reaction between several infective organisms, including *Proteus* and *Klebsiella* and the joint tissues involved in autoimmune attack in rheumatoid arthritis and ankylosing spondylitis (for long linked with previous urinary infections). In all such chronic inflammatory disorders the herbalist has through the ages instinctively looked for evidence of primary infection or toxicity elsewhere, anywhere, and has used the eliminatory remedies to help clear them up (see also 'Removal', on pp. 95–117).

So the practitioner is not tied to the present symptoms in looking to the task of removing a chronic impediment. The whole history and presentation is taken into account to see where the underlying weaknesses are and where the original intrusion began.

Cleansing options

The strategy may range from working backwards through the increments as through the layers of an onion to going directly to what appears to be the primary lesion (the most likely sites of entry are the digestive and respiratory tracts) and digging it out.

The latter may be rather more risky, especially in the debilitated, as it may dislodge more than was bargained for and new disturbances may appear. These may constitute a 'healing crisis' but probably less often than some might hope. In general the more delicate the constitution the more circumspectly one proceeds: gently ensuring the bowel is working efficiently before prescribing cholagogues and using mild diuretics before lymphatics, for example, or adding astringent and relaxant herbs to minimize disruption, may be other useful measures.

Symptom relief

As well as the primary task of resuscitating eliminatory activity there is a range of other jobs to be done. As already outlined these would be on similar lines to the treatment of acute conditions. However, there is a more pressing requirement from the patient: 'Please relieve my symptoms!'

There are many remedies with short-term symptomatic effects that might do this: ideally they should also be doing something more lasting as well, but this is not always possible and separate herbs may need to be included in the prescription for this.

Working with drugs

It is also not always possible to bring sufficient immediate symptom relief with herbs alone, especially with the small doses that have to be used. In practice most patients consulting herbal practitioners are already taking conventional medication for this purpose. This is sometimes essential for them. Much of the training of modern herbal practitioners in Britain (under the aegis of the National Institute of Medical Herbalists) is geared to informing them of medical realities, and enables them to judge what drugs are necessary and what may not be. They are also trained to keep their intentions open, and to keep the patient's doctor informed, either directly, or through the patient, about the treatment planned, if it is likely to encroach upon an existing regime.

In a world that is not ideal it remains the case that positive liaison is sometimes difficult, that practitioners may have to go ahead on their own. This is possibly the greatest source of disquiet among the medical establishment and it is to be hoped that collaboration will improve in the future to reduce risks of treatment conflict. It is certainly not a one-way street. There are times when a herbal practitioner with considerable training and practical experience can draw no other conclusion than that the patient's drug regime is either inappropriate, too long-standing or even downright dangerous; that an overworked doctor has at best not kept his eye on the ball, at worst is simply incompetent. The general practitioner, after all, has few with even a modicum of medical training to audit his or her performance: it is no wonder that those who have do occasionally discover howlers.

Whatever the situation the practitioner will proceed very carefully. It is possible to work around most conventional drug regimes: the aim of the herbal prescription is usually so radically different that the two treatments rarely clash. There are however cases where the effect and dose of the drug are so finely tuned that any extraneous pharmacological effect might be risky (antithrombosis drugs, insulin and heart stimulants are notable examples) and the options for concurrent herbal treatment are much more limited. Even in apparently the most redundant medication, the approach is one of gradual weaning off, reducing dosage only in steps, taking monitoring measurements where possible, always making sure everything is stable before proceeding, and prescribing such herbs as will help bridge the gap.

All this can make treatment for chronic conditions a tricky business. For those untrained in medicine the advice must be to restrict any active treatment except simple symptomatic relief to only the mildest and least risky solutions, and avoid life-threatening ones altogether. Fortunately at least 80 per cent of chronic disease is of the former type.

RESTORATIVE TREATMENTS

Few of the above cautions apply to the second category of treatment for chronic illness. Restorative measures can usually be applied by anyone for any condition. It may be the most important treatment of all, even if it is usually the slowest. However, before we look at the appropriate herbs for the job a wider look at restorative approaches is necessary.

Convalescence

This is a word almost lost from the medical dictionary. Yet in former times it was assumed that every illness took a lot out of the body and that rest and recovery were needed to put it back. The recuperation was an essential part of the treatment. The more serious the illness the longer the time necessary to recoup one's energies.

The discovery of new miracle drugs has obviously inclined doctors to the belief that they are curing the problem directly. The pace of modern life has conspired with this view: few people feel able to take a week off after the flu, or three months off after glandular fever.

The neglect of convalescence may yet prove to be one of the most serious mistakes of modern medicine. It is most probably one of the major contributors to the general increase of low-grade chronic illness. Herbal practitioners are most familiar with seeing how, when going back through a patient's history, the saga of ill health appears to have started with a substantial illness, obviously not adequately recovered from. Glandular fever (infectious mononucleosis) is the most common.

In many such cases, and especially in the most obvious, post-viral syndrome, the practitioner may well decide to take the patient back to the original illness and start convalescence all over again, reasoning that everything since has remained suspended at that point.

Even in other conditions, as we have seen, the state of debility reached demands that the restorative remedies used in convalescence be applied as the major therapy.

So let us consider the main principles of restoration, the principles of convalescence, applied either immediately after an acute disease or much later:

Rest

This is much the most important principle. At its most extreme, clinics that cater for convalescence will sometimes prescribe continuous sleep for many days, followed by bedrest for weeks. It is a sobering thought. While an intense daily rhythm is bearable, even stimulating, in reasonable health, it can quickly become unbearable for someone well into exhaustion. It can prove very difficult to correct a debilitated chronic condition while this rhythm is kept up. The patient should sometimes be presented with a stark choice: to carry on as before and face irreversible decline, or at the very least take sick leave, an annual holiday or a sabbatical to invest in a chance for recovery (not ruled out is a change of job). The point bears repeating: modern medicine has conspired to con us that rest and recovery are incidental – there are many times when they are mandatory.

Most often fortunately the rest component can be set less dramatically. It may be a question of helping the patient to achieve more or better sleep, or of him or her taking a few days out at the start of treatment.

It may even be something to insert into the active day. It is possible to approach work in at least two ways: by driving obsessively through each job in turn, or by keeping several tasks on the run at a time, moving back and forth between them. On the principle that a change is as good as a rest, this might be preferable both for reasons of health and for getting the work done better.

Exercise

This sounds like a contradiction to the preceding, but it isn't. A measure of physical activity is sometimes essential to clear constrained adrenal overactivity. Even in the most restful regime a daily element is usually prescribed. It helps prevent inner tensions disrupting rest and sleep.

In the more active, increased physical activity, up to but not beyond the body's limits, is often to be recommended in a restorative regime. A simple guide to maximum levels is the pulse test. Subtract your age from 220 and that is your absolute maximum safe pulse rate. A good pulse rate for (aerobic) exercise is between 60 and 80 per cent of that level. Exercising for 5 to 15 minutes at this level (it is self-correcting: a fit body takes more exercise to reach it than an unfit or debilitated one) can be a useful recommendation.

The very weak may be encouraged to take a gentle stroll (this may well take the pulse up to the above levels anyway); only in extreme cases should exercise be forbidden altogether.

Dietary change

The priority is to choose foods that will help the recuperative process and to avoid those that will hinder it.

Restorative foods: Without going into the extraordinary confusion of dietary advice one can safely draw up a list of foods that are most likely to have restorative effects. Individual recommendations will obviously vary, taking genuine intolerances into account, for example, but some of the wilder doubts and conflicts generated in the popular literature can be safely ignored. One can thus use the following foods as a foundation:

> root vegetables (e.g., carrots, parsnips, turnips, beetroot)
> cereals, notably oats (for the gluten-sensitive: rice)
> fish
> chicken (free-range: there is a difference!)
> potatoes
> natural yoghurt (preferably goat's or sheep's)
> eggs (free range)
> almonds

These will be elaborated later. Other foods can be added in moderation. In the summer a Mediterranean-style diet is often to be recommended: lots of good raw vegetables, seafood, olive oil, garlic, lemon juice, lean meat and rice. In winter a rustic fare of good stews with vegetables, potatoes and rice has its merits. Organically grown food is easier for the weary metabolism to handle. Supplementation with naturally extracted vitamins and minerals might be important here although its necessity otherwise is not always certain.

Eliminating foods: Almost always *not* to be recommended are sweets and other refined carbohydrates, a high additive intake (an unknown extra metabolic strain), rich fatty foods, caffeine and anything other than minimal alcohol (and this banned if the liver is involved). Smoking is a severe provocation but if attempts to give it up have to be too strenuous they may be more disruptive than it is worth.

Other foods will be eliminated for individual reasons. In many people debility manifests primarily as a sensitive digestion and getting them a diet they can tolerate may be the major achievement. Digestive herbal remedies will help (if they can be tolerated!).

Fasting has been used as a healing strategy in health clinics. It has its benefits, if conducted carefully and preferably under expert supervision, but it is not to be confused with restoration. Its role is cleaning the body out, perhaps prior to restorative regimes. Sometimes the extra vitality it appears to engender is of the short-lived, misleading variety.

Diet is important, but views need to be moderated. A stable, nutritious base is what is required here. Fads are not. To quote one of Britain's most perceptive physicians, Dr Peter Nixon, one not noted for conservative views, referring to the saturated-fat hysteria in relation to cardiovascular disease (*Sunday Times*, 17 Sept. 1989):

Proselytizing by the dietary evangelists, none of whom are practising cardiologists, has pre-empted understanding of the causes of heart attacks to a degree that has interfered with patient care.

I see patient after patient who need rest and sleep, and to learn how to handle themselves better in the uncertainties of today's world. They are exhausted to the point of despair, perhaps starting to get chest pain – and they have been told to diet!

Restorative remedies

The reason for placing these last is to emphasize that if serious recuperation is required the preceding measures are essential, whatever the herbs prescribed. It may be, of course, that the need for restoration falls short of the more drastic regimes, but even then an eye should be kept on the principles above.

A common feature of the most widely used herbs is that apart from any active effects they also have restorative properties. This is in line with the fundamental position of the physiomedicalists, outlined earlier. This restorative role is sometimes general, often limited to a particular area, but in each case the effect apparently complies with the simple definition of such a remedy: a restorative remedy is one which has health-enhancing effects that remain after treatment.

Good healthy food obviously complies with this definition, and it is with food that we must start this review. The dietary items listed earlier all have their own reputations as particularly nourishing, supportive or restorative in debilitated conditions. They would all earn the description 'sweet' in Chinese pharmacological terms.

Foods as tonics: A bowl of oatmeal is an excellent restorative breakfast (that also lowers blood cholesterol, stabilizes blood-sugar levels and is a gentle aperient); a herbal preparation of oatstraw (the whole oat plant, *Avena* spp.) is one of the surest restoratives in nervous debility, fatigue, 'neurasthenia', neuralgia, herpes, depression and similar complaints.

Carrots, beetroot and the like are sources of minerals and other nutrients most readily assimilated by a debilitated digestion. As raw juices they are effective cholagogues, diuretics and alteratives. Potatoes are a useful treatment for gastritis (especially raw!) as well as being an excellent food (surprisingly good-quality protein and considerable vitamin C).

Fish provides a most assimilable protein, but also fish oils which are an excellent resource for the cardiovascular system and tissue repair.

Eggs have an ideal balance of essential amino-acids as well as considerable lecithin to neutralize the cholesterol that so concerns people (no creature, herbivore, carnivore or fish, will turn down an egg if it finds one).

Chicken soup has been well attested to for centuries for its excellent nourishing properties and for its beneficial effects on respiratory disorders.

Yoghurt provides a naturally processed form of milk, easily

assimilated and with potential benefit for the bowel flora; its assimi-lability may be improved by avoiding the relatively undigestible protein of cow's milk.

In the Mediterranean countries almonds were thought to be food from the gods!

Tonic herbs: Apart from oatstraw, herbal remedies like vervain (*Verbena officinalis*), St John's wort (*Hypericum perforatum*), and saw palmetto (*Serenoa serrulata*) are useful general restoratives, with non-dynamic, food-like effects on the constitution. Most are covered in depth in Part II.

Other remedies have individual reputations for specific re-storative actions.

The oil of evening primrose (*Oenothera biennis* and spp.) provides a fatty acid metabolite, di-homo-γ-linolenic acid (GLA), normally produced from arachidonic acid in the body and important in prostaglandin metabolism: it is possible that some individuals oper-ate a deficit in GLA and it does seem that certain inflammatory and nervous conditions respond to this remedy, effectively a food supplement.

Hawthorn (*Crataegus* spp.) both gently dilates the coronary circu-lation and stabilizes heart muscle activity: it is sometimes referred to as a 'heart food'.

Ground ivy (*Nepeta hederacea*) seems to leave the respiratory mucosa in better shape after a range of respiratory problems.

Couch grass (*Agropyron repens*), corn silk (*Zea mays*) and barley (*Hordeum vulgare*) water surely soothe and ease many painful conditions of the urinary tract.

Meadowsweet (*Filipendula ulmaria*), Iceland moss (*Cetraria islan-dica*) and slippery elm (*Ulmus fulva*) will rebuild a battered stom-ach wall.

Helonias root (*Chamaelirium luteum*) and agnus castus (*Vitex agnus-castus*) have remarkable effects in stabilizing the menstrual cycle, an effect carried over after treatment.

Valerian (*Valeriana officinalis*) was used as a heal-all long before it was ever used as a tranquillizer.

Mullein flowers (*Verbascum thapsus*) have a broad balancing effect on pulmonary function.

Psyllium seed (*Plantago ovata*) and linseed (*Linum usitatissimum*) can genuinely help to re-educate a disturbed bowel function.

Liquorice (*Glycyrrhiza glabra*) is known to support adrenocortical functions, and has been used for its restorative effects on stomach wall and pulmonary tract.

These remedies would all have been classified as 'sweet' (or, in the case of the diuretics, 'bland') in Chinese pharmacology. They are slow in their supportive role, but the result of taking them is likely to considerably outlast the treatment: that is the mark of a true restorative.

The active restoratives: Other more active remedies have restorative properties as well. By definition, as we have seen, their use should be restricted in severely debilitated patients.

Thus bitters cool by increasing assimilation and nourishment at the digestive tract; one of them, dandelion, has a persistent reputation around the world as a tonic for liver function.

Some of the warming remedies are also administered for their restorative effects: angelica and elecampane (*Inula helenium*) for the stomach, garlic for the bowel, lungs and bloodstream, and echinacea for the body's defences.

An important contribution to this subject comes from Chinese medicine. There are many intriguing, often saponin-rich, general tonics, which have been carefully classified for the type of support they provide. Thus *yang* tonics and *qi* tonics – including ginseng (*Panax ginseng*) – are warming, *yin* tonics and *xue* tonics cooling. This also gives them contra-indications as well, a point that establishes these remedies as active as well as restorative. Again details of these and all other remedies above are provided in Part II.

In a Nutshell

It may now be possible to conclude Part I by drawing together the various stories so far, to distil from them something of the essential qualities of herbal remedies.

To summarize, there are four essential therapeutic approaches that characterize herbal treatment, in effect four choices available for the herbalist when faced with anything other than the most superficial ailment.

THE FOUR PILLARS OF TREATMENT

In referring back to Fig. 1, on p. 28, it is possible to insert herbal archetypes as influences on each process. An attempt is made in Fig. 9, on the next page. Most of the terms have been introduced in this part; the pharmacological terms are defined in more detail in the first section of Part II.

There are four processes which herbal remedies influence above all others:

Assimilation

The primary site of action of all herbal remedies consumed orally is the digestive tract. A majority of plant constituents with pharmacological activity act on the mucosal lining or sensory receptors of the gut wall, some (e.g. tannins, mucilages, resins) solely so. It is actually proposed in this text that a central mechanism for the effects of herbs on the body is through reflex response from stimulus at the gut wall. As the process of absorption and assimilation is also mediated primarily by the gut wall in the first instance it is not surprising that herbal remedies are widely credited with a range of effects in this area.

The action of constituents that interact with the mucosal membranes is to either:

> *reduce assimilation* by limiting absorption directly (as with the effect of tannins on food), or by increasing peristalsis (e.g. *laxatives*); or

> *increase assimilation* by reducing irritability and slowing peristalsis (e.g. the effects on this problem of *tannins*, *mucilages* and *carminative volatile oils*), or by increasing blood flow to the gut wall (e.g. *acrid principles*, *volatile oils* and *resins*).

Digestive tonics

Apart from such likely topical influences there are two major herbal strategies that are widely used to increase assimilative functions

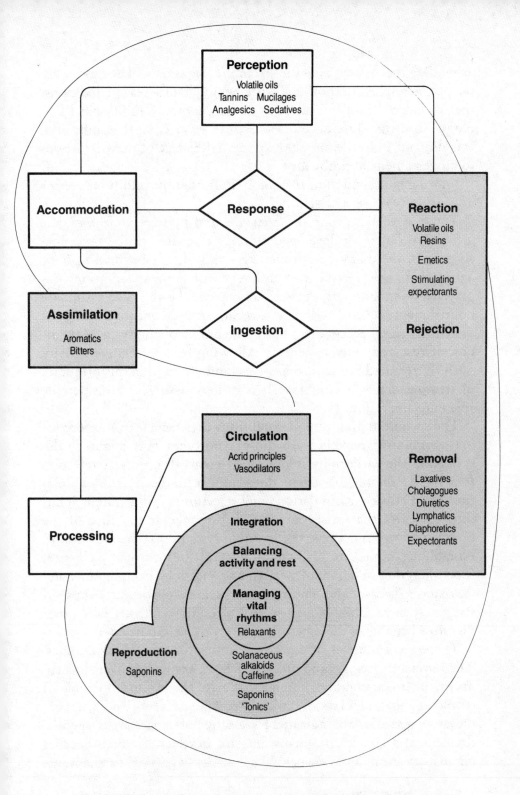

Fig. 9 Herbal influences on the essential living processes

generally: the *bitters* and the *aromatic digestives*. The first were seen to be applied to 'hot' (and specifically 'damp-heat') conditions, the second to 'cold' problems (see the chapter 'Traditional Pathology') and this difference does seem to have clinical significance. It is difficult to overestimate the potential benefit of these strategies to modern medical problems.

Improving assimilation is notably indicated, in traditional terms at least, in two areas of disorder.

The first is that group of *deficiency* and *fatigue syndromes*, the growing problem of developed cultures discussed in the preceding section. In the many case-conferences this author has had in New York where the treatment of sufferers with fatigue conditions has played a dominant part, the need to improve the ability to assimilate nourishment has cropped up as a recurrent prerequisite to progress (given the prior acceptance, but often impracticability in Manhattan, of rest and convalescence!). Allowing for the relative activity of the bitters and aromatic digestives (and the caution this presumes in treating deficient conditions), they may assume a considerable role in recuperation.

The second main group of conditions that benefit from prescribing assimilative remedies are those syndromes that might be described in the earlier physiological review as disorders of rejection (see Fig. 1, on p. 28). There does appear to be a see-saw relationship between assimilation and rejection as illustrated. Thus those diseases that arise out of a disturbance at the core of the body's resistive functions, the *immune system*, may be indications. Notable examples are allergies in general (but especially classical food allergies), inflammatory vascular conditions like migraine and Raynaud's disease, and autoimmune diseases (particularly those of the gut such as Crohn's disease and ulcerative colitis, where other digestive benefits of these herbs are likely to be important).

There are a number of other indications for the digestive tonics. The bitters are, as is elaborated elsewhere, applied to liver disturbances and toxic conditions judged to arise therefrom, to problems of blood-sugar regulation, and to managing fevers. The aromatic digestive remedies are indicated for a range of congestive dyspeptic, flatulent and colicky problems and are incidentally often used as circulatory stimulants (see below) as well as 'warming' expectorants

226   Therapeutics

for congestive respiratory conditions. Both types of remedy are of course applicable to disabling lack of appetite.

Explanations for what might otherwise be seen as a grandiose list of indications are developed throughout this book.

Circulation

Reference has been made at length in this book to the universal preoccupation among herbalists with the heating of the body as a defence against disease (see 'The early view', on pp. 92–4, 'Thomson and the four elements', on pp. 154–8, and especially 'The Temperaments of Plant Remedies', on pp. 174–83).

The strategy will not therefore need rehearsing, but it is sufficient to emphasize that in spite of not having to tackle the illnesses of their forebears modern herbalists find that the application of *circulatory stimulants*, *peripheral vasodilators* and the *aromatic digestives* (see above) remains a vital part in their range of treatments. This is particularly so where the syndrome can be classed as 'cold' under the terms set out in the chapter 'Traditional Pathology', notably congestive catarrhal problems, oedematous conditions and where circulation is obviously deficient.

It can be said that one of the first decisions in traditional herbal medicine was to assess the temperament of the patient in his or her illness. If 'hot', cooling herbs, especially the bitters, were prescribed, if 'cold', these circulatory remedies were the first choice. Such a choice is still likely today, allowing for the complications of modern syndromes outlined earlier.

Elimination

Under this category come the three linked processes in Fig. 9 (see p. 225) starting with 're': reaction, rejection and removal. Again the principles of the herbal view of elimination have been discussed in detail (see 'Reaction', on pp. 42–3, 'Rejection', on pp. 53–73, 'Removal', on pp. 95–117, and the discussion of therapeutics earlier).

The robust attitude to 'toxicity' held in the past, the frequent use of emetics and purgatives, and the ignorance about infective organisms have occasioned some mirth in modern times, along with a frequent feeling that this was a chapter in human history best forgotten. Yet as this text hopefully clarifies, there are new applications for such approaches that deserve to be taken seriously.

It certainly seems that herbal remedies have qualities that lend themselves to the treatment of problems of chronic inflammation in a very different way from that of conventional medicines. It is still the case that the modern herbalist will look far beyond the immediate symptoms for signs of congestion, failure of detoxification or elimination, or undue toxic intrusion, and apply remedies appropriately.

The herbalist's high reputation for the treatment of chronic skin disease, arthritis, inflammatory bowel disease and other such recalcitrant conditions almost certainly derives from such strategies.

Integration

The use of tonics, adaptogens and restoratives, discussed as a measure in the treatment of chronic disease above, and also under the heading 'Integration' in the chapter 'Physiology' see pp. 126–9, is the fourth uniquely herbal strategy for modern clinical conditions.

Again it is true that the traditional need for such remedies was different from that of the modern practitioner. It is probable that most modern herbal prescriptions contain a significant 'tonic' element, whereas in ancient times such remedies were clearly an afterthought, applied mainly when the patient had reached old age and in cases of extreme infirmity.

Part II
BRANCHES

5 Research

How Do We Know Whether Herbs Work?

Who asks the question?

In the later pages of this section some attention is given to the activity of medicinal plants and their chemical constituents. References are cited for a considerable amount of research work into the pharmacology of medicinal plants, reported particularly in European scientific journals. Much of this is of a high academic calibre and does much to reassure that there are in herbal remedies many constituents with real effect on the body.

It will also be clear that what is lacking is any substantial scientific research into the effect of the whole herb on the human being. If it is accepted that the plant is a vast complex of pharmacologically active chemicals, then it will be obvious *that the whole package will have different properties from that of any single constituent acting alone.* Knowing the action of the latter will not itself be predictive of the effect of the former, particularly if the experimental evidence is based on work done on laboratory animals. If proponents of herbal medicine make such claims, it is fair to ask why they have provided so little evidence of genuine clinical effects.

The obvious point to make, of course, is that a great many people have already found herbal medicines effective,* and all those using them will have strong anecdotal evidence of their apparent benefits. Compared with the experience of most modern drugs, the human use and approval of most herbal remedies is awesome. The

---

*In one survey of 2,000 people in Britain, 12 per cent of those asked had claimed to have used herbal remedies, more than any other alternative medicine, and of these almost three-quarters expressed satisfaction with that experience ('Herbs are patients' favourites', poll by RSGB reported in *Journal of Alternative Medicine*, July 1984).

requirement by the medical and scientific establishment for research to 'prove' that herbs are effective is not found among the population at large. It is almost certain that the recourse to herbal remedies as a popular option will outlive the current era of inquiry.

Nevertheless, a challenge has been thrown down: 'If what you say is so valuable and powerful, then it should be able to stand up for itself in any forum.'

It is quite possible, of course, that the herbal lobby might question the validity of the forum, might comply with it only as far as necessary ('render therefore to Caesar the things that are Caesar's'), or might even call down a plague upon its head, but it should at least have the strength to face the debate on its own terms.

It is in this spirit that the following review of the prospects for research into herbal remedies is offered.

The difficulty of questioning

The simplest point to make in introducing a review of herbal science is that those practising herbal medicine have not usually understood the requirements for research. Sir Peter Medawar's exhortation to young scientists – 'You must feel in yourself an exploratory impulse – an acute discomfort at incomprehension'[1] – emphasizes the unusual qualities demanded of those who would submit observations to the rigours of scientific inquiry. It is apparent that by contrast most ordinary mortals are, to use Sir Karl Popper's image, happy to accept that swans are white because all swans which they have seen are white. It was after all unnecessary for a long time to question the obvious impression that the sun rotates around the earth provided that its movements were charted as well as possible.

The development of medical practice has generally been marked by a disinclination to subject acquired truths to the rigours of independent assessment. In medical history, periods of innovation and challenge have been occasional and brief, marking periods of cultural ebullience, such as the Ch'in and Han dynasties in China,[2] the era of Hippocrates, Dioscorides and Galen, and its renaissance in Islam in the ninth and tenth centuries. By contrast there have been overwhelmingly long periods of apparently quiet acquiescence to orthodoxies formed often centuries, or even millennia, before. The modern era is unusual in the extraordinary level of research activity which has followed the marriage of medicine with rationalist science and technology.

The community of those who practise herbal medicine has been no exception to this general rule. Only recently, for example, have practitioners in Britain become sufficiently organized to generate the impetus for stringent research from within their own circle.†
Knowledge within traditional medicine has generally been in the form of received wisdom moulded to the individual needs and prowess of each practitioner. Such means of acquiring healing skills seem temperamentally suited to most practitioners, herbal and conventional, even today. Their interest in inquiry for its own sake, with secure truths up for constant possible refutation, is understandably secondary to their concern to survive in practice.

Fortunately some practitioners in the modern era are increasingly realizing that an attitude of inquiry is an advantage in improving the performance of their therapy. At its heart research is a process by which it is possible to select, sort and clarify the information available about a healing technique, to answer the fundamental question: 'Is this treatment likely to make the patient well or not?' As C. R. Rogers put it, 'Scientific methodology needs to be seen for what it truly is: a way of preventing me from deceiving myself in regard to my creatively formed subjective hunches, which have developed out of the relationship between me and my material.'³

There are, however, practical problems in pursuing good clinical research. The first is that to produce results carrying sufficient statistical weight is very expensive and laborious. Herbal medicine in the West can boast no teaching hospitals or research institutes, nor funding by a wealthy industrial sector. The necessary infrastructure is lacking.

The second practical point is that there is considerable doubt about the applicability of the conventional technological/engineering model of scientific pursuit and analysis to the healing event in general and to herbal practice in particular. To the extent that

†Notable is the activity at the School of Herbal Medicine (Phytotherapy) near Hailsham, and at the Centre for Complementary Health Studies, University of Exeter.

healing involves an element of purely human contact – the healer stepping outside his or her own position and into the life of the patient – it is not an event assayable by independent observers or cold analysis, nor predicated by the general conclusions which one might be tempted to draw from such an exercise. Current medical research generally concerns itself only with measuring events and data divorced from the human being, ignoring the latter's immensely powerful forces for change and development in defiance of the clearest signs to the contrary.

How do you measure an experience?

These are problems generally aired in regard to medicine elsewhere, but it may be possible to illustrate the problem with specific examples from the world of herbal medicine. One might start with a question originally put by Molière and rehearsed by Bateson concerning a substance no longer used by medical herbalists in the West, but which is relatively well understood by many: 'State the "cause and reason" why opium puts people to sleep.'[4] One of Bateson's students replied triumphantly that it was because opium contained a sleep-inducing principle! The qualities of this substance have been very well investigated by medical science. For over a century the active constituents of the white poppy (*Papaver somniferum*) have been known, as well as something of their effects on the body. It is well known that morphine is both analgesic, depressive and euphoric, as well as tolerogenic and addictive, that it depresses the respiratory, vasomotor, coughing and vomiting centres in the brain stem, as well as ACTH and gonadotrophin secretions, yet stimulates the chemoreceptor centre and ADH production; that codeine has similar but lesser effects; that thebaine produces seizures in low doses; that papaverine potentiates morphine but also relaxes smooth muscle; and that noscapine suppresses the cough reflex. There is also a lot of intriguing information about interaction with opiate receptors in the nervous system.

In spite of this information, however, we still understand most of the actual effects of opium itself from the personal testimony of Albrecht von Haller, Thomas de Quincey and others, as well as the diverse medical and social literature of anecdotal accounts of those observing in reality the complex effects of opium consumption and withdrawal.

To take an example more relevant to the modern medical herbalist: in the case of feverfew (*Tanacetum parthenium*), the British herbal profession was faced with a sudden media-induced public demand for an apparently effective migraine remedy without much personal experience of its use. In a short time an appreciable amount of research work was done in conventional medical and scientific settings on the pharmacological characteristics of the plant, including clinical trials.[5] In spite of this work the therapeutic character of the remedy has remained elusive for any practitioner not simply prescribing symptomatically for migraine or whatever, and trying to assess the most advantageous circumstances in which to use feverfew for any particular patient. Good clinical experience with case histories is still required (some clues are perhaps to be seen in its essentially vasodilatory (warming) effect: most migraines are accompanied by vasoconstriction of blood vessels, a significant minority are not; sufferers of the former often obtain relief by applying hot packs to the head and are probably more suited to feverfew than those of the latter).

The public good

Although real insights into the characteristics of remedies come from practical clinical experience, there is a need to reassure the public and legislature that herbal remedies are at least safe, and preferably effective. In Britain this has been a concern pursued by the herbal industry and profession in discussion with Government under the terms of the Medicines Act 1968. It happens that for treatment of minor self-limiting disorders remedies have been allowed to be sold directly to the public on the basis of bibliographic evidence of traditional usage alone, and the authorities have not significantly encroached upon the right of the herbal practitioner to use whatever remedies he or she considers appropriate (unlike growing budgetary encroachments on such clinical discretion among family doctors). Nevertheless, the licence to market herbs as medicines for what are considered moderate to severe conditions is dependent on providing conventional clinical evidence for such a claim. The double-blind clinical trials and experiments on animals, to name two areas of contention in research, will remain essential as evidence as long as legislative and medical authorities consider them so.

This causes herbal practitioners real concern. Apart from the cost of mounting effective clinical trials it is galling to know that the legal future of a remedy is more likely to rest on the results of its intraperitoneal injection into rats than on the testimony of patients and practitioners. Although there are signs that the patients' assessment may be increasingly used in calculating efficacy in clinical research, it is most likely that the great weight of scientific and medical opinion will insist on playing by the same rules as before. Put simply, if herbs are to have a place in the modern system they will have to establish it on that system's terms.

There is, of course, a role for conventional clinical trials in assessing herbal remedies. The double-blind random-selection methodology is a very powerful weapon indeed. In brief, a number of patients with the same condition is arbitrarily divided into two or more groups. One group will receive the treatment being tested, the other(s) will get either another known treatment or a placebo, in other words an inactive material. No one will know who is receiving what, neither subjects nor researchers: the test is thus 'double-blind'. (A code is usually held by a third person not party to the trial; this is broken only when all the results are in.)

This sort of research gives unparalleled evidence for the efficacy of a remedy for a named and classified disorder for the population as a whole. It is moreover more flexible in its application than many of its opponents imagine. Nevertheless, it is limited in two substantial ways: its assumes homogeneity in both the pathology it is targeting and above all in the subjects who are being treated. Knowing that a remedy has a statistically significant effect on a defined problem does not help decide when to prescribe it in any individual case.

Towards a Herbal Research Policy

Back to the human being

There are three main responses that those using herbs could adopt to the questions so far raised. Firstly they could retreat from the skirmish altogether, relying on the strength of the bedrock of herbal use through history and around the world to outlast any such modern officiousness. Undoubtedly many, without the inclination for the task, will follow that path. History may yet prove that the most sensible choice!

On the other hand it is possible to muddle along, rendering to Caesar the techniques and the evidence that are Caesar's where possible, and relying on popular support for the rest. Or, finally, attempts could be made to develop coherent and consistent new models of research which better reflect and illuminate therapeutic realities, but also have the authority to convince the public's guardians of their validity.

There have been fortunately some considerable efforts in constructing appropriate methodologies of sufficient weight.[6] These generally rely on improving the monitoring of individual case histories rather than on comparing treatment and control groups.

Where n = 1

The main charge against single-case studies is that they cannot credibly select real effects from confusing variables, treatment effects from placebo effects and so on. The following scenario for such research, however, shows both that it can have more credibility than might be supposed, and that it is not a soft option.

The criteria for validity of such trials have been well reviewed by Peter Reason and John Rowan:[7] they are challenging, even daunting. They include ensuring that the perceptive faculties of the researchers are constantly and clearly sharpened, providing as many points of view as possible, clarifying these perspectives, and recycling observed data around the researchers for checking and possible refutation. At stake is the need to ensure that, while denying the possibility of a truly objective view, we do not confine ourselves to the subjective, aiming instead to create a perspective which transcends the two.

Each observer makes a unique map of any territory, and all such maps are selective, idiosyncratic views of a phenomenon that cannot be reduced. To the extent, however, that maps are necessary for the exchange of information, the more that observers can submit their own maps for re-evaluation by others, the more likely it is that a real consensus, a common map, will emerge, and the more likely it is also that outsiders will understand the territory portrayed.

Such a research design would draw data about a particular treatment from:

> the *patient*, acting as co-researcher and with a uniquely intimate, though of course slanted, view of the internal landscape;
>
> the *practitioner*, with sufficient competence and clinical experience to provide both an informed and empathetic account of the encounter;
>
> a third person acting as *co-ordinator* and *observer*.

The account of each participant would be assembled individually, and then brought back for a case-conference editorial discussion at a later date to cross-check and combine so as to produce a final report of the treatment. Each such report can be examined by the co-ordinating researcher or assistant, applying a form of inquiry similar to that proposed by Diesing in the social sciences.[8] In other words, *themes* of disturbance and incapacity are elicited, then used to construct the working *case history*, both steps being subjected to re-evaluation by all co-researchers. As each case is thus graphically characterized, it can be used for comparative purposes with other cases to see whether a *pattern* occurs and can be sustained.

Truth emerges from such an exercise as a consensus, with individual judgement constantly subjected and re-subjected to scrutiny by others. Inherent validity is, of course, no greater than when a number of people agree among themselves that 'all swans are white', but it can still be argued that this is a fair basis on which to base practical predictions and applications (it would be considered very sound intelligence in the business world). It has the advantage that all conclusions are based on real experiences and can have a more thorough and meaningful clinical application.

Such an exercise would be best conducted in the environment of a training clinic, where there is likely to be a more overt climate of inquiry and debate, and extra administrative labour. It could allow for a useful database of reliable case histories to be assembled over the years, as both an educational and a research exercise.

Another way to explore the action of a herbal remedy that is sympathetic to its claimed activity is to apply a different form of measurement of pharmacological effect, a different clinical pharmacology.

The measurement of transient clinical effects

Herbs have traditionally been applied in a qualitatively different way from conventional drugs. Whereas the latter are primarily designed to directly affect a specific disability without regard for the context in which that disability occurs, herbal remedies have been directed to supporting the individual's recuperative capacities, where the chief complaint is seen as only one feature in a wider and unique pattern of disturbance. The character of the remedy reflects this broader, interactive and often supportive action. Its apparent clinical effect is not entirely measured by purely analytical investigative method, whether that be chemical fractionation or clinical trial conducted on groups of patients rendered homogeneous by random assortment and by reference entirely to isolated symptoms.

The herbal practitioner insists on the uniqueness of the individual patient, and on the right to provide a unique mixture of remedies in each case. Apart from this objection to taking part in randomized blind trials, there is the impression that herbs to a significant degree are interactive with the patient, i.e. their actual effect varies with the nature of the disturbance treated. This impression is consistent with the view that many herbal remedies act to encourage self-correcting processes. Other traditional views of herbal remedies emphasize their primary influence on transient body functions: they may be classed as diaphoretics, expectorants, circulatory stimulants, diuretics, digestive stimulants, laxatives and so on (see the chapter 'Remedies'). In other words, contrary to common belief, *most herbs can have almost immediate effects on the body.*

The requirement is to devise a process by which such an approach can be verified. Clearly conventional models for testing drugs are insufficient. Rather than aiming for conclusions about isolated pharmacological actions divorced from individual variation it is necessary here to chart changes within individuals, using such parameters as are relevant, useful and non-invasive.

Emphasis shifts too from the isolated observation to the simultaneous recording of several parameters of change. Synchronous events mutually influence each other: they are thus all equally related to each other and to the 'effect' that is observed from their operation. It is precisely this interdependence, this inductive relationship, that leads to their exclusion in conventional trials as distracting variables. Acceptance of these variables as important data is a key feature of such work and must therefore profoundly change the nature of the information gathered.

Instead of trying to eliminate all variables that might cloud the specific issue in question ('Is it drug A that reduces inflammation in this organ or other factors?', for example), the aim of the 'functional assay', as it might be called,‡ is ideally to define all factors which determine the medicinal substance's influence on the course of disease ('What, in fact, is drug A actually likely to do in this individual?'). The task would in some ways resemble the homoeopathic 'proving', in other ways take advantage of modern computerized and multi-level diagnostic techniques known as 'metabolic profiles'. Such information will for example be better suited to systems, rather than causal analysis, and any conclusions drawn from it will be qualitative rather than quantitative: relationships

‡After Professor Porkert; in an unpublished text ('The contribution of Chinese medical theory towards positive methods in the assay of drugs and therapies' (1983)) he has argued convincingly for the 'functional assay' in the assessment of traditional therapies like herbal medicine, developing particularly the view that pathological disease represents an accumulation of functional disorders over time, and that a more accurate assay of the effects of treatment should be in terms of immediate changes in function.

are induced rather than causes analysed. The process will, not unfittingly, more resemble anthropological than conventional medical research. It could of course augment the collation of exhaustive case histories as described above.

The demonstration of transient effects will not in itself lead to predictable changes in pathologies, representing as these do the somatic accumulation of previous functional disorders. However, many clinical presentations are wholly functional (e.g. acute inflammations, asthma, migraine, digestive disorders, and the whole range of psychosomatic disorders) and it should be possible to draw useful implications from functional responses for the treatment of even the strictly pathological.

Thus it might be more valid to say that a herb, in certain individuals at least, changed the constitution of phlegm, of urine, or altered circulatory activity to one or other tissues or over the body as a whole, for example, rather than that it is statistically likely to be effective against bronchitis, urinary stones or other disease state.

Pharmacological and pharmacokinetic research

Something of the present state of knowledge about the action of plant constituents is reviewed in the section following this, and it may be apparent that these raise specific questions. The following might be investigated:

> In what ways are plant constituents likely to interact to affect bioavailability and action (obvious interactions are between tannins/alkaloids/saponins/minerals/complex carbohydrates)?

> To what extent are activities of plant constituents localized to the digestive tract, given that many of them are not absorbed into the body fluids; what physiological/pharmacological models are there to explain referred or systemic responses to gut wall stimulation?

> Is it possible to apply other new physiological models to improve the understanding of the effects of plant constituents (possible leads are cell-receptor function, neuropeptides and other transmitter agents, local controls of circulation and the inflammatory response, prostaglandins and lipid metabolism)?

What is known of hepatic action on plant constituents such as would help clarify the results of the 'first-pass effect' and enterohepatic recycling?

Following from the above is it possible to assess what plant-derived constituents are likely to reach the systemic circulation (an answer to this question is an essential requisite for meaningful tissue culture experiments)?

Is it possible to assess broadly to what extent plant variability affects median pharmacological and pharmacokinetic activity?

How do changes in pharmaceutical preparation affect the bioavailability of constituents? For example, do alcoholic tinctures and fluid extracts have significantly different actions from the aqueous extracts generally predominant in traditional practice?

Experimental research

Apart from clinical trials already discussed, the question of research models for studying the action of herbal remedies is the most difficult. Ethical considerations inhibit the use of some options, impracticality others. The following presents some of the alternatives:

Cell, tissue and organ cultures
As part of the modern move to find alternatives to animal experimentation, increasing attention is being paid to techniques for assessing the effects of drugs on cultures of cells, tissues and organs *in vitro*. Conventional drug research is switching to this direction for preliminary screening in drug discovery programmes, and there is a lesser move for at least initial toxicological testing.

The advantages are in the opportunity for the direct observation of the action of an agent on target cells with some reduced ethical difficulties (although the sacrifice of animals is often necessary to supply short-lived organ and tissue samples).

The problems are the limited application of such observations to the *in vivo* situation and the need to confirm any *in vitro* findings anyway; from the point of view of herbal research there is the additional problem that it is impossible at this stage to reproduce the balance of plant constituents that will actually reach internal tissues (after digestion, absorption and the 'first-pass' hepatic effect). Difficulties are increased by the desirability of using tissues most closely mimicking the real situation, i.e. mammalian organ cultures (rather than the easier-to-culture amphibian tissues, or the less sophisticated cell lines).

Nevertheless, *in vitro* techniques could provide valuable supplementary information to other research, as in the following suggested projects:

> The influence of herbal extracts on epithelial tissue cultures (e.g. gastric, enteric and tracheal tissues; unfortunately the former two decline rapidly in culture); this represents a point of genuine tissue interaction with herbal remedies and might add much to pharmacokinetic research.

> Observations on the biotransformation of plant constituents using liver cultures (again short-lived, and a technically difficult operation, but one that is well established in conventional pharmacological research).

> Alteration in the migratory behaviour and internal metabolism of macrophages as a result of exposure to herbal extracts (much is made in herbal explanations of claims to improve resistance to infections by a general enhancement of defensive mechanisms; looking directly at macrophage response is an established screening technique).

> The influence of herbal preparations on microbiological cultures (direct antiseptic action for some plant constituents has been established, notably by Dr Belaiche in France, but there are still many questions remaining unanswered).

> Non-specific observations (as in gerontological research) on cell migrations, length of interphase, longevity and other pointers to *in vitro* cell health.

It would also be worth considering conventional screening techniques for the assessment of individual plant constituents, to be applied particularly where a remedy needs closer examination (say for legislative purposes). The wider application of such findings would be limited, but they might provide useful peripheral information.

Animal experiments

There can be no doubt about the problems of using animals to support research into herbal remedies. Apart from the difficulty of applying findings to the human situation, there are extremely strong ethical objections from almost all those who support the use of herbal medicines, at least in Britain.

Nevertheless, the subject cannot be dismissed entirely. In the first place, much phytotherapeutic research in Europe involves animal experimentation and the findings have entered everyday debate about the action of herbal remedies. Secondly, it is quite possible to devise trials that involve no pain or discomfort to the animals involved, as is the obvious practice in gerontological research (animals live longest when well treated). It is recalled that herbal therapy aims to support vital functions (in China the worth of any therapeutic practice is determined by how successfully its use appears to encourage a long and healthy life!). If the intention of any trial was to assess the effects of herbal medication applied in approximately therapeutic doses adjusted for body weight and metabolism, there could be little complaint that the animals would be harmed, and they would in fact be likely to actually benefit. Advice is that the Home Office in Britain, responsible for issuing licences for such research, would consider such trials as indistinguishable from keeping animals as pets, and no licence need be obtained.

Feasible trials might include observing behavioural and social changes after administering 'relaxants' and 'nerve tonics', monitoring the effects of posited 'adaptogens' on life expectancy, stamina and reproductive capacity, and the effects of antimicrobial remedies on normal resistance to disease among large populations, and observing changes in digestive and urinary performance (as judged by changes in excretion, appetite and weight). As the common laboratory animal with a metabolism closest to the human being the humble rat would probably be the creature of choice.

It might also be valuable to have the results of careful observations of the use of herbs in veterinary practice, where many of the limitations attending patient-practitioner interaction can be minimized.

Nevertheless, the net contribution of such trials to a useful understanding of the effects of herbal remedies on human beings is not sufficient to justify the risk of offending strong sensibilities on this issue.

Conclusion

At the time of writing the foregoing methodologies are largely suggestions for further work that might appropriately test many of the claims made by those using herbal medicines. Only a handful have actually been translated into action. As the momentum in developed societies for using herbal remedies grows apace, it is inevitable that the scientific spotlight will be cast ever brighter on this subject. Most of the scrutiny, in fact, will be inspired by those whose role it is to act as medical advisers to Government.

It is the experience of those who have debated the subject on the national scene that politicians, like most of the public, have a relatively detached view about both scientific arguments in general, and the demands for research proof in particular. As long as public safety is seen to be protected, then the public guardian will be seen to have discharged his duty.

The drive for evidence comes principally from those who see themselves as the medical guardians of the public good, the large lobby of advisers who help a politician declaim in this area. At best they may see themselves as facing, in herbal medicine, both a fiendishly complex and dubious and antiquated form of medicine full of hidden perils for the unsuspecting public; at worst they are simply protecting an established, wealthy and powerful medical interest. The experience of such counsel is that it can be uniquely harsh in its requirements for evidence.§

If such scrutiny is to grow, then herbal medicine will need to develop a research manifesto similar to the one outlined above, or else retreat to the hills and the marshes, and wait for another day.

§ In 1986 the British Medical Association (BMA) produced a report (*Alternative Therapy*, Report of the Board of Science and Education) on 'alternative medicine', after an inquiry that heard almost no expert witnesses, allowed no cross-examination and was subject to no informed peer review. Not surprisingly its findings were largely inaccurate and its conclusions were hostile. Fortunately it was widely dismissed as biased by the media and public.

Are Herbs Safe?

Safety in numbers

It is a conventional medical assumption that any medicine that is effective must also be a risk, that it is impossible to have effects without side-effects. The living body is so complex, so intricately interwoven, that any intervention at one site is likely to spark off reactions at other sites, either because of functional or structural connection or because of some similarity in sensitivity. The common response of the medical establishment to claims that herbs are free from side-effects is that they cannot then be effective at all.

Yet it is a persistent popular belief that herbs are safe. Possibly the main reason why patients first turn to herbs, apart from desperation at their prospects after conventional treatment, is that they see them as free from side-effects, 'not like those drugs'. Many who write about or advocate the use of herbal remedies often emphasize the same point. They refer to the uninterrupted use of the most established remedies by millions of consumers over many centuries or even since prehistory. This vast experience must surely have ironed out the wrinkles: if the remedies were not safe, they would surely have been exposed as such at some time in history. Even today the major herb formulations available in health-food shops sell in millions of units per year. This must provide an unparalleled screening for safety.

Are they right? If they are, how can claims for efficacy be squared with the absence of toxicity?

Poisonous plants

The first point to make, of course, is that not all plants are safe. In a publication for the Ministry of Agriculture, Fisheries and Food,

M. R. Cooper and A. W. Johnson review the published literature on the toxicology of plants growing in Britain.[9] Adverse effects after their consumption by animals or humans are reported for a high proportion of Britain's natural flora. Nevertheless, most reports concern damage to livestock after undue or excessive grazing, and clear harm done to humans is seldom reported. In very few cases are plants seen to be poisonous in low doses. The authors conclude that while many plants in Britain are known to be poisonous, few are dangerously so, and cases of severe poisoning in animals or humans are relatively rare.[10] They go on to point out, however, that the full effects of toxic constituents of plants are difficult to assess and leave open the interpretation that many plants, including ordinary foodstuffs, might have low-level toxicity that would be very difficult to isolate.

Thus it is that plants should not be considered absolutely safe: if we are honest we must say that the whole definition of toxicity is unclear. In frankly assessing the risks of consuming herbal remedies at normal therapeutic dosages we have to make a balanced judgement from all known factors.

Poisonous food

To consider the toxicity of plants for humans those that humans frequently eat must be examined first. Many ordinary foods contain theoretically poisonous constituents, not as artificial or natural contaminants, but as part of their chemical make-up. This is incidentally quite separate from such known narcotics as tobacco, alcohol and tea and coffee.

A review of natural toxins in foods – as, for example, in the list below – might surprise some readers (the chapter 'Traditional Pharmacology' elaborates on many of these factors).

> Wheat, rye, barley and oats contain a protein gluten that is hydrolysed in the digestive system to yield a peptide α-gliadin, a well-established and occasionally dangerous intestinal irritant.

> Lettuce contains in its sap a latex product, lactupicrin, that has many of the sedative and toxic properties of opium alkaloids.

Apple seeds, and the kernels of apricots, plums and other stone fruits, as well as bitter almonds, contain significant quantities of cyanogenic glycosides that yield cyanide on hydrolysis, a process that also occurs in the digestive system.

The cabbage family, which also includes mustard and horseradish, contains glucosilinates that yield goitre-causing thiocyanates and toxic nitriles.

Potatoes are members of the deadly nightshade family: when the tuber turns green under the influence of light it produces the same poisonous alkaloids.

Many common household pulses, like soya bean, red kidney bean and haricot bean (as in baked beans), contain various toxins, notably lectins called phytohaemagglutinins as well as trypsin-inhibitors, that can only reliably be neutralized by boiling for at least 30 minutes.

The oil from rapeseed, widely grown in temperate climates as a cheap vegetable oil, contains erucic acid, which is known to cause heart damage in experimental animals.

The point of this list is not to alarm the public about the hidden dangers of eating. Of course, under almost all circumstances the foods listed above are completely safe to eat. The real point is to show how difficult it is to predict the toxicity of a plant only from the presence of toxic constituents. As with other pharmacological questions, the action of the whole plant, and the way in which it is normally consumed, count for more than any individual constituent list.

Poisonous herbs?

An example of the issues of toxicity and herbal medicine can be found in the current state of the debate in Britain. One concern is that the information about herbs from other parts of the world is rarely so well charted.

From time to time herbal remedies are identified as containing known toxic constituents. Some such plants are known poisons, as in the following:

251   Are Herbs Safe?

aconite (*Aconitum* spp.)
arnica (*Arnica montana*)
belladonna (*Atropa belladonna*)
foxglove (*Digitalis* spp.)
heliotrope (*Heliotropium europaeum*)
hemlock (*Conium maculatum*)
henbane (*Hyoscyamus niger*)
jaborandi (*Pilocarpus microphyllus*)
jimson weed (*Datura stramonium*)
mandrake (*Mandragora officinarum*)
may apple (*Podophyllum peltatum*)
poison oak (*Rhus toxicodendron*)
ragwort (*Senecio jacobaea*)
white bryony (*Bryonia alba*)

Under the terms of the Medicines Act 1968 herbal practitioners are permitted to use a few of these plants up to statutory maximum dosages, but they are not permitted for general sale. They are in any case only used by a minority of practitioners and for near-allopathic treatment strategies.

Other remedies are often referred to as 'poisonous' because they provoke vomiting or catharsis, a property, however, for which they used to be highly valued in the heroic days of traditional herbal medicine – see Part I. These include:

bloodroot (*Sanguinaria canadensis*)
jalap (*Ipomoea jalapa*)
lobelia (*Lobelia inflata*)
morning glory (*Ipomoea purpurea*)
quebracho (*Aspidosperma quebracho-blanco*)
spindle-tree (*Euonymus europaeus*)
wahoo (*Euonymus atropurpureus*)

Of these, only lobelia, and to a lesser extent, bloodroot, find current use among herbal practitioners, the former for its relaxant rather than its emetic properties. All these remedies are restricted under the terms of the Medicines Act.

On the other hand, lists of dangerous herbs have sometimes included plants for which evidence of any realistic toxicity in normal human usage is practically non-existent. Lists emanating from medical or popular publications in the USA are among the worst offenders here, reflecting a more than usual ignorance of medicinal plant chemistry among medical authorities in that country. Herbs listed have sometimes included the following:[11]

> burdock (*Arctium* spp.)
> hawthorn (*Crataegus* spp.)
> horse chestnut (*Aesculus hippocastanum*)
> St John's wort (*Hypericum perforatum*)
> wormwood (*Artemisia absinthium*)

Although there is nothing certain in this world, these plants should present no problems when taken as herbal prescriptions under the appropriate circumstances (see 'Sensible Measures', below).

A number of herbal remedies have been charged on the basis of more tangible evidence but have been defended by those using them. Each has been the subject of particular discussion between legislative authorities and the herbal lobby in Britain in recent years; most have been withdrawn from general sale, but the evidence for genuine toxicity from normal consumption of the herb at therapeutic dosages is often lacking. These include:

> comfrey (*Symphytum* spp.)
> male fern (*Dryopteris felix-mas*)
> mistletoe (*Viscum album*)
> sweet flag (*Acorus calamus*)
> yohimbe (*Corynanthe yohimbi*)

The best advice that can be given is that the consumer should avoid using such remedies, assuming that they are obtainable at all (for example by picking from the wild, or buying from other countries), unless the jury returns with a final verdict of not guilty. The case of comfrey is a particularly contentious one, as is elaborated in the section on individual remedies.

Wild cards

From time to time there have appeared in medical journals accounts of apparent side-effects from the consumption of herbal remedies. Recent reports have pinpointed comfrey,[12] mistletoe[13] and, most recently and alarmingly, valerian.[14]

In most cases it must be said that the force of the evidence presented is not overwhelming. (In the valerian case the imputation was based on no evidence at all!) Most often little regard is held for the full botanical and chemical definition of the medicine implicated, leading to one case, that of the comfrey report, resting on the evidence of a label list of constituents only, when in fact the suspected herb had just been withdrawn from the formulation.

In other cases incidental variables were poorly documented, ancillary evidence was faulty, and no attempt was made at all to unravel the actual constituents of the formulations suspected.[15] This is not to deny the possibility of either idiosyncratic, perhaps hypersensitive, reactions to herbs, as to anything else, or even of low-grade problems arising through long-term treatment with some. These are possibilities that are always present, as they are in food, for example, and it is to be hoped that fair and full investigations will increasingly cast light on this area and lead to clearer quantification of the risk.

Recent experience of the muddled thinking about risks in food does not give one much cause for optimism on this front, and the potential user of herbal remedies is best guided by a code of practice, observance of which should make the use of herbs generally safe.

Sensible Measures

How to use herbs safely

For those who wish to use herbs for their own consumption or that of their families or friends, the best policy is to stick to the following principles:

Use herbs that are widely recommended in popular herb books, or where there are statutory controls, as in Britain, use those passed as suitable for general sale. They at least have a long track-record of popular use.

Be cautious about unusual or new foreign remedies that have not stood the test of long-term use by the society for whose ills they are being offered (a new Brazilian miracle-herb might once have been wonderful in the heroic management of dysenteric fever but may be wholly unsuitable as a long-term tonic for a modern chronic debility).

Never persist with any herbal remedy after a moderate period of time (preferably no more than several weeks, a couple of months at the outside) if it is not clearly improving the condition concerned. Contrary to popular belief, most herbs do not take months to work: it is the condition that sets the pace; if it is going to take months to correct, professional advice would in any case be preferable (see below).

Always challenge a treatment: if after several weeks it is thought that the herb is useful, or even if there are doubts, stop the herb for a period and see if it is still necessary.

Refer any complicated question to a well-trained herbal practitioner. The National Institute of Medical Herbalists in Britain only accepts as members those who have studied for four years at their approved course and it has members in other countries of the world (recognized by qualifications MNIMH or FNIMH). Other training around the world is unfortunately very patchy, not least among doctors who claim to prescribe herbal remedies (the phytotherapists in Europe, for example), but there are encouraging signs of rapid improvement in training standards.

Pregnancy: the special case

It is a persistent medical principle that one should refrain from giving medicines to a pregnant woman unless absolutely necessary.

Fortunately, the issues are less worrisome for the use of herbal remedies than they are for conventional drugs. Nevertheless, herbal practitioners still refrain from medicating where possible, and then prefer herbs that are positively vetted as good, like chamomile

(*Matricaria recutita*) or black horehound (*Ballota nigra*) to help relieve nausea and morning-sickness, bulk laxatives like linseed (*Linum usitatissimum*) or psyllium seed (*Plantago ovata*) for constipation, or dandelion (*Taraxacum officinale*) for fluid retention or liver distress.

Although other herbs have been used safely, they should be particularly reserved in the crucial first trimester, when organ development in the foetus is under way.

There are a number of herbs which should be avoided altogether because they can damage the foetus or provoke a miscarriage. In many popular herb books the term *emmenagogue* is found, widely but erroneously, having come to refer to a gynaecological remedy. In fact, the effect of an emmenagogue is to bring on a delayed menstruation: it takes little imagination to realize that the most common reason for a delayed menstruation is pregnancy and that the emmenagogues are thus *abortifacients*. The following should be included in a list of this type of herbs:

> arbor-vitae (*Thuja occidentalis*)
> barberry (*Berberis vulgaris*)
> black cohosh (*Cimicifuga racemosa*)
> bloodroot (*Sanguinaria canadensis*)
> blue cohosh (*Caulophyllum thalictroides*)
> cinchona (*Cinchona* spp.)
> cotton-root bark (*Gossypium herbaceum*)
> golden seal (*Hydrastis canadensis*)
> greater celandine (*Chelidonium majus*)
> juniper (*Juniperus communis*)
> male fern (*Dryopteris felix-mas*)
> marjoram (*Origanum vulgare*)
> meadow saffron (*Crocus sativus*)
> pennyroyal (*Mentha pulegium*)
> poke root (*Phytolacca decandra*)
> rosemary (*Rosmarinus officinalis*)
> rue (*Ruta graveolens*)
> sage (*Salvia officinalis*)
> tansy (*Tanacetum vulgare*)
> thyme (*Thymus vulgaris*)
> wormwood (*Artemisia* spp.)

All anthraquinone laxatives (see 'Anthraquinones', on pp. 288–90) should also be included. It goes without saying that all those plants mentioned as toxic earlier should be avoided as well.

For those who might see this list as including herbs to be tried for procuring abortions it must be pointed out that their use for this purpose has always been seen as difficult, traditionally left to individual women with particular skills in this area. The real risk is that they may cause foetal damage rather than abortions.

The inclusion of some culinary herbs does not rule out appropriately flavoured meals: the therapeutic dose of any herb is far in excess of its dose as flavouring.

The Therapeutic Perspective

Contra-indications rather than side-effects?

There is a wider argument to be rehearsed on the subject of herb safety. We need to return to the medical assertion that if a medicine is effective it must have side-effects. How can herbalists claim the one while minimizing the other?

In fact, herbal practitioners are very familiar with the notion that herbs can be contra-indicated for certain conditions, that is, that they may be so unsuitable for a condition that they may worsen it. Professional training is needed partly to point to where *not* to prescribe remedies. There is no doubt that many herbs are active remedies, and due caution should then be observed when using them.

This is not the same thing, though, as a herb having 'side-effects', as the term has come to be applied in modern times. The strong impression is that, given the enormous popularity of herbal remedies around the world, side-effects such as are often linked with drug use are very rare.

There are three possible explanations for this. Firstly, the remedies used represent only a tiny proportion of available plant species around the world. It is not too outlandish to assume that humans through the ages moved inexorably to using those plants that were effective with a minimum of toxic or other adverse consequences. The remedies that emerge through the mists of history are thus well honed by regular human experience, benefiting from an unsurpassed positive vetting. The untrained consumer can be reassured that those plants most likely to be encountered in the health-food or herbal shop, or within the pages of popular herbal books, are particularly well tolerated.

Secondly, the benign qualities of the plants arise from the very complexity for which they are dismissed by conventional pharmacologists. There are numerous examples, some detailed in the latter part of this section, where the existence of tannins, mucilages, saponins or other constituents seems in different ways to buffer or modulate the effect of primarily active constituents. It is after all the essential feature of herbal pharmacology that the whole package has potential that no isolated principle can mimic. This seems especially so in questions of safety: the whole plant so often seems to effect a broad brush-stroke of actions, rather than cut a fine scalpel incision.

The third explanation follows immediately from the second. A reading of Part I will have shown that the whole thrust of treatment in herbal medicine is different from that of conventional chemotherapy. The herbs are ideally used *to provoke a healing response by the body rather than to directly home in on the symptoms or pathology*. Their claim for action is thus lesser than that of drugs, their trust in the body's recuperative reflexes is paramount and their manipulation of intricate physiological functions minimal.

If the body is provoked in the wrong direction, then the effect will be counter-productive. This is very different from the problems that arise by burrowing into a complex tissue function and changing it without regard for the wider body condition. Contra-indications are not after all the same as side-effects.

6 Traditional Pharmacology

Introduction

Charting responses

An essential component of herbal medicine is that its healing agents are material substances.

The drying and preparation of the herbs devitalize the plant and we may assume that little putative 'vital energy' survives to become a factor in assessing any effects, as is the case with remedies. (It was the attempt to capture that energy which inspired the move towards homoeopathic medicine, with the use of fresh plant material and its 'potentization': briefly it was assumed that the more material that could be discarded – by precisely determined methods – the more potent would become the immaterial essence left.) Fortunately we need not be concerned here with the value or otherwise of the homoeopathic position, or even feel regret that the average herbal prescription is so lifeless.

The point touched on in the review of physiology (see 'The healing reflex', on p. 40) is that the herb acts essentially as an *agent provocateur*, with the greatest importance being laid on the *body's response to the stimulation* rather than on the nature of the stimulus itself. The obvious comparison is with the response to the needling that provides us with what we know as acupuncture. Similarly it is the body's whole and vital response to contact with the material substance that determines the therapeutic effects of herbal medicine.

The study of the effects of drugs on the body is called pharmacology. The spirit of this fascinating exploration has been dominated by modern medical science, so that pharmacology has come entirely to denote a narrowly fragmentary investigation. Nature is effectively disintegrated so that the action of an isolated chemical on an isolated piece or function of the body or a neutered anonymous crowd of people can be observed as precisely as is possible in a variable world. These observations are then stuck together to make a jigsaw picture of the effect of that substance on the body, and it is this picture which is the basis on which that drug is given to real people. This is an inevitable product of the rational scientific method but it is not necessarily the best way to deal with real life. It was after all the admirable Dr Frankenstein who in good faith tried to assemble life from its pieces: that the actual results of such a creation turn out to be somewhat different from prediction should not surprise us.

Any pharmacology suited to the application of traditional medicine must be a creature different from this. At no time must the view of the whole be lost (on the persistent traditional axiom that the whole is much more than the sum of its parts, and in fact actually determines them). A traditional pharmacology must start with the human experience of an agent, a well-charted catalogue of effects on mind and spirit as well as body.

Its role thereafter is to draw from these observations such messages as may enable the practitioner better to predict the action of each remedy in the infinitely variable circumstances that will be encountered in practice.

A crude chemical brew

The relationship between herbalist and modern pharmacologist has other specific features of conflict. The allopath has always asked that any drug be standardized and predictable in action so the manipulative and invasive action of the remedy on the human can be controlled as tightly as possible.

A medicinal plant consists of an immense array of chemical constituents (never all identified), each liable to be interacting with the others, most with little known pharmacological action and, worst of all, each individual plant sample has its own unique blend of constituents. Faced with this fiendish complexity and almost infinite variability, the pharmacologist has for long hungered for an identifiable 'active principle', something that, whilst reflecting the useful action of the plant, was yet amenable to isolation, characterization, and ultimately separate synthesis. (There is another very practical factor: one can patent synthesized medicines but not plants.)

So we have digoxin from the foxglove, aspirin from willow bark, quinine from cinchona bark, anticancer drugs from a periwinkle, anti-ulcer drugs from liquorice, morphine and codeine from the opium poppy, colchicine from the autumn crocus, atropine from the deadly nightshade, pilocarpine from jaborandi, ergotamine from ergot of rye, and so on. From this perspective the claims of the herbalists are seen as a quaint but irrational relic from the dark ages: how can we justify the use of a constantly changing chemical soup in place of the cleanly extracted, precisely measured active principle?

Yet clinical pharmacology has already discovered that as far as the patient is concerned predictability is an illusion. From any one dose of digoxin, for example, different patients get widely different responses, and the final prescribed dosage has to be individually tailored as a result, a familiar practical concern in medicine. Such real-life variation makes the idea of the 'standard dose' less meaningful and increases the impression that modern medical scientists often cling to the bastions of predictability in the face of the evidence, probably because they simply fear the alternative.

That alternative accepts that life is variable, following the discipline of *pattern* rather than measurement. It predicts that if one tries to impose a measured regime on life it struggles free and eventually kicks back; that the way to keep afloat in life is to learn to recognize and respond to its patterns; that *a therapeutic agent should be rated on its ability to provoke a pattern of vital healing responses in the body*, whether that agent be a crude botanical preparation, the stimulation of an acupuncture point, the movement of a spinal or muscular tissue, or the touch of a hand or a smile, rather than on its ability to force change on a fragment of a body.

The herbalist sees the best remedies as providing a number of constituents which provoke vital responses, all wrapped up in a package which has on experience been found to produce few extraneous toxic side-effects. Although there is variability, it is within workable limits, and quality control can reduce it even further. Moreover, in recording the action of the remedies the herbalist constantly renews the impression that the whole plant is much more than the sum of its parts. We shall see many examples where plants contain constituents that interact to produce the final clinical effect.

It is therefore suggested that in this context a herbal pharmacology becomes the following:

> the *interpretation* of the observed action of the remedy in practice;
>
> the process of developing the character of each remedy so that it can be used more creatively and informatively in support of healing processes, rather than searching for the actions of constituents *per se*.

This is not a familiar perspective even among texts on herbal medicine. Most of these appear to be in awe of the current pharmacological wisdom and see little choice but to view herbs entirely in such terms. This is accompanied by what is often a depressively symptomatic view of the remedies. No attempt seems to be made to really find out what each remedy is actually doing for the person taking it, perhaps because it is still very rare for an accomplished practitioner to go into print.

There is, of course, a fundamental conflict in using the results of reductionist research into the pharmacology of fragments to create a case for a new system-oriented discipline. The compromises are the more frequent as a result of the dearth of research into the action of the whole plant.

It is therefore necessary to build up a picture of the herb from different sources. For each remedy the primary source is *practical* experience, which forms the bulk of the information in the chapter 'Remedies'. The aim of this pharmacology exercise is to add to that information and make it meaningful.

The key is first of all to ensure that *all scientific observations are subservient to experience*. The herbalist is suspicious, for example, of claims for herbs that rely entirely on finding an active constituent that looks as though it *might* be useful. The recommendations that carry most weight are those of practical and clinical experience. If a scientific insight allows such practical use to be better understood, then that is sufficient justification for it. (In modern pharmacology, of course, the process is quite different: for new drugs clinical predictions are built up entirely from scientific data.)

By picking frequently encountered constituents it is often possible to highlight major themes, or archetypes, that correlate well with clinical reputation and with traditional pharmacological terms (such as the European 'hot, cold, dry and moist', and the Chinese five *Tastes*).

The major chemical groups that are seen as particularly archetypal will be marked as such in the following text (by an asterix). Their characteristics recur frequently in discussion of the medicinal action of plants as a whole and many remedies can be classified in relation to such characteristics. Some plants are notably astringent and tannin-rich; others are mucilaginous, or aromatic (rich in volatile oils); those containing saponins often exhibit interesting pharmacological properties as a result; the action of bitter-containing plants is usually predictable, and so on.

The archetypal constituents are also sometimes apparent to taste, smell or by colour and so have figured in traditional views of pharmacology. The presence of tannins and mucilages, volatile oils, bitters, saponins and acrid principles are obvious to taste or smell, that of the anthraquinone laxatives soon after ingestion! This means, of course, that it is possible to predict much about a strange plant from a simple assessment of such constituents before it is more exactly analysed.

The Archetypal Plant Constituents

Introduction

In looking at the most frequently encountered plant constituents the purpose of the exercise should be clarified. Any assumption about the action of a plant that relies solely on the basis of the action of a constituent should be resisted. It should always be recalled that the action of the whole plant is more than the action of its parts. We look at constituents, archetypal or otherwise, for the following reasons:

> to provide possible explanations for the already perceived action of the whole plant;
>
> to point to possible actions, beneficial or harmful, that might have been missed because of the context of traditional use (cardiac benefits and certain long-term toxic effects, for example, may both have escaped notice in the past);
>
> to find any evidence for the particular therapeutic approach traditionally applied to the use of herbal remedies – particularly for the claim that they provoke recuperative responses (see Part I);
>
> to illustrate the full diversity of plant pharmacology.

In the following, text is inserted in smaller type for those literate in the chemical and medical sciences. It is not central to the information given but will help provide a sounder base for such readers.

Plants will be mentioned that will not be elaborated in detail, but as many as possible will be discussed later in the materia medica section. When they are covered in the materia medica there will be provided a known list of constituents so that referral back to this section may be made.

As with the review of physiology in Part I most of the material presented is already in the public domain of pharmacological knowledge. New or contentious statements will be supported by appropriate references, but most will not.

Particular information may be had from the following texts:

Books:

The British Herbal Pharmacopoeia (1990) and *Compendium* (in press), The British Herbal Medicines Association, Bournemouth, UK

The British Pharmaceutical Codex (1949), The Pharmaceutical Press, London

The British Pharmacopoeia (1914 and 1948), London

Evans, W. C. (1989) *Trease and Evans Pharmacognosy* (13th edition), Baillière Tindall, London

Fluckiger, F. A. and Hanbury, D. (1879) *Pharmacographia*, MacMillan & Co., London

Harborne, J. B. (1988) *Introduction to Ecological Biochemistry* (3rd edition), Academic Press, London

Heywood, V. H. and Harborne, J. B. (1974) *The Biology and Chemistry of the Compositae*, Academic Press, London

Martindale The Extra Pharmacopoeia (25th edition onwards)

National Academy of Sciences (1975) *Herbal Pharmacology in the People's Republic of China*, Washington DC

The National Dispensatory (1906), Washington DC

Perry, L. M. (1980) *Medicinal Plants of East and Southeast Asia*, MIT Press, Cambridge, Massachusetts

The Pharmacopoeia of the United States of America (5th edition) (1873) *et seq.*

Progress in Phytochemistry (1970–72), eds. Rheinhold, L. and Liwschitz, Y. (vols. 1–3), John Wiley & Sons, London

Recent Advances in Phytochemistry (1970–78), eds. Steelink, C. and Runeckles, V. C. (vols. 1–9), Meredith Corp. and Plenum Press, New York

Thomson, W. A. R. (ed.) (1978) *Healing Plants – A Modern Herbal*, McGraw-Hill, London

Wagner, H. and Horhammer, L. (eds.) (1971) *Pharmacognosy and Phytochemistry*, Springer-Verlag, Berlin

Wagner, H. and Wolff, P. (eds.) (1977) *New Natural Products and Plant Drugs with Pharmacological, Biological or Therapeutic Activity*, Springer-Verlag, Berlin

Waller, G. R. and Nowacki, E. K. (1978) *Alkaloid Biology and Metabolism in Plants*, Plenum Press, New York

Weiss, R. F. (1988) *Herbal Medicine*, A. B. Arcanum, Sweden; reprinted by Beaconsfield Publishers, Beaconsfield, UK. Translation of *Lehrbuch der Phytotherapie* (1985), Hippokrates-Verlag, Stuttgart

Wren, R. C. (rewritten Williamson, E. M. and Evans, F. J. (1988)) *Potters New Cyclopaedia of Botanical Drugs and Preparations*. C. W. Daniel Co., Saffron Walden, UK

Journals:
Journal of Ethnopharmacology, Switzerland
Journal of Natural Products (formerly *Lloydia*), USA
Planta Medica, Germany

Acids (and their salts and esters)

Weak acids constitute a prominent fraction of all plant material, although relatively little exist in free form (so most plants do not taste particularly sour). Most acids are found in the form of their salts, esters or amides, and as such in a more active and fat-(lipid)-soluble form (see 'Pharmacokinetics', on pp. 332–46). Although, like many other types of plant constituents, they have been largely ignored by chemists concerned with extracting more powerful chemicals, their activity is often appreciable in the context of a total herbal prescription, and is a particular factor too in the effects of consuming fruit and vegetables.

Plant acids are most often carboxylic acids with a general formula RCOOH. There are four main groups to consider:

1 Monobasic (monocarboxylic) acids: straight-chain (aliphatic) acids containing up to 26 carbons per molecule. They include formic and acetic acids, and the saturated and unsaturated fatty acids, as well as valeric acid from valerian and hops.

2 Polybasic acids: containing more than one carboxyl (-COOH) group; very widely found in plant material; they generally have a slightly laxative effect as well as their own particular

properties. They include oxalic, succinic and fumaric acids.

3 Hydroxy acids: these include both a pair of carboxyl groups and one hydroxyl (-OH) group, giving them the properties of alcohols (q.v.) as well as acids. They can thus 'auto-esterify' and form polyesters, but their most significant pharmacological property is their ability to sequester and effectively neutralize cations, such as the ions of calcium, copper, manganese and iron. They include citric, malic and tartaric acids.

4 Aromatic acids: these are cyclic acids mostly based on benzoic and cinnamic acids.

benzoic acid   cinnamic acid

These acids and their derivatives are found widely in nature, but particularly in resins (q.v.) and balsams. Derivatives of benzoic acid include salicylic acid and the phenols, and the tannins (all referred to later); one derivative of cinnamic acid is umbelliferone from the parsley family.

Taking those plant acids with the most significance to the action of our remedies we find the following:

Unsaturated fatty acids

These are universally found in plants, more so than in animal tissues. The most notable are linoleic and arachidonic acids found mostly in seeds and other reproductive tissues of the plant, and linolenic acid found especially in growing green tissues. It is now known that these and a number of other polyunsaturated fatty acids (PUFAs) are vitally necessary in the diet (i.e. they are 'essential fatty acids', EFAs). They are needed to build and repair cell structures, such as the cell wall, and notably tissues in the central nervous system, and to form the raw material for prostaglandin production. Inflammatory and other chronic diseases are noted for exhibiting a deficiency of PUFAs in the bloodstream.

A notable application of this material in recent times has been the use of one PUFA, normally produced by the body from arachidonic acid, di-homo-γ-linolenic acid (GLA), a major component of the oil of the evening primrose (*Oenothera biennis* spp.), which is used in the treatment of a range of inflammatory diseases. These have included eczema and rheumatoid conditions as well as premenstrual syndrome: all such conditions would presumably be based on a deficit of innate production of GLA by the person involved.[1]

Although not likely to play a major part in the action of most herbal remedies, the fact that all plants contain these constituents is likely to augment their overall effect on the body. PUFAs are one of many groups of constituents that can be thought of as actual adjuvants to the main pharmacological actors. Many of these adjuvants share a restorative or nutrient action which bodes well for the overall blend.

Formic acid

Of interest mainly for its historical use as one of a number of agents employed as local irritants for treating chronic joint inflammations. As the smallest organic acid (formula $HCOOH$) it is also the most corrosive and when brought in contact with the skin it produces its own inflammatory reaction. It was used as one of a number of *counter-irritants* and blistering agents (*vesicants*) that in a less harmful way can divert damage away from the congested joint (as explained in Part I).

It is used little in modern practices, being too drastic, but formic acid (originally prepared from the red ant, *Formica rufa*) is a key component of the sting of the European stinging nettle (*Urtica* spp.), exposure to which has traditionally been associated with a reduced incidence of arthritic disease (the Romans suggested beating with bunches of nettles over affected joints!). However, formic acid is quickly oxidized to carbon dioxide and water and does not survive cooking or other preparation: it thus plays no part in internal herbal medicines.

Acetic acid

The main principle in vinegar, it is rarely encountered in any quantity in the fresh plant. However, in traditional medicine vinegar preparations of medicinal herbs were common, allowing liquid remedies to be preserved for long periods. In Chinese medicine at least such preparations were considered to have different properties from other forms of a remedy. There is a relatively modern idea that vinegar as such is beneficial for several 'toxic' states, but this is poorly articulated and explained.

Oxalic acid

This forms notably insoluble salts with such metals as calcium and in this form is found in the dock and rhubarb families (*Rumex* and *Rheum* spp.) especially, but also in many common foods (tea, spinach, beet and parsley) and in small quantities in many other plants. The main potential problem with oxalates is in some types of urinary stones, formed by precipitation of excessive oxalates in acid urine. For cases of kidney stones determination of their constitution will allow sensible avoidance of high oxalate foods to be made.

Succinic acid

An intermediary in basic metabolic processes in the body, it acts as a stimulant to tissue oxidation, and has been used allopathically with salicylates for arthritis and as a counter to barbiturate poisoning. Tissue oxidation involves increased blood flow and can often be seen as desirable, especially in degenerative conditions. Succinic acid is a variable constituent in all plant materials.

Tartaric acid

A fruit acid found notably in tamarinds but widely throughout the plant world as well. It is not broken down by digestion and metabolism so is excreted whole in the urine, so that unlike other fruit acids it actually increases acid levels in the body. On the other hand it is not easily absorbed and functions well as a gentle osmotic (water-attracting) laxative.

Citric acid

This is found widely in fruit and berries, especially the citrus fruits. It plays a key role in metabolism, with succinic and related acids, and gives its name to the citric-acid or Krebs cycle that is involved in producing useful energy from carbohydrate.

On ingestion it quickly breaks down itself into bicarbonates and is thus paradoxically an alkaline food source (hence the value of some, though not all, fruit for 'acid' conditions such as arthritis and degenerative diseases). Similar paradoxical results are seen in the mouth where contrary to expectations it reduces the tendency to acid-dependent tooth decay. The main points to its action here are its ability to check bacterial populations in the mouth directly, but more importantly it reflexly stimulates salivary secretions, a flow that ensures the beneficially alkaline and bacteria-inhibiting saliva has flushed the mouth clean of food material.

It appears that along with other sour-tasting materials citric acid also causes increased bile flow from the liver, an effect mediated by stimulation of the sour receptors in the mouth. The effect probably explains the traditional use of large quantities of lemon juice (with olive oil) to flush out bile stones. Like tartaric acid citric acid is a gentle osmotic laxative and diuretic. When the effects of vitamin C and the *bioflavonoids* are taken into account all this lends reinforcement to the view of fruit as a particularly cleansing food.

Benzoic acid

It is the central component of gum benzoin, found in high levels in Tolu and Peru balsams and also in cranberries. It is a local antiseptic in quite low concentrations; in higher dosages it becomes a local irritant. Internally it has the same effects, acting as an intestinal disinfectant and potential irritant. On absorption it acts as a powerful antipyretic comparable to or even exceeding salicylic acid. It increases metabolic rate and protein utilization in the body. It is excreted in the urine as a metabolite *hippuric acid* that is diuretic and likely to help phosphate urinary stones.

The local actions of benzoic acid and the benzoates are often utilized in the form of inhalants and throat remedies, and in such preparations as Friar's Balsam it is found to clear upper respiratory catarrh and to have antiseptic, soothing and astringent properties.

Carbohydrates Taste: SWEET

We are familiar with the main types of dietary carbohydrate such as glucose, fructose, starch and cellulose, and it is obvious that these exist in herbs as in all plants. We are concerned here with lesser-known examples that play a useful part in several remedies.

Carbohydrates are built up from basic units called sugars. They are classified according to the number of sugars they contain as follows:

1 *Monosaccharides*: single sugars such as glucose, fructose, galactose (from milk and in a rare isomer, from agar-agar), the wood sugars xylose, ribose and arabinose, and a wide variety of others such as apiose from the parsley and celery family, and hamamelose from witch hazel and the primroses. They have no known pharmacological action, and most are metabolized through normal carbohydrate processes.

2 *Disaccharides*: two-sugar units including sucrose (glucose + fructose), maltose (glucose + glucose) and lactose from milk only (glucose + galactose). Most are quickly broken down to monosaccharides, although several, such as raffinose, found in many plant tissues where it seems to have an 'antifreeze' effect, are likely to contribute to the undigested carbohydrate residue we call 'roughage'.

3 *Polysaccharides*: multi-sugar units and often extremely large molecules. The group includes the amyloses that constitute

glucose storage molecules like starch and glycogen (in animals), cellulose and inulin (a fructose store found in all parts of the Compositae family such as dandelions and marigolds). The group also includes molecules containing other components besides sugar units, most frequently glucuronic and galacturonic acids. This category includes the *hemicelluloses*, pectin, and the important *gums* and *mucilages*.

Immuno-stimulating polysaccharides

Recent work has revealed that a number of water-soluble, acidic, branch-chained heteroglycan polysaccharide molecules, with molecular weights in the range of 25,000 to 500,000 or even higher, show significant immuno-stimulating properties at least *in vitro*. Most attention has been paid to those of the North American herb, echinacea (*Echinacea angustifolia*), to which further reference is made in the section on individual remedies, but similar molecules have been discovered in chamomile (*Matricaria recutita*), marigold flowers (*Calendula officinalis*), wild indigo (*Baptisia tinctoria*), saw palmetto (*Serenoa serrulata*) and Siberian ginseng (*Eleutherococcus senticosus*).[2]

The obvious point to make about such molecules is that on oral consumption their effect would be largely confined to the gut: polysaccharides are either broken down on digestion or else very poorly absorbed. It may, of course, be in the body's attempt at absorption that immunostimulation occurs (see the discussion on dietary allergies in Part I).

By contrast, the primary medicinal reputation of the polysaccharides has resulted from this very indigestibility and their physical properties in solution.

Hemicelluloses

These are polysaccharides found, like cellulose, in the plant wall, which provide a variable proportion of dietary roughage. Unlike cellulose which consists of very long chains of glucose molecules, the hemicelluloses are a heterogeneous mixture of different sugar and uronic acid derivatives. Because of this heterogeneity and the resultant fact that they are very difficult to isolate and characterize they do not lend themselves easily to conventional pharmacological research.

They nevertheless influence the characteristics of plant fibre considerably, providing a particularly soft bulk to the stool. The fact that they tend to be leached out in the commercial preparation of bran provides one possible reason why bran can be too irritating for many bowels. The hemicelluloses therefore contribute considerably to the beneficial softness of whole cereal and vegetable fibre. Because of their relative insolubility in water, however, they probably play little part in the average herbal prescription.

Pectins

These are complex galacturonic-acid-based carbohydrates found in the plant cell wall particularly of roots and fruits. They are originally produced as the insoluble protopectin; however, during fruit ripening and on other occasions they tend to change to become the gelatinous and water-soluble pectins. The same conversion takes place in boiling water (as in jam making) and possibly in the acid environment of the stomach. In the digestive tract as a whole pectin is a valuable bulk laxative and healing agent in intestinal disorders such as diarrhoea and dysentery. This latter healing property can be demonstrated locally by the use of pectin as an antiseptic and healing paste for indolent ulcers and deep wounds. As a constituent of dietary fibre pectin has demonstrated that it is exceptionally beneficial, working well, for instance, in slowing glucose absorption from the gut and thus helping to support pancreatic blood-sugar control. Pectin also reduces the levels of cholesterol in the bloodstream after meals, a fact which should be of interest to those with cardiovascular disease. Like the hemicelluloses, pectin is not found in any quantity in the average fluid herbal preparation, but is likely to feature in capsulated or tableted prescriptions.

Seaweed gums

Found in the cell walls and intracellular regions of algae and seaweeds, these gums have different structures from others in the plant world. They tend to be particularly good bulk laxatives, having the astonishing ability to expand when combined with water. Among notable examples is agar-agar, which forms an effective gel in concentrations in water of as low as 1:200. A similar agent is carrageen, derived from Irish moss. Algin is the most common seaweed gum commercially, and exhibits the usual properties with the noted extra benefit of selectively binding the heavy metal strontium so as to prevent its absorption into the body. In Japan seaweeds play a large part in the diet and medicine, though most certainly for other reasons than just the benefits for the bowel.

Reference could be made in this context to the discussion of remedies with a 'salty' taste in the Chinese view of pharmacology (see 'Salty', on pp. 188–9): the idea that such remedies moisten and soften indurated congestions like constipation can be easily appreciated.

* GUMS AND MUCILAGES

The gums and mucilages are extremely common constituents of plants that have been almost universally ignored by modern pharmacists. Nevertheless, they have several very important functions central to the action of many herbal prescriptions.

Gums and mucilages have traditionally been distinguished by their physical properties, the first 'tacky', the second 'slimy'; however, there is no clear chemical distinction between the two groups and they are best considered together here, especially as they are most often found together in plants. If there is any distinction to be made, it is that gums tend to be used as thickening and bulking agents in pharmaceutics, and they play a less obvious part in most plants. Once swallowed, their actions are no different from those of the mucilages.

The essence of the action of these constituents is physical rather than chemical. The gums and mucilages are made up of uronic acid and sugar derivatives, and even if they are broken down on digestion these can have no great pharmacological effect. As it is these molecules are very resistant to the digestive juices and many survive to reach the bowel. Yet plants containing them such as marshmallow root (*Althaea officinalis*), coltsfoot (*Tussilago far-fara*), slippery elm bark (*Ulmus fulva*), plantain (*Plantago major*), or comfrey (*Symphytum officinale*), all have predictable effects on digestive, respiratory and urinary systems, the last two quite remote from any conceivable local effect. In fact, the phenomenon of the action on the body of the mucilages raises important principles about the effect of herbal constituents in general.

The key action of the mucilages is on the surface with which they come in direct contact. They produce a coating of slime that acts to soothe and protect any exposed surface. Thus the mucilaginous plants have been used primarily and universally as wound remedies, soothing pain, irritation and itching, and in their drying also often acting to bind any damaged tissue. The overall action is referred to as *demulcent* or *emollient*.

The demulcent action is continued down the lining of the digestive tract, so explaining the use of mucilaginous remedies for gastrointestinal inflammations, lesions and ulcers, and for reducing the irritant results of excessive stomach acid or digestive juice secretions. (Slippery elm powder, for example, is a very popular remedy for relieving the effects of acid dyspepsia or the ingestion of food that disagrees with the digestion.)

Yet there is more to this than soothing a passive tube lining: the digestive tract is a vitally responsive neuromuscular organ, one of the most complex structures in the human body, with even its own ('enteric') nervous system, a vast hormonal system, and a surprising autonomy from higher control. It depends for its minute-by-minute responses on the messages passed in from receptors in the walls of the tract, and on the feedback from its own subsequent actions.

Irritation, for example, of the receptive nerve endings in the lining, as in infection or inflammation, will lead to reflex increased motility of the tract, both in the region and, by further reflex, in other passages of the gut (diarrhoea most often follows irritation high up in the small intestine or even stomach). Symptoms of irritation include dyspepsia, colic, spastic bowel, flatulence, reflux regurgitation, vomiting, diarrhoea, dysphagia (difficulty in swallowing), as well as many cases of abdominal pain, especially in children. To the extent that mucilages soothe the irritation that may be behind such symptoms, then they will also reduce those symptoms.

This is not a cure, of course, and it comes more under the heading of management, but use of mucilaginous remedies can provide an invaluable aid in the treatment of digestive disorders.

We now turn to the two other areas in which mucilaginous remedies are often used, the *respiratory* and *urinary* systems. Here initial incredulity is forgivable for, as we have seen, no useful part of the mucilages actually reaches these two regions of the body. The solution to what might have been an embarrassing problem is provided by the reflex associations between the digestive tract and the bronchial tree and urinary tubules: in the embryonic development of the body the tissues of these systems have a common origin (the bronchial tree develops as a diverticulum of the gut) and it seems as if their respective nervous supplies retain connections afterwards. Thus agents that affect the lining and the wall of the digestive tract can *by reflex* influence the function of the bronchial and urinary ducts.

Thus we find that mucilaginous remedies have soothing properties for the bronchial and urinary ducts, acting to calm irritable coughs, increase the fluidity of bronchial secretions if they are excessively dry, and reduce the spasm in the asthmatic condition (this suggests their use for dry nervous coughing and breathlessness); they reduce the renal colic due to urinary stones, and the symptoms of urinary or bladder infections. Again we are looking at management rather than cure, but these conditions present many opportunities where such an approach may be very useful. We may draw some important general propositions about the action of herbal constituents from the example of the mucilages.*

---

*In traditional European (Galenic) terms the mucilaginous remedies were considered 'moist', increasing fluidity and lubrication, and soothing; as such they tended to have a neutral temperament, for if the remedy were 'hot' it would dry up its 'moisture', whereas excessive 'cold' is congealing. We can agree that mucilaginous remedies are notably mild and agreeable, acceptable to even the most delicate patient.

In Chinese medicine the association of mucilages with the bland effect or 'taste' was discussed in Part I (see 'Chinese Pharmacology', on pp. 183–94).

Propositions:

many important effects can be demonstrated with parts of the plant rejected by the orthodox pharmacologist;

these responses are often produced through mediation of the reflex-programmed response.

Phenols

A large number of important plant constituents are based on the phenolic molecule. We shall be dealing with most types under their separate headings; they include the following:

> simple phenolic compounds and their glycosides
> tannins
> coumarins and their glycosides
> anthraquinones and their glycosides
> flavones and their glycosides

SIMPLE PHENOLS

Phenols are molecules in which a hydrogen of an aromatic nucleus is replaced by an hydroxy group:

OH

phenol

This hydroxy substitution can occur more than once, so that with isomers there are three possible dihydroxybenzenes, and three possible trihydroxybenzenes, respectively catechol, resorcinol and hydroquinone, and pyrogallol, benzenitrol and phloroglucinol.

The hydroxy group confers on the molecule the property of an alcohol, but although phenols can thus be considered as tertiary alcohols, the fact that the hydroxy group is attached directly to an unsaturated carbon nucleus (the so-called 'enolic' grouping) means that after all the phenols are weak acids.

Most phenol derivatives (as listed above) are polycylic molecules, formed from more than one ring, and this affects basic properties fundamentally. The simple phenols discussed below are mostly formed by the substitution of other radicals for one or more of the hydrogens. When these radicals are alkyl groups, as in eugenol or thymol, the substance is particularly bioactive, with increasing toxicity.

In general phenols are bactericidal, antiseptic, anthelmintic (toxic to gut parasites), and in isolation caustic, vesicant (including blisters), and anaesthetic. The antimicrobial effect is probably due to induction of structural damage in the membranes of cell walls and internal structures. Unfortunately, like all antibacterial agents, they inhibit leucocyte activity (this is far more a problem with antibiotics like penicillin), and although many plants containing phenols may also contain compensatory leucocyte-stimulating agents, the association of antimicrobial remedies with a simultaneous weakening of the body's own defences should not be forgotten.

Phenol itself is used as a standard for other antimicrobial agents.

Salicylic acid

The well-known basis for the aspirin group of drugs, salicylic acid, is found freely or as its ester methyl salicylate in a number of plant families. It contributes the active (aglycone) element to the following glycosides: salicin from the willow (*Salix* spp.) and poplar (*Populus* spp.) families, and from cramp bark (*Viburnum opulus*) and black haw bark (*Viburnum prunifolium*); populin from the poplar family; gaultherin from wintergreen (*Gaultheria procumbens*), birch (*Betula* spp.), and Indian pipe (*Monotropa uniflora*). Methyl salicylate is also a prominent constituent of the meadowsweet (*Filipendula ulmaria*). (Aspirin was given its name from the former botanical name for meadowsweet: *Spiraea*, thus a-Spiraea, 'from meadowsweet'; salicylic acid itself was named for the fact that it was first isolated from the willow bark.)

Salicylic acid is a strong antiseptic, a property following from the fact that it is a carboxylated phenol:

OH

COOH

salicylic acid

Esters and salts are somewhat less active, and they are less irritating to the lining of the stomach, for example. The form prepared commercially, acetylsalicylic acid, was found to have the least irritating properties. A central component of the function of the salicylates is an action inhibiting the potent mediators of inflammation, the prostaglandins, implicated too in the clotting process.

The salicylates are pharmacologically very active. Externally, they are weakly antiseptic and irritant, though in small concentrations (as found in many plants) they stimulate regeneration of epithelial tissues.

Internally, they are strongly antipyretic and act to increase peripheral blood flow and sweat production, by a direct action on the thermogenic centre in the hypothalamus (but see other ways to manage fever: 'Rejection', on pp. 53–79). Temperature is lowered only in those individuals with pyrexia: in the normal balance salicylates actually increase body heat production so compensating for the heat loss.

They act on the hepatocytes (liver cells) increasing the volume and concentration of bile.

They are catabolic (leading to increased breakdown of protein in the body), so urinary urea and sulphur excretion are increased; in addition the concentrations of uric acid are increased, and this, combined with the competitive inhibition of uric acid excretion at the kidney, means that salicylates are contra-indicated in gout (although they may appear useful in the short term). They also have a slight diuretic effect.

The analgesic action of salicylates is well known: this may be a central effect on pain perception or may involve their action on prostaglandin metabolism, or it could be a combination of both actions.

Conversion of salicylate derivatives to salicylic acid itself is known to occur in acid conditions: this provides useful increased antiseptic effects in such situations as arthritic joints and in the urinary tubules.

The anticlotting properties of the salicylates have been used recently as a prophylactic treatment for thrombotic conditions. This aspect so far is little investigated, and we can draw few conclusions about the applicability of salicylate-containing plants for this.

Methyl salicylate, as found notably in oil of wintergreen, has additional external uses as a local rubefacient and is very well absorbed through the skin: it is thus a useful application for an inflamed joint – reducing the inflammatory process while at the same time painlessly increasing the blood flow itself.

The most well-known side-effect of the salicylates is their ability to produce multiple gastric submucous haemorrhages, especially when given in concentration. They can in fact be relied on to produce some stomach bleeding in almost everyone, although this is only occasionally so serious as to provoke concern. In this context it is worth noting the use of meadowsweet to *heal* damage to the stomach wall, a paradoxical action probably produced by the combination of mucilages and tannins usually discarded in conventional exploration of medicinal plant chemistry.

Eugenol

Obtained from the oil of cloves (*Eugenia caryophyllata*), and found also as the active constituent (aglycone) of gein from avens or cloveroot (*Geum urbanum*), and as a major component in cinnamon oil (*Cinnamomum zeylanicum*, not *C. cassia*).

This substance exhibits the natural anaesthetic and antiseptic properties of the phenols, so that oil of cloves has long been used as a remedy for toothaches and as an antiseptic mouthwash. Eugenol no doubt contributes to other properties of clove oil, externally rubefacient and counter-irritant, internally stimulating secretion of saliva and gastric activity by reflex as well; in the lower intestine it acts as a carminative or antispasmodic.

Thymol

Derived from oil of thyme (*Thymus vulgaris*) and found in other aromatic labiates, particularly horsemint (*Monarda punctata*). It is an effective antifungal agent and has been used topically at concentrations of 1–2 per cent (thyme oil contains 20–30 per cent). It is also used for oral and intestinal infections where its other antiseptic properties are evident (it is 20 times stronger as an antiseptic than phenol) and it is also an effective anthelmintic.

A useful bonus is that although it is so much stronger than phenol it exhibits far less the mucosal irritating properties of the group. It is very poorly absorbed into the body fluids, so finds its main use within the gut or on the surface of the body. It makes an ideal basis for toothpastes and mouthwashes.

Hydroquinone

The aglycone of arbutin found widely in the heather family (the Ericaceae) and in the Rosaceae. The medicinal plant that most notably contains arbutin is the uva ursi (*Arctostaphylos uva-ursi*). This is used as a urinary antiseptic. The reason: arbutin is converted, mainly in the urine, to hydroquinone. This has antiseptic effects, particularly against *Klebsiella* and *Escherichia coli*.

*TANNINS   Taste: SOUR

Tannins make up a large group of polyphenols found very widely throughout the plant world. Their role in the plant is a matter for speculation, but their particular concentration in those tissues lost from the plant, e.g. old and dying leaves, outer cork, heartwood and galls, suggests they might represent metabolic waste products. On the other hand there is evidence that they also act to deter insect and fungal attack (in the oak increased tannin production in the leaves in late summer is closely correlated with a diminished insect attack on them; oak galls, the richest source of tannins, are themselves responses of the tree to insect attack).

Whatever their role they have been used for millennia by man to 'tan' animal hides and convert them to leather. This practice is an application of their basic property of precipitating proteins into insoluble complexes, combining with these complexes and rendering them resistant to proteolytic enzymes.

Such a property, applied to living tissues, constitutes the term 'astringency'; the taste this refers to is that resulting from puckering of the protein lining the mouth and tongue. Beyond this as acids their overall taste is sour and we have seen that there is a good description of their properties in Chinese literature under the qualities of that taste.

There are two groups of tannins: the hydrolysable and the condensed tannins. The first are derivatives of simple phenolic acids such as gallic acid or ellagic acid. When heated in acid they yield pyrogallol, an antiseptic and caustic substance that is also hepatotoxic. Plants that contain large quantities are thus less suitable for use over open wounds. Hydrolysable tannins turn brown on exposure to air, and are largely responsible for the brown colour of many plant tinctures.

Condensed tannins or nonhydrolysable tannins are more resistant to splitting and hence analysis. They are related to the flavonoid pigments (see 'Flavones', on pp. 291–4) in that flavins and catechins combine in their biosynthesis. When heated in acid they tend to polymerize to form red insoluble substances called tannin reds or phlobaphenes (these are the reddish deposits that are seen to form in tinctures and fluid extracts of some plants on long standing, especially in light; their presence is indicative of a high level of condensed tannins in the plant). The phlobaphenes give a characteristic red colour to some plant tissues, e.g. roots of tormentil (*Potentilla erecta*). The final breakdown product after heating for all these condensed tannins is catechol. They show little evidence of hepatotoxicity or any other ill effects, and their use is thus to be favoured.

Other related examples of polyphenols are arbutin from uva ursi (*Arctostaphylos uva-ursi*), rugosin-D from meadowsweet (*Filipendula ulmaria*), and sanguin H-6 from raspberry leaves (*Rubus idaeus*).

All tannins have a number of properties in common:

> they are soluble in water and alcohols, but not in organic solvents;

> they form precipitates with proteins (especially proline-rich proteins like gelatine and salivary proteins), nitrogenous bases, polysaccharides, some alkaloids and a few glycosides (they have been used therapeutically as antidotes to alkaloidal poisoning on the basis of their ability to form insoluble tannates with them – incidentally only dilute solutions of tannins are necessary for this job);[3]

> much of the tannins ingested remains unabsorbed in the gut but a variable proportion reaches the body fluids as soluble tannate and is excreted by the kidney as such.

These properties bear significantly on the application of tannin-rich plants as remedial agents. These have been popular in most traditions, particularly for treating wounds and burns. Here their ability to complex with exposed tissues to form a tough imperme-able 'leather' film has obvious advantages in protecting the wound from further harm and infection and hastening underlying healing. With third-degree burns the use of very strong tannin sources is the most effective traditional technique for preventing septicaemia and saving life. Pouring a strong decoction of tannin-rich material on the open flesh produces a sealing 'eschar' that provides almost a temporary new skin. The technique is still applied in rural China as part of the primary health-care system, and it is recommended as a first-aid measure where emergency services are defective. The technique involves repeated washings with the tannins. A useful bonus is provided by the fact that bacteria are killed by such exposure, so that tannins can be considered locally antiseptic too.

Tannins are also used externally as haemostatics to check haemor-rhaging, and to subdue exposed inflammations. They have notable benefit applied to mucosal surfaces lining the orifices, so that tannin-containing herbs are used as eyewashes, mouthwashes, va-ginal douches, snuffs, and as treatment for rectal problems.

Taken internally, these properties are carried to the wall of the gut: tannins 'curdle' mucus secretions, and contract or pucker the exposed cell walls of the lining epithelial membranes and so further inhibit cellular secretions. With the slender boundary between outside and interior found in the gut wall, the tannins' anti-inflammatory effect (involving lymph stasis and neutralization of autolytic enzymes) is more pronounced so that it finds particular application in controlling the symptoms of gastritis, enteritis, oesophagitis and inflammatory bowel problems.

The traditional application of tannin remedies for controlling diarrhoea is an example of this: in rural circumstances most diarrhoea (and this symptom is the main proximal cause of death in most of the world) is caused by inflammation or irritation in the small intestine – enteritis. The diarrhoea, of course, involves the large bowel but this is a reflex response originating higher up and designed to remove the offending material as speedily as possible. Although diarrhoea in this sense is a healthy response, it can, if prolonged, lead to dehydration and death very quickly. To control its ferocity, the use of good astringent remedies is indicated, and these work, not by 'stopping up' the flow, but by reducing the inflammation up in the small intestine.

In modern developed societies looseness of the bowel is often due to other causes than small-bowel infection, and these can include bowel spasm and degenerative inflammatory disease of the small or large bowel. Clearly the uses of tannins may be limited in such cases: however, as long as there is some local irritation involved, there is the chance that tannins will reduce the intensity of the reflex intestinal hurry. Although the application is a purely symptomatic one it differs from the use of such agents as kaolin and morphine by actually encouraging healing of the affected bowel wall, and some checking of any unwelcome pathogenic population.

Such beneficial effects of tannins in the bowel should be balanced against possible problems in their widespread use. It was noted that tannins form precipitates with all proteins. These include dietary proteins, of course. Once precipitated such protein-tannin complexes are far less likely to be absorbed into the bloodstream as they become resistant to the action of digestive enzymes. This fact should limit the time in which tannin-rich remedies are used. More importantly it casts a shadow over the widespread use of coffee and particularly tea. The astringent taste of over-steeped tea is familiar, and it is generally recommended that tea should be taken only lightly brewed. The whole picture is typically complex: caffeine, as an alkaloid, is also complexed by tannin – this means that it is less available to the body in the more tannin-rich tea than in coffee. There may even be advantages in the tannin effect: it is known that milk added to tea permanently changes its quality. This involves the formation of complexes with the milk proteins; for those allergic to cow's milk this may mean that milk taken in tea is acceptable (however, this should not be taken for granted); conversely, adding milk to tea's tannins effectively engages them so that they can do less to other proteins in the digestive tract.

Interference can also occur between tannins and alkaloidal and other pharmacological constituents: one must therefore expect some reduced activity in some plants if they contain high levels of tannin or if tannin-rich remedies are added to them in the same mixture.

Tannins are like mucilages in that they work as astringents only at point of contact, on the surface or on the gut wall. They have no appreciable astringent action on internal organs or tissues, although astringent plants may contain other constituents with this function.†

COUMARINS (and their glycosides)

This is a group of substances found very widely in plants but little studied pharmacologically. Coumarin itself is found particularly in the foliage of members of the pea family (e.g. clover) and in the grasses (where it gives the scent of new-mown hay). It is known mainly for its tendency to produce bloating in livestock grazing on pasture too rich in clover, and, extracted commercially from the tonka bean, as a perfume and perfume fixative.

The coumarins are derivatives of benzopyrone, where a pyrone ring is attached to the basic phenolic structure:

†In Galenic terms the tannin-rich remedies are described as 'dry', acting to 'strengthen', 'bind' and 'stop fluxes' (meaning discharges), but able, if taken inappropriately, to 'spoil the nourishment'. The connection with the points discussed above is clear, especially given the preponderance of diarrhoea as a symptom. There is connection too with the Chinese tradition although tannins were included in a much broader category, the 'sour' influences (see 'Chinese Pharmacology', on pp. 183–94).

coumarin

The fermentation product of coumarin itself, dicoumarol, found naturally in spoilt sweet clover, is a potent anticoagulant (the basis of warfarin rat poison) that eventually produces haemorrhage. Several coumarin derivatives have since been used as anticlotting agents in modern medicine: their similarity to the structure of vitamin K has led to speculation that they work by competing for that substance in the formation of the clotting factors prothrombin and factors VII, IX and X. This view is reinforced by the finding that the action of coumarins in this regard is counteracted by vitamin K.

It is the presence of anticoagulant coumarins (as well as the haemolytic *saponins*) that prevents safe injection of plant material directly into the bloodstream. Fortunately, the coumarins are neutralized to harmless derivatives in the digestive tract and normally present no difficulty on consumption. For these reasons they are not used as anticoagulants in herbal medicine (in fact, no such therapeutic category is found there).

Coumarin has some antibacterial properties: those of the mouse-eared hawkweed (*Pilosella officinarum*) have been found to be the most active agent in the traditional and apparently effective use of that plant in the treatment of undulant fever in goats.

Other derivatives of coumarin are known: the antifungal umbelliferone found in the Umbelliferae or parsley family and in many other individual remedies; the aglycone of the valuable vascular healing agent aesculin from horse chestnut (*Aesculus hippocastanum*); scopoletin from the deadly nightshade family; and the potent vasodilators khellin and visnagin from the Middle Eastern plant khellin (*Ammi visnaga*). Another well-known coumarin is bergapten, derived from bergamot oil, and used controversially as a sun-screening agent in many modern suntan lotions.

*ANTHRAQUINONES (and their glycosides)
Taste: BITTER

Plants containing anthraquinones have been used for millennia as dyestuffs and purgatives. This important commercial dual function led to an early isolation and characterization of the active principles, which were shown to be derived from, or related to, the substance anthraquinone. Notable dyestuffs include madder (*Rubia tinctorum*) and the insect-derived cochineal. Familiar laxatives include senna pods (*Cassia angustifolia* or *C. acutifolia*), cascara sagrada (*Rhamnus purshiana*), alder buckthorn (*Rhamnus frangula*), rhubarb root (*Rheum palmatum*), yellow dock (*Rumex crispus*) and aloes (*Aloe vera*).

There are a great many varieties of anthraquinone derivatives, found in several plant families. They all share the same basic molecular configuration:

anthraquinone

They tend to be found in the form of their glycosides (the aglycone or active part combined with one or more sugar molecules) which, because of the variety of possible sugars, increases the range even further. Direct anthraquinone derivatives include the following aglycones:

Rhein from *Rheum*, *Rumex* and *Cassia* spp.
Emodin from *Rhamnus* spp.
Aloe-emodin from *Rheum* and *Cassia* spp.
Chrysophanol from *Rheum* and *Rumex* spp.

There are also many reduced derivatives that polymerize to produce compounds like the sennosides of *Cassia* spp., and the reidins from *Rheum* spp. In addition there are biosynthetically distinct, but closely parallel, glycosides from aloes, of which aloin is the most notable.

From pharmacological investigation we know that the action of the anthraquinones is dependent on the presence in the gut of bile and on the fact that they are ingested in the glycoside form. The role of the bowel flora has also been firmly implicated (for example, it has been established that sennosides are hydrolysed to sennidins in a step-wise fashion via sennidin-8-monoglucosides, then reduced to rheinanthrone, a purgative active principle).[4] The isolated aglycone is inactive if ingested although it is potently active if ingested intravenously. All this suggests that bile and the sugar moiety are both necessary for the absorption of the anthraquinone from the gut, but that it is the aglycone alone that is active. Once in the bloodstream the aglycone is absorbed into the internal machinery of as yet undefined target cells and processed there (probably to emodin in all cases). Here it affects the protein biosynthetic pathway, probably leading to the formation of enzymes (all this is supposition based on the 8–14 hours it takes for an ingested dose of anthraquinone to be active: this is a typical time lag for protein or enzyme synthesis to be effected).[5] The final result seems to be the release of prostaglandins of the PGE series, which increase the irritability of the smooth muscle cells of the bowel wall (possible mechanisms for the 'irritation' include the stimulation of local cyclic AMP production and the inhibition of Na^+/K^+-ATPase).

The anthraquinone laxatives essentially irritate the bowel wall, provoking increased muscle contractions and peristaltic movements.

One must be careful here. Many people use anthraquinone laxatives as a daily ritual, finding that they cannot move their bowels without them. This is an increasingly irreversible condition. The general rule in herbal medicine is that the prolonged use of a stimulant leads to increasing loss of tone of the tissues stimulated: in other words, the underlying atonicity becomes worse. The only justified use of the stimulating laxatives then is as a short-term measure, to move an ongoing congestion or as part of a broader programme of bowel re-education (an effective approach is to use one part of an anthraquinone-containing remedy with two parts of chamomile and four parts of psyllium or linseed for a period of up to six months: even the most atonic bowel can have its tone restored with such a mixture – see the discussion of cascara sagrada in the materia medica section for more information).

There is another danger. By no means all constipations are brought about through atony of the bowel. Mass movements may be inhibited also by excessive tension of the bowel muscle. In the classic form as nervous or spastic colon, or 'mucous colitis', tension is transferred from the wider nervous system, leading to either bowel looseness or constipation, especially in response to external stresses or anxiety. In general any constipation that is made worse in periods of tension, alternates in any way with bowel looseness, is associated with the passage of small nut-like stools, or is found in children or adolescents, must be accepted as being due to excessive bowel tension and *must not be treated with stimulating laxatives*. (Visceral relaxants, such as are found frequently among herbal remedies, are the indicated therapy, coupled as always with a high level of gentle roughage – not bran.)

Looking at the remedies more closely, we note that anthraquinones, by their stimulating action, have a tendency to induce griping, manifested more in some remedies than others. Some, like alder buckthorn, are 'cured' by storage for a year or more, reducing the griping tendency. Most contain variable quantities of tannins that act to limit the intensity of the laxative action – and in the case of some like the docks and English rhubarb root (*Rheum palmatum*) actually lead to a use in cases of diarrhoea. In general one must assume other interactions between constituents in individual remedies, as always.

There are other influences too: the anthraquinone derivative rhein is significantly antiseptic and is especially toxic to the enteric pathogen *Shigella dysenteriae* as well as to *Staphylococci*.[6] Further, the general bitterness of the anthraquinones means, as we shall see when discussing the bitters as a group, that they stimulate digestive secretions, bile flow, and the upper digestive system as a whole.

It would however be unusual to give anthraquinone laxatives on their own: the general rule is to provide calming 'carminative' remedies such as fennel, dill (*Anethum graveolens*) or aniseed with them to stop any tendency to griping and to generally placate the bowel. For most prescriptions any laxative intent is part of a broader treatment anyway.

FLAVONES (and the flavonoid glycosides)
Taste: BITTER/SWEET

These are the most widely found of the phenols in the plant world. They occur in living tissues only as flavonoid glycosides (the aglycones are toxic to the plant and are isolated as such only from dead wood). They are found especially in flowers, fruit and leaves. Their colour (*flavus* means yellow) enables them to play a part in attracting pollinating insects, etc., but they are toxic to many insects and also appear to play a part in deterring insect predators. They are also thought to have growth-regulating properties in the living plant. Their taste is interesting: they can be either bitter or sweet. Modern chemical experiments show us that it takes only minor adjustment in the construction of any particular flavonoid to convert it from a sweet to a bitter substance or vice versa. This suggests that the receptors for bitterness and sweetness on the tongue are close together and structurally similar, a point that is relevant to our discussions on these two tastes elsewhere.

One may expect to find flavonoids in every plant, though their concentration varies widely, with some, like citrus fruits, buckwheat (*Fagopyrum esculentum*), and all white and yellow flowers, showing significantly high levels.

There are in fact four main groups of flavonoid aglycones based loosely on the flavone model:

flavone

1 Flavones
   e.g. apigenin in celery seed and parsley
   luteolin in *Equisetum* spp. (the horsetails)

1a Isoflavones (isomers of flavones with steroidal properties)
   e.g. genistein in clover, gorse and other legumes (a pro-
   oestrogen with oestrogenic properties)
   rotenone in derris (the basis of the well-known organic
   gardener's insecticide)

2 Flavonols
   e.g. quercitol (glycoside: rutin) in buckwheat, rue, and over half
   all plants tested
   kaempferol in around half all plants tested
   myricetin in woody plants only

3 Flavonones
   e.g. eriodictyol ⎫ together make up 'citrin' of citrus fruit
   methyleriodictyol ⎬ glycoside: hesperidin)
   liquiritigetol in liquorice

4 Xanthones
   e.g. gentisin in gentian

Flavonoids have several important pharmacological properties. Many are diuretic, some are antispasmodic, anti-inflammatory, antiseptic and even antitumour; all these qualities will be discussed in connection with the individual remedies in due course. However, the predominant action of the flavonoids as a group is on the vascular system. This has been highlighted in particular by the work done on the so-called *bioflavonoids* or 'vitamin P', principally hesperidin and rutin. In 1936 Albert von Szent-Gyorgyi discovered that ascorbic acid on its own was not sufficient to heal all cases of deficiency-induced scurvy (*purpura haemorrhagica*), and that lemon juice and extracts of red pepper were beneficial in these cases. A crystalline flavonoid fraction was isolated as having the particular effect, and given the name 'citrin'. Later this was found to be made up of a mixture of glycosides, of eriodictyol, and of methyler-iodictyol (later called hesperidin).

These components have the effect of decreasing capillary fragility and permeability. A third component was later discovered by chromatographic means as having the properties of quercitol, and was confirmed as rutin. This reinforces the effect on the capillaries but is in addition effective in lowering blood pressure. Rutin has thus been used allopathically to treat the capillary symptoms of hypertension, diabetes, salicylate and arsenic poisoning, and allergic conditions. It has found a modern application in the control of radiation-induced haemorrhage. Buckwheat is used by the modern herbalist for much the same problems, and there are many other remedies high in these flavonoids that are also applied. One may take particular note of yarrow (*Achillea millefolium*), elderflowers (*Sambucus nigra*), and lime or linden flowers (*Tilia* spp.).

In sum, we may view the presence of significant amounts of flavonoids in a plant as being particularly helpful in dealing with circulatory problems. They act as a stabilizing and calming factor in the peripheral circulation, and with additional anti-inflammatory and diuretic properties, their influence is likely to be well rounded. A plant notably exhibiting such properties is the hawthorn (*Crataegus oxyacantha*), to which full reference will be made in the materia medica.

Ascorbic acid

The example of the work of Szent-Gyorgyi illustrates a broader principle in herbal medicine. He showed that a supposed 'active principle', vitamin C or ascorbic acid, was therapeutically incomplete in isolation. When one realizes that ascorbic acid and the bioflavonoids are found together in almost all cases, it does seem that discussing ascorbic acid on its own is an unnecessary limitation.

Yet this is still the rule in modern medical debate. Trials are done on the possible value of ascorbic acid in preventing or treating the common cold, for example, without any attempt to differentiate between the effect of the isolated ascorbic acid and that of the ascorbic-acid-bioflavonoid complex, or in fact of the ascorbic-bioflavonoid-fruit-acid complex found in most fruits and berries. When the value of the bioflavonoids and fruit acids is appreciated one is surprised at this blind spot in modern medicine. In fact, this is just one of a multitude of cases where the whole plant is dissected to find out which of its constituents seems to convey its activity in a form that can be isolated, measured and patented. The whole is too crude and variable for modern analytical tastes, yet it is the infinite interactions between all the constituents of the whole that make up the action of the herbal remedy.

Proposition:

isolating active principles is not the way to capture all the qualities of the whole plant.

*Volatile Oils

The most complex and perhaps the most fascinating of herbal constituents, providing the herbal practitioner with one of the more potent aids to treatment, volatile oils are nevertheless barely recognized as useful by conventional pharmacologists.

A key feature of volatile oils is the obvious practical one. They by definition easily vaporize from their source material and in the gaseous form they stimulate the olfactory senses: in other words they have an odour. What this means is that firstly one can easily tell whether a herb contains volatile oils, and secondly that what one is smelling is escaping. Excessive boiling of remedies or their prolonged storage in adverse conditions will lead to an inevitable loss of the volatile component, a fact, of course, that can be readily appreciated by a reduction in aroma. Quality control of aromatic herbs is thus very simple although, as we shall see, there may be more to the aroma than that.

Generally speaking volatile oils are mixtures of hydrocarbons and oxygenated compounds derived therefrom. As the oxygenated form is more soluble in both water and alcohol, it is this form that on the whole determines the taste and smell of the mixture. The most common hydrocarbon is the terpene, built up by the successive accumulation of isoprene molecules (C_5H_8):

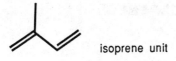 isoprene unit

By apposing different variations of this building block a wide range of substances can be synthesized, starting from the simplest upwards:

> monoterpenes $C_{10}H_{16}$
> sesquiterpenes $C_{15}H_{24}$
> diterpenes $C_{20}H_{32}$
> sesterterpenes $C_{25}H_{40}$
> triterpenes $C_{30}H_{48}$, etc.

Terpenes are synthesized a great deal in plants and include the basis for the steroidal molecule, carotenoid pigments and rubber, but we are interested here in only the smallest molecules, the mono- and sesquiterpenes, as being the only ones small enough to be volatile.

Monoterpenes are far and away the largest group of volatile oils and will dominate our discussion below. The names of the most common examples will become familiar as we go through the materia medica:

anethol	citronellal	menthone
borneol	cymene	nerol
camphene	cymol	phellandrene
camphor	fenchone	pinene
carvacrol	geraniol	terpineol
carvone	limonene	thujone
cineol	linalol	thymol
citral	menthol	

The *sesquiterpenes* are the largest group of terpenes in the plant world but only a few are volatile (notably the azulenes, bisabolol and farnesene, from chamomile and yarrow); the rest exhibit very interesting activities in other ways – some 60–70 have been found with appreciable antitumour activity, while many others are very bitter tasting and contribute to the *bitters* category we will be discussing below.[7]

We will start looking at the monoterpenes by discussing a few notable examples in more detail.

295   The Archetypal Plant Constituents

NOTABLE MONOTERPENES

Menthol

Extracted from peppermint (*Mentha x piperita*) and other members of the mint family, and existing in the crystalline state at room temperature, menthol is noticeably cooling on the skin and this is accompanied by a slight local anaesthetic action and followed by reflex local vasodilation. This combination of properties makes it a popular ingredient for liniments for muscular and joint pains.

It is also a powerful antiseptic and antiparasitic and in alcoholic solution it has been used for treating ringworm. It also appears to have some benefit in treating scaling from the scalp and any accompanying hair loss. When inhaled it checks nasopharyngeal catarrh and will bring welcome relief in nasal congestion: its use here, however, should be limited to the short term, as there is evidence that it has a cumulative irritating effect on the respiratory membranes that can help prolong a tendency to catarrh.

When ingested menthol is an effective carminative, as are most plant volatile oils, but it has captured particular attention for its apparent benefit in cases of colitis and bowel disease.

Camphor

Obtained naturally from the camphor plant (*Cinnamomum camphora*), or produced synthetically from a base of pinene isolated from turpentine, it is also likely to be found in other plants, e.g. some of the *Artemisia* spp., *Chrysanthemum* spp. (e.g. feverfew and tansy) and some of the Labiatae. It is closely related structurally to *borneol* (originally 'Borneo camphor'), found notably in rosemary (*Rosmarinus officinalis*) and shares many of its properties.

It is locally rubefacient and anti-inflammatory, producing also a menthol-like cooling (when isolated it shares with menthol and thymol the property of being solid at room temperature) which makes it slightly anaesthetic.

Internally it encourages the secretion of saliva and digestive juices, stimulates peristalsis and relaxes sphincters: it thus aids the whole digestive process. It is used as a circulatory stimulant, dilating the peripheral circulation, but it has a paradoxical action on the heart: stimulating it if failing yet dilating the coronary circulation (oil of rosemary is considered a heart tonic in Russian folk medicine).

Many of its properties can be explained, as with other volatile oils, by the reflex responses resulting from irritation of the stomach lining, but there is a direct action on the central nervous system as well: it stimulates CNS function and is an effective counter to barbiturate and morphine respiratory depression. It may under different circumstances produce feelings of exhilaration, or drowsiness and stupor. Inhaled it stimulates mucus flow and acts to cleanse a congested condition.

Thujone

Found notably in the oil of sage (*Salvia officinalis*), in which it makes up almost 30 per cent of the volatile component.

It is antiseptic and carminative like other terpenes. It is however relatively toxic, and although sage is very useful as a mouthwash and gargle, it can have unfortunate effects internally if given in quantity. It stimulates smooth muscle, and having also oestrogenic properties is contra-indicated in pregnancy and can arrest lactation.

To what extent thujone contributes to the unusual action of sage in inhibiting perspiration is not known (there is a possible general inhibition of glandular secretions through the body). It has a potentially useful effect in mental conditions, having in moderate doses a restorative and calming effect, probably in part through a visceral antispasmodic action: in large doses, however, it provokes irritability.

OTHER MONOTERPENES

Because of their relative structural simplicity, improved analytical procedures and commercial importance in the perfumery trade monoterpenes have been quite well investigated in modern times. Many of the old claims for them have been substantiated and even extended.

The antiseptic properties of monoterpenes have been confirmed. Compared with the standard phenol, the antiseptic capacity of some are as follows:

carvone	× 1.5	(the strength of phenol)
citronella	× 3.8	
menthol	× 4.0	
linalol	× 5.0	
citral	× 5.2	
geraniol	× 7.1	
thymol	× 20.0	

Some monoterpenes have fungicidal and anthelmintic effects, e.g. thymol and ascaridole, which is the major constituent of the rather toxic traditional agent for worm infestations, chenopodium oil (*Chenopodium ambrosioides*). Some monoterpenes also repel insects, e.g. citronellal.

The rubefacient circulatory-stimulating properties of such as menthol, camphor and borneol have been touched on, and many others are included in liniments and embrocations for the same reason. Internally the same properties form the basis of an expectorant action, e.g. cineol from eucalyptus oil, pinene from angelica (*Angelica archangelica*), pinene, borneol and others from thyme (*Thymus officinalis*); and of diuretic properties, e.g. diosphenol from buchu (*Barosma betulina*) and terpineol from juniper (*Juniperus communis*). In the first case the action is triggered by stimulation of the stomach lining, in the second it is a result of direct irritation of the urinary tubule wall.

Other monoterpenes act on the nervous system. The carminatives are essentially in this category, the action being spasmolytic by local reflex on the nerve endings in the gut. However, action on the nervous system is clearly more extensive than this: in-depth analysis of the action of a proprietary German preparation 'Melissengeist', extracted from the lemon balm (*Melissa officinalis*), showed that of its components some, e.g. citral, limonene, citronellol, citronellal and geraniol, had appreciable sedative activity, citronellal being the most potent. They were significantly effective at concentration down to 1 mg per kg of body weight, and some had observable spasmolytic action at concentrations comparable to the morphine alkaloid papaverine. Even more interesting was the clear effect demonstrated at the highest centres, as with psycho-autonomic problems such as are accompanied by symptoms of excitability, restlessness, headaches and palpitations. The otherwise extraneous information that the same monoterpenes are found concentrated in the hippocampus (in the limbic system) of the cat provides most interesting corroboration for a specifically central action for this group of substances.[8]

There is a further group of monoterpenes, the *iridoids* and their glycosides, which has a high level of pharmacological activity, but it is not volatile and will be considered later.

SESQUITERPENES

The sesquiterpenes, having a greater molecular weight, are much less volatile than the monoterpenes and are thus less associated with the volatile oils. The best examples of some that are come from the chamomiles (*Anthemis nobilis* and *Matricaria recutita*) and yarrow (*Achillea millefolium*).

The azulenes

These substances, for example chamazulene from chamomile and yarrow and guaiazulene from lignum-vitae (*Guaiacum officinale*), do not exist in any quantity in the natural state. They are produced as artefacts of the steam distillation process of extraction from volatile precursors in the plant such as matricin, achillin or artabsin. They will also be found in appreciable quantity after the normal process of infusion in hot water, especially if this is done in an enclosed container that allows steam rising to recondense and drain back into the liquid: to gain the full value of remedies such as chamomile and yarrow it is necessary therefore to make a hot infusion or tisane of them, and to take a measure of care in the process (see the chapter 'Remedies').

The azulenes are effective anti-inflammatory and antispasmodic agents, reducing histamine-induced tissue reactions and calming the nervous system, both peripherally, as in visceral tension, and centrally, as in anxiety, nervous tension and headaches. Their activity also extends to reducing the anaphylaxis consequent on the allergic response and they are thus indicated for conditions such as hay fever, allergic asthma and allergic eczema. They are strongly antiseptic on contact.

Bisabolol

This is a naturally occurring constituent of the volatile oil of chamomile (along with another anti-inflammatory sesquiterpene *farnesene*) and acts as partial compensation for any use of the plant that does not involve heating with water. It has been shown to reduce the amount of the proteolytic enzyme pepsin secreted by the stomach without any change occurring in the amount of stomach acid.[9] This suggests a specific interaction with pepsin activity, a possibility with great implication for the treatment of gastric and upper intestinal diseases. It has also exhibited direct anti-inflammatory action (on granulomas).

Other components

There are a great many other components of volatile oils. It is important therefore to return again to the important point that the whole should not be limited by a preoccupation with only a few of its parts. As an illustration it may be useful to quote in full the complete analysis of the constituents of the volatile fraction of cranberry juice[10] (see table below).

Given that even small volatile molecules have potential pharmacological action the conclusion of the above analysis is clear: volatile oils are complex in both constitution and effects.

Notable non-terpene constituents of volatile oils are the *ethers*. Their exact properties are reflected in the actions of the plants that contain them. Examples are anethole from aniseed (*Pimpinella anisum*) – in which it makes up 80–90 per cent of the volatile oil – and fennel (*Foeniculum vulgare*); cineole from the oil of the eucalyptus (*Eucalyptus globulus*) and cajaput (*Melaleuca leucadendron*); apiole from celery (*Apium graveolens*) and parsley (*Carum petroselinum*); and myristicin from nutmeg (*Myristica fragrans*). All these remedies have carminative, circulatory stimulant, aromatic digestive, warming expectorant and urinary antiseptic properties.

Another group of volatile constituents are those containing sulphur (such as *mercaptans* (R-SH), *monosulphides* (R-S-R¹) and

The volatile fraction of cranberry juice

Terpenes

pinene
myricene
limonene
linalol
terpineol (13 per cent)
nerol

Aliphatic alcohols

2-methyl-3-buten-2-ol
2-pentanol
pentanol
hexanol
1-octen-3-ol
octanol
nonanol
decanol
octadecanol

Aliphatic aldehydes

acetaldehyde
pentanal
hexanal
octanal
nonanal
decanal

Acids

benzoic acid (26.6 per cent)
2-methylbutyric acid

Aromatics

benzene
benzaldehyde (9.6 per cent)
benzyl ethyl ether
acetophenone
methyl benzoate
benzyl formate
ethyl benzoate
benzyl acetate
2-phenyl ethanol
2-hydroxy diphenyl
benzyl benzoate (11.9 per cent)
dibutyl phthalate
benzyl alcohol (6.0 per cent)
4-methoxy benzaldehyde

Others

diacetyl
ethyl acetate
2-furaldehyde
methyl heptanoate

disulphides (R-S-S-R^1)), which provide the *acrid* volatile components of garlic (*Allium sativum*), onion (*Allium cepa*), radish and asparagus. In the case of garlic and onion, the non-volatile molecule alliin is acted on by enzymes when the plant is crushed to produce the volatile disulphide allicin. This conveys many of the vasoactive and disinfectant properties of garlic, discussed in the materia medica.

In summary

We can now review the action of the volatile oils as a whole, picking up trends apparent from the discussion of the terpenes and putting them into a broader perspective.

Antiseptic: this property is linked in part with the ready lipid-solubility of volatile oils thus their easy entry into the interior of the pathogen. Once inside they seem to interfere selectively with the cell machinery of bacterial and fungal organisms. Some of the more toxic volatile oils are also poisonous to enteric worms, but these should be treated with caution, given the similarity of the metabolism of the worm and of its host.

The same lipid-solubility means that volatile oils are distributed easily throughout all the body compartments and into all the body excretions and secretions, so that their antiseptic action is maintained, for example, in the urinary system, the interior of the lungs and the bronchial tree, the sweat, salivary, vaginal and lachrymal secretions, and is carried in the case of the lactating or pregnant mother to the infant or foetus.

Apart from a direct antipathogenic effort, volatile oils have the side-effect of increasing the amount of white blood cells in the blood (leucocytosis): this brings them in line with other herbal 'antiseptics' in possibly supporting the body's own defences and encouraging endogenous protection as much as any direct disinfection.

Irritant: volatile oils stimulate tissues with which they come into contact. On the skin they stimulate underlying *circulation* (i.e. they are rubefacient), and this effect is observed on internal consumption as well. Many aromatic plants are associated with increasing circulation through the tissues (the remedies 'hot in the first, second, or third degree' in Galenic terms, are discussed in full in 'The Temperaments of Plant Remedies', on pp. 174–83) and the volatile oils of ginger (*Zingiber officinale*) do highlight a general tendency to provoke vasodilation, possibly by activating kinin, prostaglandins or other humoral mechanisms. This is one of the most important characteristics of the volatile oils.

The irritant effect is seen too on the lining of the alimentary tract, producing stimulation of the superficial nerve endings and reflex increases in salivation, gastric secretions and appetite, improved peristaltic co-ordination with the relief of flatulence, colic and purgative-induced griping. The so-called carminatives are particularly beneficial in these latter respects, and are referred to in this text as *aromatic digestives*. Some slightly harsher volatile oils, such as those of elecampane (*Inula helenium*), by stimulating the stomach wall a little more induce a reflex *expectoration* or clearing of any congested lungs. Similar reflexes possibly explain respiratory stimulation and even the circulatory stimulation noted above.

Relaxant: apparently contradicting the previous action, this property reflects the general influence that volatile oils have on nervous tissue. Any lipid-soluble substance will always tend to reach and affect the nervous tissues. Central effects are mostly of a tranquillizing nature, but may be stimulating in some circumstances (and include the effects on the limbic system discussed above); there is a peripheral *antispasmodic* effect as well. It is for this general action, peripheral as well as central, that the term 'relaxant' is used. We will encounter it again elsewhere. What it implies is that a state of tension can be as readily diminished viscerally, 'from the neck down', as by any sedative effect. This may be of immense value in treating and counselling a patient one is attempting to wean off tranquillizers and the unspoken assumptions about the mental state of the patient implied in their use. The body is often used as a sounding board to resonate states of tension. Although this tension is co-ordinated by the body's nervous system the term 'psycho-somatic' is not an accurate reflection of the totality of the tension's manifestation (the term somato-psychic has sometimes been used to denote this type of effect). One may often find, for example, that visceral relaxation of the stomach in nervous dyspepsia, the bowel in a spastic colon, or the bronchioles in asthmatic conditions, will not only ease the local conditions but will feed back to relieve tensions reflected in the central nervous system. The concepts that inspire the therapeutic applications of yoga are very similar. A great many aromatic plants will be found to have various relaxant effects.

The presence of volatile oils in a plant is immediately obvious by its aroma, and allowed such plants to be readily classified in traditional medicine.‡

*Resins   Taste: ACRID/ASTRINGENT

A complex group of solid or occasionally liquid substances insoluble in water but soluble in alcohol, ether and chloroform. They are produced by a number of plants either spontaneously or as a result of injury, and their role in the plant is probably to protect against the effects of insect, fungal or other infestation, or to seal the tissues against the effects of damage.

The essential resin is a mixture of resin acids, resin alcohols (resinols), resin phenols (resino-tannols), esters and inert substances called resenes. This may also be mixed with volatile oils and gums to form oleo-resins and gum-resins respectively (or compound mixtures like oleo-gum-resins). Other resins are complexed with aromatic balsamic acids like benzoic and cinnamic acids (which partially increase their solubility in water) and are referred to as balsamic resins or, if the balsamic component is large and the resin in a fluid form, simply balsams (this latter term is sometimes wrongly applied to oleo-resins).

   Resins include guaiacum (*Guaiacum* spp.), colophony (*Pinus* spp.) and dragon's blood (*Daemonorops* spp.).

---

‡The presence of volatile oils correlates principally with the rising tendency in the dynamic view of the plant (see 'The Four Tendencies', on pp. 172–4). The aroma of a plant can be clearly visualized as rising, ephemeral, an active essence of the plant. As such a force it was expected to promote upward and outward movements in the body such as expectoration and perspiration (a function we can confirm in many individual cases); it would help to disperse cold and remove obstructions in the peripheral regions, helping to repel external forces, and bringing heat from the core to the surface. The latter part of this description at least resembles closely the action of remedies 'hot in the first degree' in Galenic terms, and we may refer to the description of yarrow in the materia medica for a practical application of a peripheral vasodilator. Volatile remedies can also be 'hotter', up to 'third degree', yet with their relaxant properties their stimulant effect is often held in check.

Oleo-resins include crude turpentine (*Pinus* spp.) and copaiba (*Copaifera* spp.).

Oleo-gum-resins and gum-resins include myrrh (*Commiphora molmol*), frankincense (*Boswellia* spp.), asafoetida (*Ferula foetida*) and gamboge (*Garcinia hanburii*).

Balsamic resins include benzoin (*Styrax* spp.).

Balsams include balsam of Peru (*Myroxylon pereirae*), balsam of Tolu (*Myroxylon balsamum*) and storax (*Liquidambar orientalis*).

Apart from uses in pharmacy and industry, the medicinal effects of the resins are almost entirely as antiseptics and stimulants to phagocytic activity. In the form of mouthwashes or gargles they both disinfect the region and provoke a local increase in white-blood-cell counts (leucocytosis). It is likely that a similar effect occurs further down the digestive tract at least as far as the stomach and the duodenum.

The balsams have been used as antiseptic wound dressings for several centuries and in Western herbal medicine 90 per cent tinctures of myrrh and marigold (*Calendula officinalis*) are used as effective topical applications for infections of mucosal surfaces.

*Saponins Taste: SWEET

Deriving their name from the Latin *sapo*, meaning soap, saponins have long been implicated as that plant constituent producing frothing in aqueous solution, and in particular as the predominant principle of the European soapwort (*Saponaria officinalis*), the roots of which have been used as a rural soap substitute.

The pharmacological reputation of the saponins used to be a simple one: on injection, like all detergents, they cause lysis of the blood cells, haemolysis, and are thus highly toxic. Many arrow poisons have a saponin base. However, this has been shown to be a property of the whole molecule, a glycoside. On oral ingestion hydrolysis readily occurs, splitting the glycoside into its sugar moiety and the aglycone or sapogenin. The sapogenin does not possess haemolytic properties and is quite safe.

One thus merely has to remember that the saponins are a further reason for not injecting herbal extracts intravenously. It is interesting to note, moreover, that to fish and cold-blooded creatures saponins are always toxic in any form (and provide the basis for many fish poisons harmless to humans).

This rather negative reputation for saponins has been transformed since the 1960s by closer observation of the action of many herbal remedies, and in particular of the remedy ginseng. It is now accepted that these rather elusive substances are responsible for quite astonishing properties, and in some ways can claim to have challenged the whole edifice of orthodox pharmacology.

The high molecular weight of the saponins and their usual occurrence in groups have led to difficulties in isolating and elucidating them and their structures, but it is known that they can be divided into two categories on the basis of the structure of the sapogenin, as steroidal and triterpenoid saponins.

In both cases the sugar moiety is attached to the carbon-3 point (marked '3' above), and both skeletons are derived via the terpenoid biosynthetic pathway mentioned earlier. The steroidal form is found in the saponins of the monocotyledenous plant families (those related to the grasses) such as Dioscoreaceae, Liliaceae, and Amaryllidaceae, and, among the dicotyledons (the great bulk of plant families), in such as the foxglove (*Digitalis* spp.), nightshade families and in fenugreek (*Trigonella foenum-graecum*). They have a close structural relationship with steroid hormones, cardioactive glycosides and vitamin D, and this makes these saponins of commercial interest as starting points for the synthesis of such drugs, e.g. the use of dioscin in the yams (*Dioscorea* spp.) for the synthesis of the contraceptive hormones. Their contribution to the pharmacology of plants containing them is less notable than their triterpenoid counterparts, but the effect on the female hormonal system of fenugreek containing the sapogenin diosgenin, the effect on inflammatory conditions of wild yam (*Dioscorea villosa*) (dioscin) and sarsaparilla (sarsapogenin and smilogenin), the influence on the reproductive system of beth root (*Trillium erectum*) (trillarin) suggests that the steroidal nature of their saponins may be interacting with steroidal receptors in the body as the triterpenoids do, or may even act as *in vivo* precursors to the steroidal hormones. One important remedy we will be discussing, helonias, or false unicorn root (*Chamaelirium luteum*) has such notable clinical effects on the function of the ovaries, that such a hypothesis must be assumed. The toxic effects of the members of the nightshade family (the problems with greening in potatoes is a reminder), are due to steroidal saponins with alkaloidal properties.

The triterpenoid saponins are rare in the monocotyledons but are widely found elsewhere in the plant world, as a sort of vegetal version of the steroidal molecule. They may be present in considerable amounts, as evidenced by a tendency of the plant extract to foam in water. Most of the saponins discussed in this section – including those of remedies like ginseng (*Panax ginseng*) and liquorice (*Glycyrrhiza glabra*) – are of the triterpenoid variety.

All saponins have useful topical effects that have been largely neglected in modern pharmacology. The most notable is an effect on the respiratory system: a stimulating expectoration brought about by reflex stimulation of the stomach wall. This in turn is a result of the fact that most saponins when taken in bulk have emetic effect: their detergent action promotes elimination on the part of the stomach. When taken in sub-emetic dosages, the emetic action is sublimated to a reflex-stimulating expectoration as with such well-known alkaloidal emetics as lobelia (*Lobelia inflata*), or ipecacuanha, or ipecac, (*Cephaelis ipecacuanha*). Squills (*Urginea maritima*) is one example of an emetic-expectorant with a saponin constituent. Others include the cowslip (*Primula vera*), the common daisy (*Bellis perennis*), mullein flowers (*Verbascum thapsus*), the violet family (*Viola* spp.), snakeroot (*Polygala senega*) and liquorice (*Glycyrrhiza glabra*).

Other saponins have a less irritating effect on the digestive system, actually settling it and aiding the absorption of important minerals. The saponins of spinach, asparagus, beetroot, oats and many of the legumes are likely to have a useful action here.

Saponins are now known to have interesting systemic effects.[11] Many appear to be *anti-inflammatory*, such as those of figwort (*Scrophularia nodosa*), and the Chinese remedies *Akebia trifoliata* and *Bupleurum chinense*; others are notably *diuretic*, such as those of silver birch (*Betula pendula*) and corn silk (*Zea mays*). There is also a group of saponins with interesting prospects for the treatment of *vascular* disorders, perhaps including varicose veins, thrombotic conditions, arteritis, phlebitis and even arteriosclerosis; these have been highlighted in the vascular remedy horse chestnut (*Aesculus hippocastanum*), but as the saponin-containing remedies yarrow (*Achillea millefolium*) and limeflowers (*Tilia* spp.) overlap in their traditional applications, this may turn out to be a wider property.[12]

However, it is the peculiar characteristics of the 'Harmony' remedies that most capture attention. Formerly dismissed in the West as figments of the Oriental imagination, their worth has been confirmed in many cases, and a triterpenoid saponin content has been generally implicated. The long list includes:

> *Aralia manshurica*
> Chai Hu (*Bupleurum chinense*)
> Dang Gui (*Angelica sinensis*)
> ginseng, or in Chinese Ren Shen (*Panax ginseng*)
> Hu Mu (*Aralia chinensis*)
> jujube, or in Chinese Da Zao (*Zizyphus jujuba*)
> liquorice, or in Chinese Gan Cao (*Glycyrrhiza uralensis*)
> Siberian ginseng (*Eleutherococcus senticosus*)
> Yuan Zhi (*Polygala tenuifolia*)
> Wu Wei Zi (*Schizandra chinensis*)

These remedies are among those used in Chinese and other Eastern medicine as harmonizing tonics or 'king' remedies. We shall look more closely at the examples of ginseng and liquorice in the materia medica. It does appear that the saponin constituent has a complex interaction with hormonal receptor sites so as to provide a uniquely balanced series of relationships with the metabolism, energy economy and mood. Their remarkable 'amphoteric' properties (appearing to be indicated for contradictory symptoms in any particular area) have led to great difficulty in their being accepted by the conventional pharmacologist, but as we shall see in the case of ginseng, this can be explained quite rationally. Acceptance of such a contribution would lead to a totally new model of pharmacology, one that becomes especially applicable to the understanding of many Chinese herbal remedies. We can summarize the main features of the model as follows:[13]

> Given the extremely subtle control mechanisms existing within the living body, especially in regard to hormonal and chemical co-ordination, it is theoretically possible, by interacting with the communication channels involved (such as receptor sites), to have remedies that are *state-specific*; this means that remedies have *different actions* dependent on the prior state of the body they act upon – we may thus be forced to abandon the idea of a standardized effect.

> If a state-specific remedy acts at the site of central co-ordination in a control system it is possible that it can improve the overall *adaptability* of the whole system; the effect of those remedies that have been studied has led to researchers describing them as 'adaptogenic'.

> The adaptogenic remedies suggest a different form of treatment: instead of using remedies to correct specific faults they can be applied as part of a wider programme to maintain balance and homoeostasis, when this is put under threat; this not only allows us treatment of illness before it becomes a serious problem, but also leads to a view of the condition from the vital rather than the pathological perspective.§

§The fact that the saponins have a subtle sweet taste (and in the case of liquorice a very sweet taste) is interesting. They thus ally themselves with the nourishing and stabilizing cereals and vegetables as manifestations of the Earth in Chinese medicine. In particular they share the qualities ascribed to the sweet *Taste* of tonifying, maintaining the balance, toning the *Spleen*, acting mainly in the 'middle heater', and of being indicated in deficiency states.

*Cardioactive Glycosides

These plant constituents share with the morphine alkaloids the distinction of being the most intensively studied and used in allopathic medicine, and, in isolation, of being simple conventional drugs. We will thus see a direct action on a target tissue, with conventional side-effects and potential toxicity, and the resulting need to be more circumspect in prescription. We will however be reminded of the fact that in the whole plant there are influences that broaden the range of action of the remedy and to varying extents provide a measure of protection. Nevertheless, this constituent is the first of another breed: those that give the herbal remedy a sharp edge.

Ever since Withering isolated the action of the foxglove (*Digitalis* spp.) from the prescription made up by an English West Country herbalist for dropsy in 1785, the value of the cardioactive glycosides in supporting a failing heart and preventing the unpleasant symptoms that follow has been extremely well established. Dropsy was the only obvious sign of heart failure in former times: it is the fluid accumulation that collects due to the inability of a failing heart to adequately handle the venous return; in the case of the right heart, the resulting fluid collects in accordance with the force of gravity in the ankles, legs and lower abdominal cavity; if the left heart fails, the fluid collects behind it in the lungs, giving breathlessness on exertion or when lying down; before the role of the heart was established, the automatic procedure was to diagnose diuretics to clear the water.

The use of cardioactive glycosides by at least some herbalists is likely therefore to have been empirical good fortune. Their properties otherwise were not lost on our ancestors, however: plants with cardioactive glycosides were widely used by hunter-gatherer communities around the world as arrow poisons.

The cardiac glycosides are built up from a steroidal aglycone having very similar properties and origins to the steroidal saponins (they are sometimes found together) and thus to the steroid hormones, vitamin D, the bile acids and cholesterol. They are divided into two groups on the basis of whether the aglycone possesses a five- or six-membered lactone ring:

bufadenolide
skeleton

cardenolide
skeleton

The bufadenolides (so called from their structural similarity to constituents in toad venom), are restricted to the Liliaceae (such as squills) and the buttercup family, or Ranunculaceae (such as the hellebores). The cardenolides are by far the most common variety.

The essential pharmacological activity of the glycosides resides in the aglycone: nevertheless, the sugar moiety is relatively complex and influences the availability and distribution of the aglycone and its specific presentation to the heart tissue. This accounts for the different effects apparent in the use of the whole foxglove leaf (*Digitalis* spp.): the interconversion between glycosides that occurs as sugar chains are gradually hydrolysed in the body allows for quite a complex bioavailability in the natural mixture of glycosides.

The notable effect of the cardiac aglycones is on the heart muscle. One observed action is on the potassium-calcium balance across the myocardial cell membrane, so that potassium is lost from the cell and calcium raised, this then being better able to catalyse muscle contraction (there is also possibly a secondary effect of the aglycone on the calcium mechanism). As well as calcium accumulation in the cell, there is a relative concentration of sodium ions relative to the potassium loss, this effect being repeated in other cells throughout the body.

The cardiac glycosides of the heart have effects on two types of heart activity: inotropic (force of contraction) and chronotropic (rate and rhythm of contraction). In brief there is a reduction in the heart rate but an increase in the force of contraction: an effective increase in the efficiency of the heart's work so that cardiac output per unit of oxygen consumed is much improved. One feature of congestive heart failure is a reduced ability to utilize available energy, so that nutritional demands of the heart (and thus its coronary circulation) remain high even though it is doing less work: the result is often compensatory hypertrophy of the heart muscle and a risk of anoxia and coronary infarction. The applicability of the cardiac glycosides to this condition should be quite obvious. They are indicated too in conditions predisposing to arrhythmias, tachycardia or fibrillation, where their effect on ionic movement across the cell membrane has the effect of reducing the sensitivity of the myocardium to potentially stimulating irritations. As such problems can occur along with heart failure, this is an added bonus.

The effect of the cardiac glycosides on the heart varies with the condition of its muscle cells, and the dosage of the medication. The chronotropic effect is seen only with a somewhat higher dose than the inotropic action. Secondly, in the atrial region which includes the pacemaker site and generally more sensitive musculature, the cardiac glycosides are liable to lead to an increase in sensitivity over a certain dose range, with an increased likelihood of fibrillation and other complications. All effectively hinges on the levels of ambient *potassium*: potassium ions in the extracellular fluid are antagonistic to the action of the cardiac glycosides and exert a steadying influence. If potassium levels fall too low, the toxic effects of the glycosides become apparent at even low dosages. This used to be a major hazard in the treatment of heart failure: one of the usual practices is to give diuretics to relieve some excess fluid retention and take some strain off the heart so that it can respond more easily to stimulation; unfortunately diuretics produce an inevitable loss from the body of potassium ions. Only when this was realized were potassium supplements added to diuretics (generally indicated by the suffix 'K'), and many cases of death due to digoxin poisoning prevented.

The herbal practitioner in Britain using cardiac remedies regularly uses the leaves of dandelion (*Taraxacum officinale*) as an accompanying diuretic: this has been shown to have unusually high levels of potassium, enough to lead to a net gain of potassium in the body after the diuresis has resulted.

312   Traditional Pharmacology

The use of cardiac remedies is not to be recommended by those clinically untrained. If heart failure is a factor, there is probably a digoxin prescription being taken already and the main question is whether this can be compatible with other treatments being considered. In those cases where heart failure is diagnosed *de novo* in the course of treating with herbs, then it would be obviously foolhardy to plunge into an attempt to control it without previous experience. In Britain the favourite cardioactive remedy among medical herbalists is lily-of-the-valley leaves (*Convallaria majalis*) that have a particularly selective action, low toxicity, and an unusual mixture of cardiac glycosides that ensures a slow-onset effect in total (interestingly the plant is almost ignored by modern pharmacologists as no single glycoside stands out as notable).[14]

Other remedies containing cardiac glycosides should be treated as toxic (except where stated). They include:

> black hellebore (*Helleborus niger*)
> figwort (not at all toxic) (*Scrophularia nodosa*)
> foxglove (*Digitalis purpurea, D. lanata*)
> green hellebore (*Helleborus viride*)
> hedge hyssop (*Gratiola officinalis*)
> kombe, or strophantus (*Strophantus kombe*)
> ouabain (*Strophantus gratus*)
> pheasant's eye (*Adonis vernalis*)
> squills (not toxic in careful use) (*Urginea maritima*)

*Cyanogenic Glycosides

Taste: BITTER

This group is so called because after hydrolysis (breaking down to sugar and aglycone in the presence of water) the aglycone converts to hydrogen *cyanide* (prussic acid). In any quantity, therefore, these glycosides are extremely toxic. Most of us are familiar with the fact that bitter almonds and other stone-fruit kernels (peaches, apricots, plums, etc.) contain these poisons, and that the smell of bitter almonds (in fact, the smell of benzaldehyde, an intermediate in the formation of the cyanide) plays a part in many of the quainter detective stories. Apart from the stone-fruits, cyanogenic glycosides are found in many other plants, some like clover, flax and elder, hawthorn and other members of the Rosaceae, used quite freely for other medicinal uses without risk. They are found in large amounts in the South American Indian staple food cassava, or manioc, preparation of which thus involves careful boiling and leaching (incidentally an astonishing example of the intimacy traditional humans have with their local flora).

In small quantities the cyanogenic glycosides confer useful therapeutic properties. Plants containing them are *antispasmodic* and *sedative*, as seen in the antitussive properties of wild cherry bark (*Prunus serotina*), a popular cough syrup. They *increase activity in the parasympathetic nervous system*, so by increasing vagal tone they slow the heart rate and improve digestion (hence the habit of eating almonds and almond desserts after meals in the Middle East).

They are excreted rapidly through the lungs, where they have the effect of transiently increasing respiration (wild cherry bark again). They contribute to the therapeutic effects of hawthorn (*Crataegus oxyacantha*), yarrow (*Achillea millefolium*), and chamomile (*Anthemis nobilis* and *Matricaria recutita*), some of the safest plants in the materia medica, which demonstrates again the inadvisability of condemning a plant or vegetable solely on the basis of its lists of constituents. However, excessive consumption is clearly dangerous in any case: poisoning episodes with excess almond consumption (especially if adulterated with bitter almonds), and plum cherry liqueurs are recorded.

The apparent tendency of the cyanogenic glycosides to damage first those cells that are actively dividing has led to attempts to harness the toxicity to the inhibition of tumour cells. This is possibly one explanation for the benefit of red clover flowers (*Trifolium pratense*) taken in quantity for such conditions. The most notable example, in recent years, however, has been the use of the cyanogenic glycoside amygdalin (found in almonds, all stone-fruit kernels, and widely through the Rosaceae) obtained specifically from apricot kernels. This is a prominent component of a new health-remedy variously labelled 'laetrile' or 'vitamin B17', which is sold as a remedy against cancer. This remains a highly controversial treatment and the remedy is almost certainly overrated, but it is not inconceivable that it might have a selective toxicity against malignant cells. The irony is that, even if it was to benefit cancer, this would be on conventional chemotherapy terms rather than on the 'natural health' basis claimed for it. Laetrile is essentially toxic.

Mustard Oil Glycosides Taste: ACRID

The mustard oil glycosides, or glucosilinates, are pungent components found almost only in members of the cabbage family, the Cruciferae; around 60–70 different examples have been isolated from members of the group. They are found distributed through the plant, but particularly in the cortex of the stem and the seeds. The active pharmacological agents are as always the products of hydrolysis, the aglycones, in this case highly irritable isothiocyanates, thiocyanates, nitriles and thiourethanes.

The volatile isothiocyanates are the basis for the acrid vapour produced when the plant is damaged, while by far the most toxic constituents are the nitriles, produced particularly by subjecting the plant to water at very high temperatures.

As with some other acrid constituents the key factor in the formula of the glucosilinates seems to be the presence of sulphur. Their general formula can be expressed as follows:

$$(R)-C \overset{S-\!\!\!\diagup\!\!\!\bigcirc-\text{sugar}}{\underset{N-O-SO_2-OH}{\big|}}$$

The glycosides are readily hydrolysed, mainly, in fact, on damage of the plant because of the liberation of an enzyme myrosinase. The whole glycoside is thus rarely encountered as such.

Plants containing these glycosides are primarily irritant to the membranes they contact. They are much used externally as *rubefacients*, to provoke local increase in blood flow, and even as *vesicants* (producing blisters), in the form of poultices for inflamed joints and other inflammations. Mustard plasters are the most common examples of this approach.

In this and in all other examples the mustard oil glycosides share the properties of a larger category of acrid constituents considered below. A special consideration in this case, however, is the inadvisability of using water above 45°C (113°F) to make the poultice, so that a minimum of toxic nitriles is produced.

There is one other individual factor that distinguishes mustard glycosides from other acrid constituents: they are *goitregenic*, that is they depress thyroid function. The effect is only noticed when the plants are consumed in quantity, but it is a clear epidemiological factor where cabbage is a major staple, or where milk is drunk from cows fed large quantities of Cruciferous plants like kale, shepherd's purse or charlock; in all cases a low intake of iodine (as in inland communities) is a necessary co-factor. Although unlikely to be significant in normal therapeutic use, this effect does make the Cruciferous plants contra-indicated in cases of hypothyroidism (as should be the consumption of excessive brassica vegetables). Incidentally, one may note that boiling cabbage does produce low levels of toxic nitriles: however, this is one plant toxin that no one seems to be worried about!

The following are some Cruciferous plants all containing mustard oil glycosides:

> black mustard (*Brassica nigra*)
> cabbage, cauliflower, kale, broccoli, kohlrabi (*Brassica oleracea*)
> charlock (*Sinapsis arvensis*)
> horseradish (*Cochlearia armoracia*)
> nasturtium (*Tropaeolum majus*)
> radish (*Raphanus sativus*)

rape (*Brassica napus*)
scurvy grass (*Cochlearia officinalis*)
shepherd's purse (*Capsella bursa-pastoris*)
turnip (*Brassica rapa*)
wallflower (*Cheiranthus cheiri*)
watercress (*Nasturtium officinale*)
white mustard (*Sinapsis alba*)

*Miscellaneous Acrid Constituents   Taste: ACRID

The mustard oil glycosides represent only one group of irritant, pungent constituents used in herbal medicine. Primary among the rest are the acrid *alkaloids* such as capsaicin found in cayenne and chilli peppers (*Capsicum minimum*), and the miscellaneous components (including *volatile oils*) found in other spices, notably ginger (*Zingiber officinale*). Also to be included are the *sulphur-containing constituents* of the onion family, notably garlic (*Allium sativum*). They all share pharmacological characteristics with the mustard oil glycosides.

The main action of the acrid agents is to stimulate the circulation. This is an extension of their general irritable nature which involves provoking a low-grade inflammatory response from living tissues. The action can be evoked after both external and internal application.

Externally the acrid constituents are widely used in the form of poultices or ointments as *rubefacients* and *vesicants* over inflamed organs or tissues, particularly arthritic joints, in a paradoxical action referred to as *counter-irritation*.

The explanation proffered is that such remedies provide a therapeutic inflammation without the mediation of painful and possibly destructive inflammatory agents like histamine. They certainly provoke the necessary dilation of blood vessels in the area (like a mild burn), making the patch appear quite red, and a consequent increase in blood flow to the affected tissues. If the role of inflammation is seen to be essentially positive (see 'Inflammation', on pp. 58–63), then a mechanism that can provide its benefits with minimal side-effects can be justified. The traditional view was that in making the inflammatory process less essential, it was possible to diminish its intensity.

If left on for an extended period, a strong acrid poultice will stimulate the vasculature to such an extent that the blood-vessel walls start to leak, and local blistering occurs. Herbalists of the old school would produce blistering as a matter of course, then lance and drain it, to produce apparent miracles of relief in severely arthritic joints for some appreciable time thereafter. Their explanation was that the technique allowed locally accumulated toxins to be drained off, thus relieving the inflammation of its major task. (It is strongly recommended that those without practical training in the technique should leave it well alone, and confine themselves to producing a mild erythema instead!)

The stimulation of circulation at a local level touches on wider considerations of central importance to the practice of herbal medicine. These are well illustrated by the internal applications for the acrid remedies. On ingestion the irritant action of these agents is continued, first on the mouth and oesophageal mucosa and then on the stomach wall leading to the increased production of gastric acid (see below). Whether from reflex from such mucosal irritation or after absorption into the bloodstream, the vasculature is provoked, leading to a material *increase in blood flow* through all the tissues in the body. The sensations that follow are familiar to all who have eaten a hot spicy meal: there is flushing of the skin and increased perspiration, with an overall feeling of warmth and resistance to cold. In short the acrid remedies appear to *generate heat* in the body.

In general one can conclude that increased circulation is reflected in an increase in tissue temperature. The body produces heat as a 'waste product' of its metabolic processes and then attends closely to its adequate dispersal. The bloodstream is the main heat channel from interior to exterior: arterial blood carries heat with it. The fact that ingestion of acrid constituents produces more heat was the key observation in ancient times and the association is still a key part of herbal therapeutics.

How the acrid constituents effect these changes is still not clear, but one important example, the alkaloid capsaicin from cayenne, has prostaglandin properties and it is quite possible to speculate that a direct action on the potent vasodilatory mechanisms operating in all body tissues is involved. However, in addition to dispersing circulation more effectively, the acrid remedies also clearly add to the body's total quota of heat: it must be assumed that they also have a stimulating effect on aspects of heat-producing metabolism.

We can see how the 'hot' remedies were applied in traditional practice in Part I (see 'The Temperaments of Plant Remedies', on pp. 174–82). The idea, in modern terms, was to induce a 'therapeutic fever' in those cases of febrile disease where vitality was seen to be depressed or debilitated. This assumed a completely different view of the value of fever from that prevailing in establishment circles, where the primary objective was to staunch it and the distress and possible harm it caused as effectively as possible. Seeing fever, like inflammation, as an attempt by the body to repel pathogenic influences, the traditional practice was to nurture and manage the process so that it would be allowed to complete its task with the minimum of trouble. The other effects of the acrid remedies can be appreciated in this context: increasing sweat production, maintaining the circulatory effort throughout the body, improving the ability of the digestive system to denature any gut contents, and in most cases disinfecting and increasing elimination from the lungs (see below).

In modern times demands for fever management are far less pressing than they were in traditional times, when febrile diseases were the main cause of death. Thus the importance of increasing heat has also diminished. However, the acrid remedies are still indicated whenever there is an apparently sluggish circulation, or when the sensation of cold is a feature of a syndrome. In such cases they may bring apparent relief beyond that expected by their immediate pharmacological actions.

The acrid remedies have other specific applications. They stimulate the secretion of stomach acid, they tend to settle digestion in the lower gut, and many are sterilizing expectorants.

Stomach acid is one of the most important defence mechanisms in the body. When secreted adequately it ensures that food is sterilized. It is difficult to contract enteric infections, like cholera, typhoid, dysentery, or others less critical, if the stomach secretions are maintained. Maintaining these secretions is thus the main priority where enteric diseases are endemic. Strong acrid remedies *stimulate stomach acid production* and in such areas eating spicy foods is the norm. It is a practice to be recommended to visitors to such areas as well, and to public health programmes as a cheaper and less harmful alternative to mass vaccination.

The gastric action, however, does provide one major contraindication for the acrid constituents: they should not be used where there is peptic ulceration or other problems of gastric hyperacidity.

The effects of the acrid remedies lower down the digestive tract are relaxing rather than stimulating. They tend to have a *carminative* action: reducing flatus, colic and other signs of poor digestion. Along with the action to stimulate gastric acid they thus make ideal condiments, especially with meat and other rich foods.

Many acrid constituents are removed from the bloodstream through the lungs. For this to occur the constituents must be volatile and as such they are simply breathed off. The volatile oils of ginger and garlic and the volatile isothiocyanates of horseradish are the main examples. As the acrid constituents are harmful to pathogens and the volatile oils doubly so, pulmonary excretion effectively disinfects the lungs, from the lowest regions upwards (garlic has exceptional properties here). They also act as *expectorants*, improving the flow upwards of bronchial mucus, and in their usual way actually warm the lungs. They are thus ideal for bronchial and pulmonary infections and other examples where the lungs are affected by 'cold' catarrhal congestion.

The case of the acrid remedies highlights further principles that could characterize herbal pharmacology.‖

‖There is broad agreement between traditional European and Chinese views on the pharmacological action of the acrid remedies. In Galenic terms they open the pores, promote perspiration, 'soften tough humours' (humours or toxic accumulations that are 'congealed or cold'), and encourage their elimination; they raise the vital heat of the blood and help to fend off injurious cold (a Galenic metaphor for all disease).

Propositions:

in certain presentations a simple remedy can effect profound recuperative changes in the body;

in a different presentation the same remedy can be counter-productive.

*Bitter Principles   Taste: BITTER

This group of constituents is probably even more central to herbal therapeutics than the acrid constituents are, especially in modern times. Most herbal prescriptions have an element of bitterness to them, and this is the quality most remarked on by those taking them for the first time. It is that quality that most characterizes herbal medicine and sets it apart from other therapies.

Comprised chemically of the most diverse array of molecular structures, the bitter principles have in common the ability to stimulate the bitter receptors inside the mouth, and thus evoke the taste of bitterness. Unlike other taste effects that of bitter stimulation seems to involve no electrical event on the surface of the cells: the conclusion is that each bitter molecule acts on cell membrane receptors to produce intracellular biochemical changes. The immediate result is a rise in the concentration of calcium within the cell: this is likely to initiate the signal to the gustatory nerve.[15] All the pharmacological effects that shall be discussed follow from this simple stimulation.

The largest group of bitter substances are of terpenoid structure, in particular the monoterpene iridoids and secoiridoids and the sesquiterpene lactones.

Iridoids comprise the main bitter constituents of the Gentianaceae, chicory (*Cichorium intybus*), wild lettuce (*Lactuca virosa*), dandelion, quassia bark, and valerian root (*Valeriana officinalis*).

Sesquiterpenes are responsible for the major bitterness of the

Artemisia, or wormwood genus, blessed thistle (*Cnicus bene-dictus*), and ginkgo (*Ginkgo biloba*).

There are also diterpene bitters, as in white horehound (*Marrubium vulgare*) or columbo root (*jateorrhiza palmata*), and triterpenoids have been found to be responsible for the toxic bitterness of the Curcubitaceae (including colocynth, the bryonies, pumpkin, cucumber and marrows).

Many alkaloids are bitter, notable among these being the proto-berberine isoquinoline alkaloids of *Berberis*, and golden seal (*Hydrastis canadensis*), the morphine alkaloids, the purine alkaloids (e.g. in coffee) and the quinoline alkaloids of quinine and angostura.

There are many miscellaneous compounds with bitter taste. For example, the strong bitterness of hops is due to a mixture of ketones and amino-acids.

A glance through the list of bitter plants above will pick out many articles used commonly in social contexts. Dandelion and chicory roots are used with coffee beans (*Caffea arabica*) to provide a pleasant after-meal bitter drink. The drink vermouth gets its name from the bitter plant wormwood (*Artemisia absinthium*) and is widely used as an appetite-stimulating aperitif; the same principle underlines the digestive action of traditional bitter beer brewed with hops (*Humulus lupulus*). It is still a common practice to inquire of the bar if a tot of Angostura Bitters (*Cusparia angustura*) is available to settle a hangover. All these uses are manifestations of a universal cultural experience that bitters are excellent adjuncts to food (especially when eating richly or in quantity) as well as being the basis of the best tonics. Repeatedly, in the records of traditional plant medicine, we find that bitter remedies are referred to as the 'true stimulants', a notion surviving in the modern idiom that 'nasty-tasting medicines are the best for you'. How can all these reputations be explained?

Our comprehension of the action of the bitter remedies has moved far in recent years. We know that they are only effective in the stimulation of the bitter taste receptors (although many have additional pharmacological actions in their own right as can be seen later) and have no effect, for example, if administered in capsule form or by intra-gastric tube. It is thus the bitter receptors that mediate the responses witnessed, a classic example of a reflex response where a small stimulus provokes a complex patterned reaction. It is now known that the immediate result of bitter taste bud stimulation is the release of the gastrointestinal hormone *gastrin*.[16] By looking at the known physiological action of gastrin, we find a close match with the traditional applications of the bitters. This permits boldness in interpreting the action of bitters, and to make useful correspondences with traditional concepts.

We find that the action of gastrin is to increase the following:

> gastric acid and pepsin secretions
> pancreatic digestive secretions
> intestinal juice production
> hepatic bile flow
> hepatic bicarbonate production
> Brunner's glands secretions
> intrinsic factor secretion
> insulin, glucagon and calcitonin secretions
> muscle tone of lower oesophageal sphincter
> muscle tone of stomach and small intestine
> cell division and growth of gastric and duodenal mucosa
> cell division and growth of the pancreas.

By using this information we can elaborate the usual indications for bitters in the herbal tradition.

Bitters increase appetite: gastrin is among several known factors that increase appetite, either by acting directly on appetite centres in the hypothalamus, or indirectly through increased stomach motility. Bitters too have been used as the basis for aperitifs or to induce appetite in convalescence. In modern practice they may find use in helping anyone in whom anorexia is perceived to be hindering repair or recovery. Sometimes, of course, a lack of appetite is a vital protective measure preventing overloading of a body already preoccupied with other matters, but it should be possible to distinguish this anorexia from the debilitating condition that often accompanies reduced vitality, and for which bitters administration can be ideal. In cases of anorexia nervosa the use of bitters may provide a useful tool in the wider management of the condition.

Bitters increase digestive secretions: by increasing stomach and pancreatic enzyme secretions, bitters aid the body in its break-down of food material, an effect particularly significant if these secretions are chronically defective. In brief, digestive secretions are responsible for both sterilizing the stomach contents and for break-ing down protein and other large molecules that would otherwise present an antigenic threat to the body's immune system.

It is a paradoxical but critical fact that food is not only the essential nourishment for the body but that it also presents by far the greatest potential immunological challenge to it, a fact reflected in the intense investment of the digestive tract by lym-phoid tissues. It is only the denaturing of antigenic material by the digestive juices that contains what would otherwise be an almost intolerable situation (see 'The challenge of food', on p. 75).

A low rate of secretion can be inferred if there are signs of liability to enteric infections, or if there is any suggestion of antigen pen-etration through the gut wall, for example food allergies or any autoimmune problem coincident with evidence of depressed diges-tion.

A key point in herbal therapeutics is that depressed digestive secretion has immense potential for harm in the body and should be corrected wherever it is encountered. Apart from enteric infec-tions and food allergies, signs of such depression are a nauseous congested or bloating feeling after eating even a little food, or small malodorous stools.

With the increasing dietary adulteration in modern foods the risk from that source has increased considerably, so that the indica-tions for bitter remedies are likewise more common. They are a valuable resource.

The action of the bitters in increasing the destructive components of digestive secretions has led to the tendency to discourage their use in cases of hyperacidity or such problems as peptic ulcerations. Yet it will have been noticed that secretions of protective fluids, such as bicarbonate from liver and pancreas and from the Brunner's glands, are also raised. In other words, unlike the acrid constituents the bitters stimulate the totality of digestive activity. There are other reasons why bitters are not necessarily contra-indicated in hyperacidic conditions:

Bitters protect gut tissues: by increasing the tone of the gastro-oesophageal sphincter, bitter remedies help prevent reflux of corrosive stomach contents into the oesophagus in 'heartburn', hiatus hernia or oesophageal inflammation. By improving the already rapid rate of mucosal regeneration in the stomach and duodenum, the bitters may also reduce the damaging effects there of digestive juices and dietary toxins, and actually promote healing in the case of infection or ulceration. By having a similar action on the matrix of the pancreas, they may help in the recovery from pancreatic disease as well (and more speculatively, although traditional usage is supportive – see below – may also help pancreatic endocrine tissue in recovery from late-onset or toxic diabetes mellitus).

Bitters promote bile flow: bile is the excretion and secretion of the liver. Such are the fluid dynamics in the liver that each cell can be perceived as sitting in a stream – of a mixed nutrient-rich portal blood from the gut and oxygen-rich arterial blood from the general circulation. As these fluids diffuse through the cell they are subjected to the intense processing associated generally with liver function. Most metabolic products of this activity pass from the liver cell into the outgoing blood flow; some of the most significant, however, are passed into a separate exit that drains into the biliary system. The liver cell is thus essentially self-cleansing.

The organ can however be subjected to heavy toxic loads, whether as the result of an unhealthy diet, or defective digestion (see above) or general ill health, with the production or accumulation of waste material. Under these circumstances the fluid flowing through each liver cell may not be enough to keep it clean and there will be a threat to liver health, either involving obvious liver pathology or the more common range of functional disorders. To have an improved bile flow will effectively help to keep the liver free of such accumulations. Thus it is that the bitters have in every tradition been associated with improving liver function. The demand for their use in an increasingly toxic age is more than it ever was.

Their use has been considered in metabolic, allergic and immunological conditions where investigations point in the direction of the digestive system (it is known that the liver has an influence over the immunological system). One will often find, for example, that herbal treatment of migraines will include 'hepatic' remedies, most of which happen to be bitter.

There is not only a greater production of biliary elements as a result of prescribing bitters, there is also a substantial diluting of bile, possibly with an increase in bicarbonate content as well. This has benefits wherever there is gallstone formation or gall-bladder disease, connected as these are with an over-concentrated bile. Bitters are thus one of the most established treatments for these problems (along with acidic remedies like lemon juice for their effect in diluting the bile as well).

Bitters enhance pancreatic function: this is somewhat speculative, but a most interesting case can be made from circumstantial evidence. We know that gastrin helps pancreatic regeneration and also increases the secretions of insulin and glucagon, the two main hormones produced by the pancreas. It happens, however, that these two hormones are almost completely antagonistic in their action and secretion, so there may be the potential for a 'state-dependent' effect: a response to gastrin that varies depending on the state of mutual secretion of the two hormones at the time.

Interestingly enough there is a tradition of using bitters in controlling late-onset diabetes (one that can be supported in modern clinical practice, although one must be very circumspect in treating this condition), and a confirmed prediction from Chinese physiology that bitters are an effective counter to reactive hypoglycaemia (with impressive and immediate effects on its symptoms in many cases).

The tentative conclusion reached is that the bitters tend to normalize pancreatic hormone secretions, raising glucagon when insulin is relatively excessive and vice versa (although most likely to raise a hormone level when that is actually deficient). In other words it is suggested that bitters may *moderate excessive swings in blood-sugar levels*, both in the long and short term.

Bitters are 'tonics': if all the above actions are taken together, it is possible to see how the totality can be enhancing to general health. There is in short a broad-based stimulation of all upper digestive functions. This is the arena in which the body interacts with its nourishment, where it meets most material put into it, and where most metabolic and calorific processes are controlled. To the extent that the region is in the firing line in modern living conditions, then it will respond favourably to the administration of bitter remedies.

Traditionally these were invoked mainly at times of debility or convalescence, when it was desirable to improve the quality and quantity of nourishment to the body. In modern times it is possible to justify their use increasingly as illness becomes more chronic in nature, and as food becomes less familiar to digestive and assimilative functions.¶

*Alkaloids Taste: BITTER

With the alkaloids herbal pharmacology comes closest to the conventional science. These are the most potent of all plant constituents, and are the ones most investigated by modern science. Their potency extends to almost universal toxicity and it would be correct to state that the action of any alkaloid on the body is inherently stressful.

However, there are reasons why the herbalist in practice worries relatively little about alkaloids.

Firstly almost all herbs have some alkaloids in their constitution, including those with the most impeccable safety record. Once again it seems to be the case that the whole plant is more than just the sum of its parts.

Secondly in those relatively few remedies with a significant alkaloidal content, the toxicity is usually of the most direct kind. In other words exceeding the safe therapeutic dose will give rise to

¶Reference to 'Bitter', on pp. 190–91 will demonstrate the agreement about the action of bitters around the world. It will also point to a significant contra-indication to their use.

Bitters were universally considered cooling to the body. This meant they were used for the heat of fevers and inflammatory disease, and other syndromes marked by 'heat' and 'damp-heat', but were not used for 'cold' conditions (see the chapter 'Traditional Pathology'). This is still clinically important.

obvious symptoms like vomiting or diarrhoea or immediate central nervous symptoms. Rarely will plant alkaloids display the more insidious toxicity of a synthetic drug which is designed not to produce alarming symptoms. It may be, in fact, that the immediate irritation is the essential part of the provocative action of the remedy.

Nevertheless, having said all this, it is incumbent on the herbal practitioner to take especial care with the administration of herbs that contain significant levels of alkaloids. One probably significant factor is that alkaloids tend not to be very soluble in water, but they do dissolve well in alcohol. As most traditional herbal preparations were aqueous infusions or decoctions, then it can be assumed that they were relatively low in available alkaloid. By contrast, the modern medical herbalist in Britain uses primarily alcohol/water tinctures: the available alkaloidal count is certainly higher in such preparations and would have the effect of making the alcoholic tincture more potent than the infusion. Using herbs in a small way usually involves starting with aqueous preparations: this makes sense.

This opens up a wider point of importance, however: it means that the action of an alcoholic tincture is likely to be significantly different from its infused version. The traditional reputation of herbs is mostly based on work with the latter; modern clinical expertise is being developed mainly with the former. The results may be different enough to cause confusion.

The attempts to define an alkaloid chemically have never been satisfactory. The word originally derived from the term 'vegetable alkali' used to describe the alkalinity of some of the early alkaloidal isolates. In general the category can be said to incorporate alkaline nitrogenous substances with marked physiological effects. However, neither colchicine nor ricinine is alkaline, nor are mescaline, ephedrine and muscarine nitrogen-containing, and whereas alkaloids are traditionally said to come from the higher plants, both animals and lower organisms are known to produce them. Whilst most alkaloids are heterocyclic, there are others, such as mescaline, ephedrine and hordenine which are non-cyclic and are sometimes referred to as 'protoalkaloids'.

Apart from their toxicity (their main function in plants seems to be deterrence against browsing animals and herbivorous insects) the action of the alkaloids is not easily summarized: each has its own individual character. Instead a list will give some idea of their range and categories. As the individual examples provided are the most well known, and thus often the most notorious or dramatically active, a more toxic picture of the alkaloidal range may be conveyed than is actually justified.

The best approach, followed here, is to take them in groups with common biosynthetic origins. There are many other groups, but these are the significant ones. It will be seen that many of the alkaloids have a particular action on the central nervous system (more precisely on the synapses in the nervous pathways). Their general lipid-solubility is relevant to this action.

Pyrrolidine alkaloids

Originating from the amino-acid ornithine, this group includes the tropane alkaloids, atropine, hyoscine and hyoscyamine from the nightshade family (henbane, datura, Jimson weed, belladonna and bittersweet, for example). As a group these block parasympathetic nerve activity. The group also includes the 'truth drug' scopolamine and cocaine.

Pyridine and piperidine alkaloids

Derived from the B vitamin, nicotinic acid, this group includes the alkaloids of lobelia and tobacco (especially nicotine). They act to stimulate and then to block all autonomic nervous activity.

Pyrrolizidine and quinolizidine alkaloids

Both have notable toxic reputations. The first is derived from ornithine and linked with liver damage: it is found in the ragworts (potential trouble for grazing stock), borage, comfrey and coltsfoot (where evidence for toxicity is less clear).

The second group is derived from the amino-acid lysine, and provides the alkaloids that make the consumption of some plants of the pea family, notably laburnum, lupins and brooms, so dangerous.

Indole alkaloids

A complex group, founded on tryptamine, and including many of pharmacological interest. They include the 'animal alkaloids', adrenaline, noradrenaline, serotonin (5-hydroxytryptamine or 5-HT) and their ilk, the tranquillizing alkaloids of passion flower, the ophthalmic alkaloids related to physostigmine from the calabar bean, the uterine stimulants ergotamine and ergometrine from the fungus ergot of rye, and the man-made derivative of these, lysergic acid diethylamide (LSD). Also included are the alkaloids of the Indian snakeroot (*Rauwolfia serpentaria*), including reserpine, having powerful hypotensive (and in isolation from the whole plant, depressive) effects. There are several notable central nervous stimulants: strychnine, johimbine and psilocybin.

All these alkaloids have their effect on the neuromuscular system by interacting with adrenergic receptors. We might also note two new orthodox discoveries, the antileukaemic drugs vincristine and vinblastine isolated from the Madagascar periwinkle (*Catharanthus rosea*).

Quinoline alkaloids

Derived from phenylalanine, this group includes quinine and other alkaloids from cinchona bark, and also the alkaloids found in Angostura Bitters.

Isoquinoline alkaloids

Related to the above, this is one of the most significant groups. It includes several subclasses:

> Simple isoquinolines: alkaloids of mescaline cactus (*Lopophora williamsii*), notably mescaline
> Benzylisoquinolines: precursors of many below, including the opium poppy's papaverine
> Phthalideisoquinolines: including narcotine

Protopines: exclusive to the poppy family, including protopine

Protoberberines: berberine, hydrastine, canadine, etc., from *Berberis* spp., and golden seal

Morphine alkaloids: including morphine, codeine and thebaine from the opium poppy

Ipecac alkaloids: including the emetic alkaloid emetine from ipecacuanha

Purine alkaloids

Notably including caffeine, theobromine, theophylline and aminophylline from cocoa, tea and coffee, these are derived from the purine nucleotides adenine and guanine (hence their collective name: xanthines). They act to prolong the effective life of many hormones, notably adrenaline.

Terpenoid alkaloids

Having a terpene skeleton, this group includes the poisons of aconite and the delphiniums, the tranquillizing alkaloid of valerian, and a range of interesting new discoveries in the plant world.

Pharmacokinetics

Plant medicines are material medicines. There can be no long-term future for a herbal pharmacology unless it examines the processes by which the body interacts with, metabolizes and dispenses with these material substances. The name for this discipline is pharmacokinetics, the science of the movement of drugs.

The factors that influence the movement of a remedy through the body and its availability to the tissues ('bioavailability') allow the herbalist better insight into the ideal conditions in which to apply any prescription. It must be emphasized, however, that most factors are highly variable so that total bioavailability is very much an individual matter, to be assessed, if at all, only as a result of years of practical and diagnostic experience. The following therefore represents only broad trends.[17] Pharmacokinetics has generally been considered under the following headings (with references to the physiological terms introduced in Part I in brackets):

> Remedy absorption (assimilation)
> Remedy distribution (circulation)
> Remedy metabolism (processing)
> Remedy excretion (removal)
> Tissue sensitivity (perception)

Remedy Absorption

There are three main routes by which a remedy might gain access to the body fluids apart from parenteral injection (which we shall ignore in this course: it can be actually dangerous to inject herbal material direct into the tissues – haemolysing saponins and coumarins and the hepatotoxic tannins are very common in plants).

Skin

This provides a large area over which it is possible to apply medication for both topical and systemic treatments.

The most frequent indications for skin applications are local skin lesions, wounds, abrasions, inflammatory skin disease, and the like. Such healing, soothing or anti-inflammatory remedies are targeted to the immediate surface and questions of systemic absorption are of secondary importance.

External applications are also used, however, to affect deeper tissues. The toughened surface of the skin permits the application of relatively irritant ('counter-irritant') remedies, designed to provoke increased circulation in the underlying tissues, as in arthritic joints and pleural inflammations, and this is a common use for skin treatments. Other remedies are applied to influence healing of soft and bone tissues beneath the skin.

Some traditions apply systemic remedies through the skin by choice (for a useful account of such an approach one can read the books by the French herbalist Maurice Messegué),[18] and here one can note that remedies absorbed this way are not subject to immediate metabolism by the liver as they are in oral administration – this means that the action of herbs given through the skin will be significantly different from their normal reputation.

Absorption rates through the skin are highly variable. They are most rapid over areas of thin skin and particularly where there are many hair follicles and sebaceous glands (e.g. face, neck and shoulders, on arms and legs and the backs of hands). If the skin is damaged, absorption is the most rapid of all and is obviously much less selective.

The skin is generally resistant to water and aqueous solutions, but if it is soaked for a time its resistance breaks down and it becomes hydrated (the appearance is seen after a long stay in the bath). When hydrated the skin is highly permeable to aqueous solutions and this provides the most efficient way of applying remedies. Ways to induce this condition include soaking in a herbal bath (more efficient to do this in small volumes for hands, feet or pelvis), putting the remedy under an occlusive dressing (applying sticking plaster to the skin prevents evaporation of fluid from the surface and so hydrates it), or mixing it with an oily base as an ointment or cream (the oily constituent has a similar occlusive effect to the sticking plaster).

Mucous membranes

These are mostly used for local treatments, though they also have systemic applications. Those areas most used are the following:

Rectum: for local application (especially haemorrhoids) but also for those agents provoking nausea or other adverse reaction if given orally. There is also avoidance of the 'first-pass liver' effect, though herbalists do not usually consciously make use of this factor. Absorption is very variable and can be slow. There is little point in using rectal applications for treating conditions of the large bowel as there is little diffusion of material upwards. (Term used: suppositories.)

Vagina: almost always used for local problems such as vaginal infections or cervicitis. Absorption rate is comparable to that of the mouth lining. (Term used: pessaries.)

Mouth: used as the site of absorption by homoeopaths but less so by herbalists, largely because of the difficulty of holding most herbal prescriptions in the mouth long enough! There is, however, a good absorption rate, with favourable prevailing pH values, and the site has potential for its proximity to the central nervous system.

Nose: snuffs are used locally (e.g. for polyps or catarrhal disease) and for quick access to the cerebral tissues. Very fine powders are used and for these absorption rates are rapid.

Digestive tract

Oral administration of herbal remedies is by far the most common, and the digestive tract presents the surface most adapted towards absorption. There are broad influences on this process we can usefully review.

The lining of the digestive tract is in most places only one-cell thick. Moreover, because of intense folding of the lining, both macroscopically and microscopically, there is a vast absorptive area, comparable in fact to the ground area of a small house! The actual interface of absorption is therefore the cell wall facing the gut lumen, and it is molecular movement across this selectively permeable and extremely complex barrier that constitutes assimilation.

Two methods of absorption predominate. The first, *passive diffusion*, accounts for by far the greatest bulk of trans-membrane passage. It needs no energy source, and the rate of transfer is simply proportional to the difference in concentrations of that particular substance on each side of the membrane (the removal of absorbed material from the far side of the membrane by the circulation effectively maintains a high concentration in the gut).

To use this route the absorbed material must be able to dissolve in the substance of the cell wall it traverses; the latter is made up of a double layer of protein molecules with a fatty (lipid) layer in between. For most small molecules, crossing the protein layers is not a critical stage, but the lipid barrier provides a definite rate-limiting factor. For most purposes it can be said therefore that *the rate of passive absorption is proportional to lipid-solubility*.

For most substances dissolved in water (e.g. herbal extracts) the degree of lipid-solubility is directly proportional to the degree of association of the molecule: all molecules dissolved in water tend to dissociate into polar-charged ions, but this process renders the substance less lipid-soluble and thus less readily absorbed from the gut. The degree of dissociation is affected by the degree of acidity of the solution (measured as pH, where the lower the pH the higher the acidity, higher pHs reflecting increased alkalinity).

The association-dissociation characteristics of any substance are measured as its pK value, where pK is that pH at which a given substance is 50 per cent ionized. Those with low pKs are referred to as acids, those with high pKs as bases. Most plant constituents are weak acids, though a significant but variable group are weak bases. For weak acids a pH lower than their pK will lead to decreased ionization (and thus increased lipid-solubility); weak bases associate when pH is higher than their pK. In the stomach

335 Pharmacokinetics

pH is low, so that weak acids are absorbed better there; weak base absorption is favoured in the relatively higher pH of the small intestine. Thus we may say that the bulk of herbal constituents is absorbed in the stomach, very soon after swallowing, and rather earlier than most conventional drugs. On the other hand potent alkaloids are among those that, because they are weak bases, are absorbed mostly in the small intestine, perhaps hours later.

The second main mechanism for transfer of material across a cell membrane is *active transport* by the use of energy-consuming carrier mechanisms. This can pass material either against a concentration gradient (e.g. glucose, vitamin B12, and most minerals) or faster than passive diffusion down a concentration gradient (e.g. many vitamins, allopathic drugs and some active constituents of herbs).

Obviously in these cases the rate of movement is not so much dependent on available concentrations as on the carrier capacity ('seats on the ferry'). One can thus reduce such absorption by providing other substances that compete for the same carrier ('competitive inhibition'), or factors having direct influence on the mechanism itself (for example, cyanide, a product of constituents often found in plants, poisons by inhibiting many active carrier mechanisms).

The correlative of this is that substances absorbed actively do not necessarily increase their concentration in the body fluids as a result simply of increasing applied dosage: classic examples are vitamin C and those of the B group. Although some herbal constituents are undoubtedly affected by being absorbed actively, the implications of all this are not yet clear.

We may take note of several general influences on absorption rate from the digestive tract in the light of the above information.

> **Stomach acidity:** if there is reduced stomach acid (shown perhaps by a tendency to enteritis or heavy bloated indigestion), there is reduced absorption rate of weak acids, i.e. of many herbal constituents.
>
> **Food:** this generally slows absorption; the remedy will move into the circulation faster when taken well before meals. This, however, is less so for weak acid constituents, so that for the

bulk of herbal material taking a dose *just* before a meal is in order. For the most potent possible constituents, the alkaloids, the presence of food can be particularly interfering. This may, of course, be a useful bonus, but if the alkaloidal fraction is judged to be important in a treatment (in using the more allopathic remedies, for example), then a dosage longer before meals would be advisable. Net intake of material is generally the same in the long run, whatever the relationship with foods, but some interference in total absorption is quite possible through the formation of insoluble complexes, especially with cereals, and the mucilaginous and tannin constituents of plants.

Gastrointestinal motility: generally anything that promotes stomach emptying increases absorption from the intestine. As material spends most time in that tract this usually means that the absorption of most things is increased, even for those remedies normally absorbed from the stomach.

Factors that induce such an increase include fasting, anxiety, hyperthyroidism and a high fluid intake.

Factors slowing stomach emptying and tending to reduce overall absorption are bulky and fatty foods, mental depression, hypothyroidism, ulceration and other digestive inflammations. Most digestive diseases interfere with absorption.

There are many miscellaneous factors interfering with absorption or enhancing it. They include the state of the ever-changing intestinal flora (drastically affected after broad-spectrum antibiotics, for example), the formulation and other characteristics of the remedy itself, and other factors not yet quantified. The main points to note concern the mixing of remedies with food and the role of the digestive function in the broadest sense.

Remedy Distribution

Once into the body fluids the remedy is distributed to the tissues in accordance with the extent of blood flow, the ease of passage across cell membranes, and the extent of binding to plasma and tissue proteins.

Regional blood flow

The tissues of the body can be divided into groups on the basis of their share of circulation. Those most perfused by blood will also be those tissues most exposed to the action of any remedy, whilst those with little active circulation will have less chance to respond to treatment. In order of decreasing perfusion the following lists may be made:

> endocrine and other glands, heart, lungs, brain, liver and kidneys;
> lean tissues such as skin and muscle;
> fat tissues;
> bones, teeth, ligaments and tendons.

One can make some assessment about response time from knowing where particular target organs fit on this scheme. The presence of disease also plays a considerable part: inflammation can increase the blood flow to an area very considerably and improve access of remedies to that tissue accordingly. On the other hand diseases of the heart, liver or kidney, by interfering with circulatory health, can have a significant effect in reducing access to all tissues.

Another appreciable factor inhibiting access to tissues is obesity. The presence of large fat stores creates a sink wherein much remedial benefit is likely to disappear. In general, therefore, the effective dosage must be increased in the obese patient.

The membrane barrier

Cell membranes have much the same properties throughout the body, so movement through the tissues depends largely on lipid-solubility (see above). Notable is the movement into the central nervous system: here the so-called 'blood-brain barrier' lets through only those materials that are lipid-soluble. Under normal conditions this does favour alkaloids and volatile oils, which anyway have most effect here, but it does mitigate against many herbal constituents.

These principles are important in treating pregnant and nursing mothers. The placental membrane is no different from other tissues in this regard, and we can assume that any herbal remedy will reach the foetus unhindered. This does limit the amount of safe treatment in pregnancy. During breast-feeding the very high perfusion of the lactating mammary glands means that the infant receives a proportionately high dose of any remedy that the mother is taking (and in fact may be gently treated in this way) so similar care is necessary.

Protein binding

Proteins have a tendency to bind to smaller molecules floating in their vicinity. Whilst this is rarely permanent it can act as an appreciable factor against free distribution through the tissues. By far the most significant protein concerned is albumin, the main free protein constituent of the bloodstream or 'plasma protein', although other plasma proteins and proteins in the tissues themselves also play a part.

In general these proteins act a little like fat in the obese, except that the binding rates of different substances vary widely. A constituent closely bound will have a much longer effective life in the tissues, but its free levels will never get very high – it will need higher doses to compensate. Another constituent not readily bound to protein will reach high levels in the circulation and will have a short life – its dose would need to be kept in check but it would require frequent dosages.

Unfortunately, we have as yet little information on how this affects herbal constituents; however, we can appreciate how overall changes in the amount of plasma protein can affect dosage regimes. Liver disease, nephrotic syndrome (protein loss in the urine), coeliac disease and starvation all lead to sometimes severe drops in plasma protein levels. They will demand increased dosage frequency and

339 Pharmacokinetics

smaller doses. Similar changes would be necessary if there was significant competition for binding sites from other substances, as will happen in the uraemia of kidney failure or in acidosis.

Remedy Metabolism

We need not concern ourselves with the metabolic processes by which materials are transformed in the body. Most is accomplished by the liver, which has as its brief the conversion of materials from their lipid-soluble form to the polar, water-soluble products that are more easily excreted from the body (it is very difficult for the body to get rid of lipid-soluble materials: they keep dissolving their way back in!).

The fact that the liver has vast potential for altering the nature of any remedy is very significant. All material absorbed from the digestive tract has to pass through the liver before it goes anywhere else, and a large percentage of it will be metabolized immediately (the 'first-pass effect'). This is likely to contribute to the therapeutic action of the remedy, as the metabolites are often the more active constituents. However, it is clear that application of remedies by skin or rectum, for example, by avoiding the first-pass effect will lead to quite different responses in the patient. Similarly it can be seen that anything which affects liver capacity will have considerable impact on the fate of each prescription.

Increased liver metabolism will have the effect of increasing the proportion of non-lipid-soluble metabolites and of increasing loss of the remedy from the body. Thus each dose will be less available to the tissues, especially the central nervous system, and will survive for less time in the body: dosage frequency and quantity should rightfully be increased. Factors having this effect are alcohol and smoking, food additives and many chemical adulterants in the diet, as well as many drugs, notably steroids, digoxin, barbiturates and the tricyclic antidepressants.

Decreased liver metabolism will have the opposite effect. There will usually be less excretion and greater tissue availability of any remedy, leading quite easily to overdosage. Several drugs have this effect, notably the oral contraceptives, MAOI antidepressives, phenylbutazone and chloramphenicol. It is surprising that the real dangers in using these drugs are not more widely known, especially with regard to allopathic medicines where overdosage can have severe consequences. Another very important influence with the same effect on the liver is simple old age: this partially accounts for the smaller doses one uses with the elderly.

There is an extremely important relationship between liver metabolism and the actions of the bacterial flora in the gut. It has emerged after investigation of the fate of morphine in the tissues, but the same principles are known to involve cardioactive glycosides and probably a number of other important plant constituents.

Morphine is metabolized in the liver (and elsewhere) by conjugating it with an anion called glucuronate. This makes it far less lipid-soluble and ready for excretion. Being a large molecule it is excreted in the bile rather than from the kidney, and thus finds its way into the digestive tract. In the lower reaches are variable populations of bacteria, however, with enzymes that deconjugate the morphine glucuronate, freeing the morphine again. This is promptly re-absorbed to re-enter the circulation. This 'entero-hepatic' circulation has two effects: it significantly prolongs the active life of the substance concerned, and it incidentally provides nutritional support for, and thus increases further the effect of, the bacteria responsible. Thus with repeated doses of the substance a real cumulative effect is likely. On the other hand a dose of broad-spectrum antibiotics is likely to have a serious effect on a maintenance regime of morphine, heart treatment or other medication affected.

Remedy Excretion

As soon as a remedy enters the body fluids it begins to be excreted. Obviously the rate at which that happens determines very largely the overall effect of each dose. Excretion occurs at the kidneys, via the bile and bowel, and to a variable extent through the sweat glands and other body secretions.

The main loss occurs through the kidneys, perhaps after suitable metabolism by the liver. We need not concern ourselves with detailed influences on urinary excretion except for a few broad effects. The use of diuretics (and most herbs have some diuretic effect) will tend to increase remedy excretion, and the effect of coffee and circulatory stimulants in this context may be noted.

The pH of the urine can be important. In the case of vegetarians it tends to be high (more alkaline); this favours the reabsorption, and thus reduces the elimination, of weak bases, which include notably the powerful alkaloids. Thus vegetarians are likely to get a stronger response from alkaloidal herbal medicine. On the other hand, those with carnivorous appetites, or presenting with acidic urine, will have only short exposure to alkaloids in their herbal prescriptions and will instead excrete the bulk of the remedy less rapidly.

We have already seen how the efficiency of biliary excretion can be markedly reduced by the entero-hepatic circulation; this occurs less obviously for all material passed out with the bile as there is variable reabsorption of almost all biliary material from the bowel. This is much increased with constipation, and such a condition generally suggests that remedies will stay longer in the system. Other notable influences are liver and biliary disease which can stop biliary excretion in rare cases. As the bile is the main route of excretion of larger molecules and as these are usually the most pharmacologically active, the implications of these influences will be obvious.

Of the other routes of exit the sweat glands are the only ones that merit attention here. They have a passive role in excretion compared to the kidneys but share a similar basic filtration and reabsorption system. Thus we find they often stand in for defective kidney function (marked by irritation in areas where sweat accumulates) and will in these circumstances excrete a great deal. In normal conditions their role becomes important in hot climates where perspiration is high, accounting for the excretion of a relatively high proportion of any administered remedy. Thus when perspiration is high, the dosage of remedies should be raised as well as the increase in fluids.

Tissue Sensitivity

After taking all other factors into consideration, at the end of the process the actual effect of any remedy is unpredictable.

This is an inconvenient fact for conventional pharmacologists as much as for anyone else. Each individual has a unique blend of constitutional and acquired characteristics which determines the reaction to any food or medicinal material.

For example, the primary response of sensory receptors in the peripheral nervous system, the body's 'perception' of a stimulus, is influenced by the extent of previous exposure to the same stimulus (*habituation*). In the broader context there is a wide variation in the number and type of receptors involved, and in the ability of any stimulus to reach such receptors (usually reflecting the state of health of surrounding tissues).

At the humoral level enzyme profiles are completely idiosyncratic, cell-membrane receptor behaviour variable on a minute-by-minute basis, and programmed reflex responses (see 'Response', on pp. 39–44) endlessly adjusted through conditioning or learning.

Such imponderables are reflected in the results of the taste thresholds for quinine. While the majority of subjects tested first detected the taste of quinine at the 24 mM level, there were some whose thresholds were noticeably different – anywhere between 0.7 and 750 mM.

Such alarming variability might push all pharmacology, conventional or herbal, into laughable irrelevance if it wasn't the case that much of it is within broadly predictable categories. Age, nervous state and sensitivity, the nature of previous meals, medical history and concurrent disease all influence ultimate tissue sensitivity in relatively predictable ways. These are elaborated later.

Taking such factors into account is an important responsibility for anyone who would give a medicine to another. Those prescribing conventional drugs are at a disadvantage because of the critical nature of their treatments, where even small variations in effect can have substantial consequences. The herbalist, however, if he or she aspires to be more than purely intuitive in judgement, must also take these factors seriously. It is true that the nature of the herbal intervention reduces the risks a little; whether a gentle provocation or a nourishing tonic is being invoked the exact dosage is less important than the correct choice of approach. There are however cases where herbal remedies act in such a way that bioavailability becomes more critical, and appropriate care will have to be taken.

All this incidentally casts into perspective the argument often used by conventional pharmacologists that herbal remedies are essentially unpredictable. The lesson might be that predictability is itself an illusion, and that appropriate clinical experience and judgement are the most important factors in dispensing remedies. The herbalists' argument, rehearsed extensively in this book, is that the nature of their treatment incorporates and actually takes advantage of individual reactions. In treating the human as a vital whole with his or her own individual strategies for survival, resistance and recovery, and in looking for ways to support such strategies, the herbalist starts with, and takes immediate account of, individuality.

Nevertheless, all dispensers of remedies would do well to note the following factors affecting tissue sensitivity.

Age

Both the very young and the very old react to material remedies very differently from the adolescent and the adult. In the case of newborn infants there is a significant reduction in metabolizing capacity compared with the adult, so that half-lives of administered substances are up to three times longer. Dosage levels must be correspondingly reduced even before other factors of sensitivity are taken into account.

Metabolizing capacity improves rapidly and between the ages of several months and about ten the rate of utilization of remedies is the highest of any age group. This is due partly to the higher percentage of body water (up to 70 per cent compared with the adult's 50 per cent) and extracellular volume (35 per cent versus 20 per cent), and partly to the hormonally induced higher metabolic rate in this age group. Therefore although dosages are still reduced compared with the adult, an increased dose *in terms of quantity per unit body weight* is justified (up to twice the adult dose per unit body weight for the three-month-old child, 50 per cent or more for the average five-year-old).

By contrast the handling of remedies with increasing old age grows more deficient. For example, the glomerular filtration rate at the age of 90, closely reflecting cardiac output, is at least half that at prime, and this is the end process of a gradual decline in performance that begins in early middle age. A parallel degeneration in other organs and systems leads to the general rule that, other things being equal, the total dose for the over 60s is 75 per cent of the full dose, for the over 70s, 60 per cent, and for the over 80s the dose should be 50 per cent or less.

Disease

Kidney disease is an obvious example of a major influence on the disposition of remedies. As far as renal function is directly concerned, elimination of any substance is found to correlate closely with endogenous creatinine clearance, wherever the major damage lies in the renal unit. Creatinine clearance is in turn a very good indication of the extent of kidney disease and, if such figures are available, the practitioner will have a good idea of the effect on the half-life of any remedy he or she might give. Depending on the proportion of the remedy eliminated at the kidney, one might allow for as much as an eight-fold reduction in the dosage for severe kidney failure.

The other major effect of renal disease is on the extent of protein binding. In general poor renal function is associated with a reduction in protein binding, at least in the plasma. This is most likely due to a combination of reduced plasma albumin (e.g. in nephrotic syndrome) and alteration in the binding capacity of the protein remaining, possibly caused by competitive inhibition with some blood factor present in uraemia. The effect of this reduced binding is to diminish the 'storage' capacity of the blood and thus lower blood concentrations, and to increase tissue utilization and elimination, though possible impairment of tissue protein binding as well complicates the total effect. Extreme caution in kidney disease is the obvious recommendation.

The effects of liver disease on remedy availability have already been touched on. The impact of chronic liver disease on albumin and other plasma protein levels and on general hormonal activity should be additionally noted.

There are other diseases having effects on remedy disposition. Hyperlipidaemia, or raised fat levels in the blood, is known to result in competitive inhibition of albumin binding; other diseases with this effect include diabetes mellitus, hyperthyroidism and recent myocardial infarctions.

Malabsorption syndrome will lead to deficient absorption of lipid-soluble remedies from the gut. Those substances with higher molecular weight, like steroids and alkaloids, are particularly susceptible.

General alterations in blood flow consequent on heart failure, portal hypertension and shock can have significant implications on availability at the tissues. The role of the autonomic nervous system, particularly in shifting blood flow under stressful conditions, is also appreciable.

Thyroid hormone increases liver metabolizing activity and also renal clearance so that the half-lives of many remedies are likely to be increased with thyroid deficiency and decreased with hyperthyroidism. On the other hand intestinal activity is increased in the latter.

Conclusion

Even after taking all such predictable variables into account it is likely that most individuals may vary by as much as 50 per cent from expected levels in their reactions to any remedy, and that about 5 per cent of the population may react dramatically differently.

The science of pharmacology thus quickly turns into the art of clinical prescription. It must be said, however, that the second is much better when founded on the first.

7 Practical Matters

Herb Recognition and Quality Control

Introduction

A woodcarver would rightly complain if commissioned to produce a work given screwdrivers instead of chisels. Unfortunately the modern herbalist is quite likely to be given a comparable challenge. While there are many good suppliers in the business, there are others who do buy at the bottom end of the market and in the chain of supply there are many opportunities for extended or inadequate storage and even accidental substitution. The buyer of simple herbs cannot always rely on getting material of the expected standard. Although in Britain at least a combination of state legislation and voluntary policing by the trade is leading to progressive improvements in the situation, it is still the case that anyone seriously interested in using herbs to promote health should have an elementary knowledge of how to recognize their chosen remedies and how, approximately, to gauge their quality.

The situation today is very different from that in the past. Through millennia of human history most herbal medicine was applied by people at home in nature, people who would know their way around the plant world at least as well as we today would understand household implements or bus timetables. Most remedies would have been picked personally or by vendors who would have found it as difficult to pass off poor samples as a modern greengrocer would to sell an old lettuce or mouldy fruit. Everyone simply knew a lot about plants.

Even the dealers in the cities prided themselves, at least until the Second World War, on the canny ability of their staff in quality control, having much the same talents as wine merchants to this day. In Britain the herb dealers were usually family firms with long apprenticeships as their norm. In an informed market simple commercial survival depended on making good assessments of herb quality. As most stocks were imported the buying markets were generally held near the ports, like those of London and Liverpool. Literally tons of herbs at a time would be auctioned: at these events dozens of buyers might be seen taking samples from each bale or sack, eyeing them, feeling their texture, 'nosing' and tasting: all the time mentally calculating how far they could commit their firm's money to the ensuing auction. If a shipment was of poor quality, it would be left unsold. This in turn acted as a sharp incentive to the suppliers of herbs in their countries of origin to grow, harvest and store their stocks well. Unfortunately, demand for herbs slumped in the 1950s and 60s: most of the old firms contracted or went out of business; the old staff retired and were not replaced by new apprentices. Today there are only a handful of the original firms left.

What has happened, of course, is that there has recently been an upsurge in demand again. This time, however, the demand is less informed: large quantities of herbs are bought by new firms specializing in packageable formulations, taking advantage of a new type of market. Without canny quality control from the consumer, the pressure has been taken off throughout the line of supply. The general quality of herbs at point of sale has suffered. As more consumers once again become informed and selective the quality of material is improving, but for those who would use herbal remedies it is still very much the case of *caveat emptor*. It is useful to know the difference between poor and decent samples.

Pharmacognosy

As soon as the trade in herbs became established in human history, there was a need to establish standards, recognized criteria, to define the drug for the purposes of commerce and medical safeguard.

This need provided for the first form of botany and for many centuries it was the main justification for plant study. However, since 1815, it has had its own name, pharmacognosy, from the Greek *pharmakon* (a drug), and the Latin *cognoscere* (to acquire knowledge of). The name was first used in a title of a book published in that year by Seydler, *Analecta Pharmacognostica*. Pharmacognosists have since been concerned primarily with studying naturally occurring substances with medicinal action, analysing them with ever-increasing exactitude, determining their constituents, setting chemical as well as physical standards, developing techniques for the detection of contamination or adulteration of samples, and so on.

The most visible results of their work have been the pharmacopoeias, those reference works used to set standards for all medicinal agents. Until the early decades of this century most entries in pharmacopoeias were of plants or plant-derived drugs. With the increasing reliance on synthetic agents the work of the pharmacognosists has been encroached upon and they are now, sadly, a diminishing breed of academic. This is in spite of renewed interest in new species of plants as a source of new drugs for the pharmaceutical industry.

As the standard pharmacopoeias, such as the *British Pharmacopoeia (BP)* and the *United States Pharmacopoeia (USP)*, have become progressively stripped of their botanical monographs, the few remaining pharmacognosists have had to concentrate on new commissions. In Britain some have been involved, since 1968, with members of the herbal profession and leading experts in the trade to produce the *British Herbal Pharmacopoeia (BHP)*, commissioned by the trade in a unprecedented exercise in enlightened self-interest. Especially in its latest edition,[1] it provides a standard for the quality of herbal remedies that is both recognized by the legislative authorities and has inspired admiration from around the world.

What the monographs in the *BHP* provide is a standard against which the quality of any particular sample of herb could theoretically be measured. For those equipped with a microscope and rudimentary laboratory facilities it allows precise assessment of herbal quality.

For those without such equipment or skills the fact that pharmacognosists have set their standards is a reassurance: it also encourages efforts to develop basic botanical skills.

Many of those who become interested in herbal medicine as a professional option come to it from other disciplines. There is a tendency to acquire just enough skills to know when to prescribe the remedies, but otherwise to remain a conventional physician, acupuncturist, osteopath or whatever. This is unfortunate. As with all crafts it is difficult to be more than a superficial practitioner without at least some understanding of the material and its behaviour. Being entirely in the hands of the pharmacist or pill-maker does not encourage mastery of the medium. The majority of full-time herbalists prefers to maintain direct contact with the land, even if that is a tiny town garden; they will try to grow at least some of their stocks, and will also enjoy making up some of their medicines from source. This interest in practical botany is understandable.

For each of the herbs that are described in this book there are very brief pharmacognostic notes. These will allow for basic identification of the herb and be a possible taster for those interested in pursuing the subject further. As a further help a few of the most common botanical terms are defined or illustrated in the following pages.

To begin with, however, some of the fundamental criteria of herb quality can be listed.

Selecting herbs of good quality

Unless one can grow herbs personally or can buy directly from the grower it is necessary to be cautious before purchasing stock. A dried sample should satisfy the following requirements:

> Herb material (i.e. leaf and foliage) should be as near to its original green as possible; colour loss suggests sun-drying (and thus ultra-violet bleaching), excessive storage time or poor storage conditions.
>
> Flowers should be as close as possible to their original colours for the same reason.
>
> The sample should look good generally: there should be recognizable plant fragments with a minimum of dust and other obvious adulterants. Beware of powdered samples: some remedies are genuinely suited to powdering but in most cases the process simply shortens shelf-life at best; at worst it can hide many sins and reduce the scope for adequate quality control.
>
> Rub a small piece between finger and thumb and then smell

('nose') it: it should smell fresh and clean. If the plant is meant to be aromatic, the aroma should be clear and strong. If stored too long or under poor conditions, aroma will be lost or compromised by that of mould; in the latter case there will be a musty contamination.

Taste a *small* piece (this is safe in all but a very few plants) and spit out the piece after chewing it and holding it on the tongue for a moment or so. The taste should also be clear and clean; any mucilage, astringency, bitterness or local numbing qualities should be present as expected. Be suspicious of any tastes not expected.

Pieces of wood, root or bark should be tested for consistency and, if possible, snapped so that the 'fracture' can be observed (see below); incomplete drying or damp storage conditions may be reflected in an unduly spongy consistency.

Plant classification

Thanks to the strenuous efforts of Carolus Linnaeus (1707–78) and his many successors, it is now possible to get near-universal agreement on the botanical name of any plant. In an extraordinary example of human accord all cultures around the world have accepted Latin and the Linnaean convention as the common botanical language. Linnaeus developed the binomial system wherein each plant is referred to by two names, the first, spelt with a capital letter, denoting the genus of which the plant is a member. The second name, written with lower-case initial letter, is the plant's specific name. Occasionally the specific name may be followed by another denoting a variety of that species.

This may be seen in the following example, which charts the full taxonomic classification of the two common varieties of fennel. In looking down the list, particular note should be taken of the family name: this is always supplied in monographs on plants as a convenient way of placing the plant in its wider botanical context and to hint at many other botanical properties to be expected.

It will also be noted that conventionally the name of the classifying botanist is provided in abbreviated form after the specific name.

The taxonomic classification of fennel

Phylum:	Angiospermae (the flowering, as opposed to coniferous, plants)
Subphylum:	Dicotyledoneae (two-leafed embryos, as opposed to those of grasses)
Superorder:	Rosidae (the rose superorder)
Order:	Umbelales
Family:	**Umbelliferae** (the carrot family)
Subfamily:	Apioideae (the celery subfamily)
Tribe:	Apieae (or Ammieae)
Genus:	*Foeniculum* (the fennel genus)
Species:	*Foeniculum vulgare* L.
Varieties:	*Foeniculum vulgare* var. *vulgare* (Mill.) Thelung (bitter fennel)
	Foeniculum vulgare var. *dulce* (Mill.) Thelung (sweet fennel)

When herbs are discussed in this text their full botanic name is emphasized. Those who work with herbs professionally often prefer to use botanic names to avoid the confusion that often arises in the use of common names, which can vary widely.

The reference to the family name helps in anticipating some of its qualities. For example, the members of the Labiatae are generally aromatic, with considerable volatile oil content (they include peppermint, rosemary, sage, hyssop, oregano, marjoram and lavender); the Liliaceae, or lily family, often contain steroidal saponins (and include the North American gynaecological herbs); the Cruciferae include the mustards and brassicas which all contain circulatory-stimulating mustard oils; the Rosaceae, or rose family, tend to contain cyanide-forming ingredients; the Compositae generally store their carbohydrates in the form of inulin; the Umbelliferae are closely related to the interesting genus the Araliaceae, which include ginseng, and so on.

Plant Structures

The nature of the remedy, its mode of preparation and its determining characteristics depend on the part of the plant which is used. A few comments about each can be helpful.

Leaves and tops ('herbs')

These consist of the stems (often limited in their girth by 'official' – i.e. pharmacopoeial – requirements) and leaves frequently associated with flowers and young fruits. They may be summarized as those non-woody parts of the plant found above the ground with the usual exception of seeds. (These are often found in herb samples, though this may be a sign that the plant was harvested too late in its development: most herbs are at their best collected just before the flowers open.)

Where possible the structure of the sample supplied should be examined. In most dried samples the plant has been broken too far for its appearance to be gauged, but where large pieces are found they may be described in conventional botanical terms of leaf and stem size, shape and appearance (see Fig. 10).

Flowers

Flowers are the reproductive organs of the plant and consist of four basic parts.

> *Calix*: the protective, usually leaf-like sheath out of which the flower opens.
>
> *Corolla*: the petals that act as an attracting organ for pollinators (and humans!).
>
> *Androecium*: the collective parts of the flower providing *pollen* (the male gametes in fertilization); they are usually called *stamens* (made up of *anthers* and *filaments*).
>
> *Gynoecium*: the female organs containing the *ovules* (the female gametes in fertilization) within the *ovary*, the *stigma* and *style* making up the *carpel*.

Leaf shapes

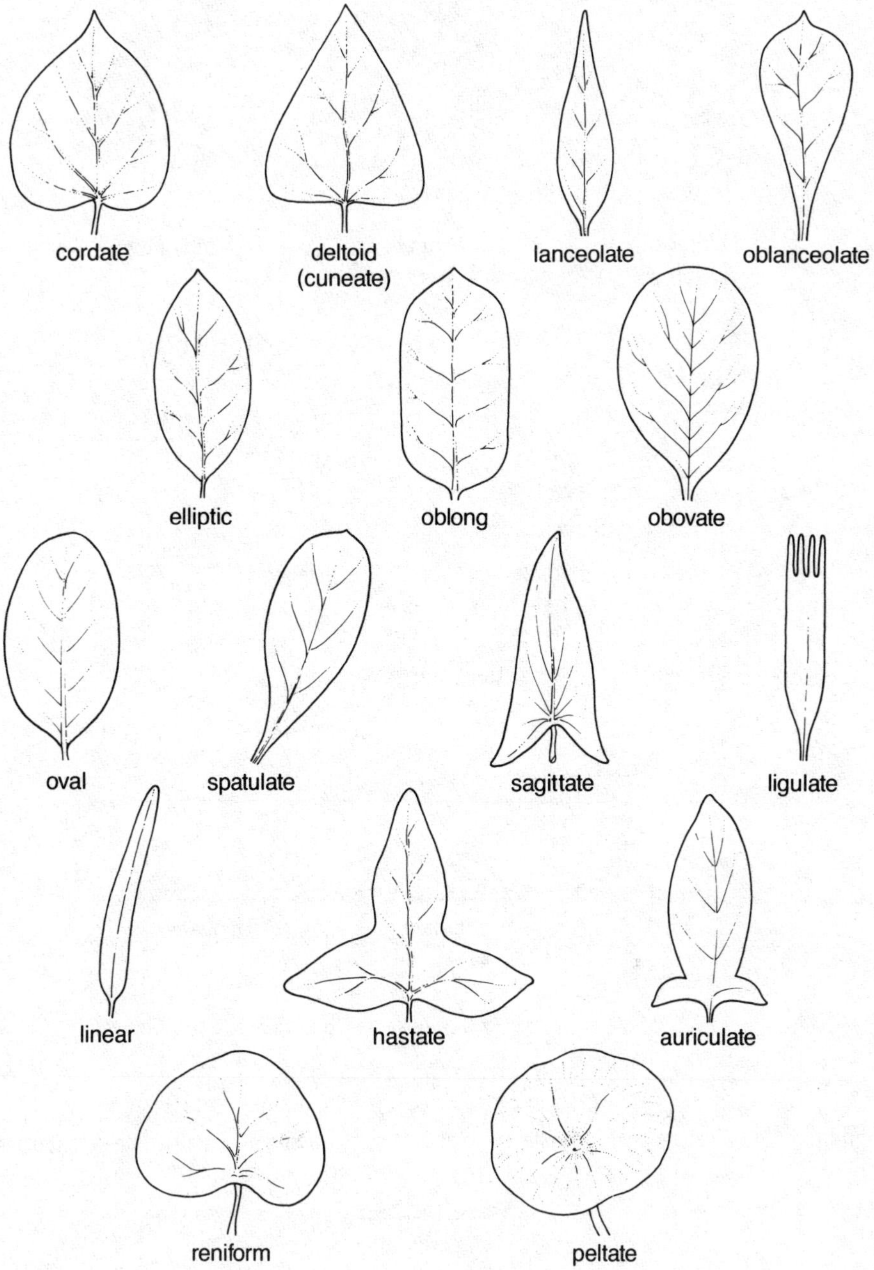

cordate

deltoid (cuneate)

lanceolate

oblanceolate

elliptic

oblong

obovate

oval

spatulate

sagittate

ligulate

linear

hastate

auriculate

reniform

peltate

Fig. 10 Leaves and tops

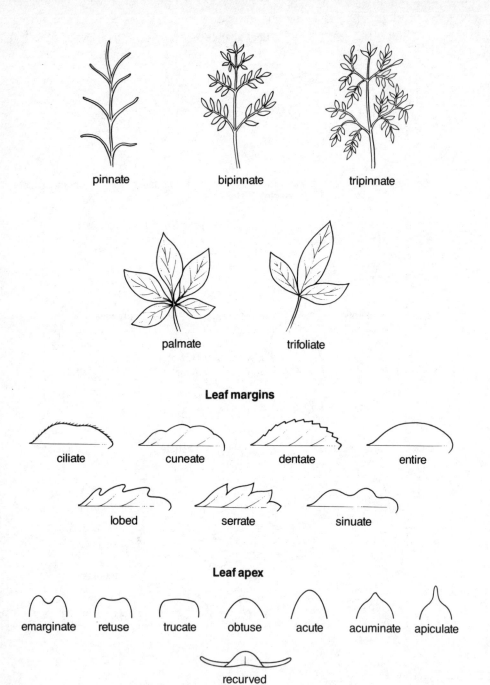

pinnate   bipinnate   tripinnate

palmate   trifoliate

Leaf margins

ciliate   cuneate   dentate   entire

lobed   serrate   sinuate

Leaf apex

emarginate   retuse   trucate   obtuse   acute   acuminate   apiculate

recurved

Fig. 10 Leaves and tops (*continued*)

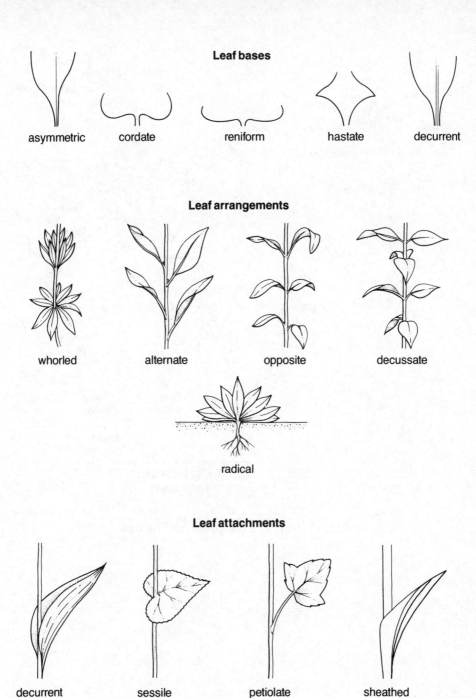

Leaf bases

asymmetric　　cordate　　reniform　　hastate　　decurrent

Leaf arrangements

whorled　　alternate　　opposite　　decussate

radical

Leaf attachments

decurrent　　sessile　　petiolate　　sheathed

Fig. 10 Leaves and tops (*continued*)

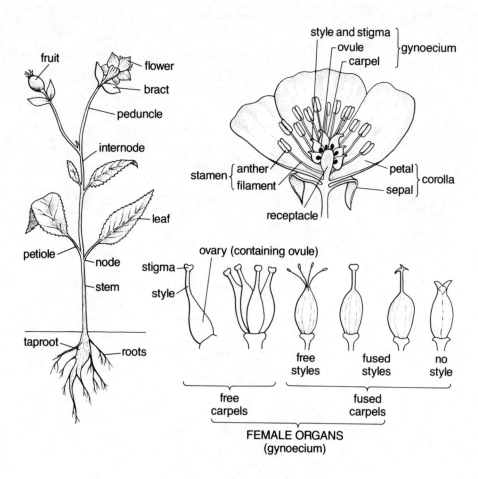

Fig. 11 Parts of the plant and flower

Except in cases where flowers are single, they are arranged in inflorescences: these vary in their structure in predictable ways (see Figs. 11 and 12).

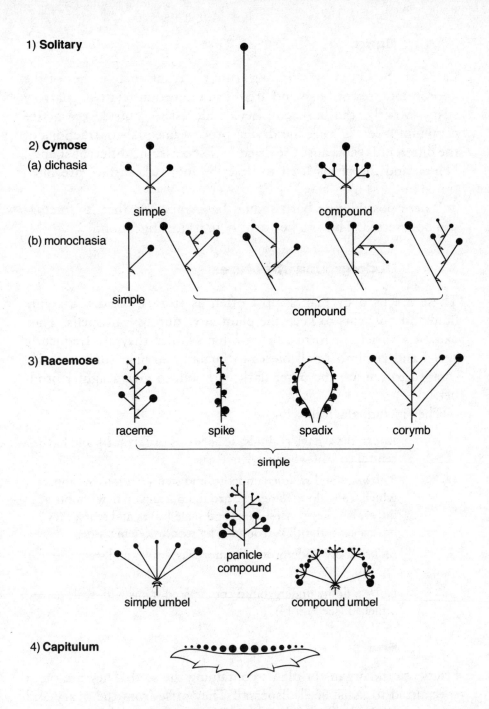

1) Solitary

2) Cymose
(a) dichasia
simple   compound

(b) monochasia
simple
compound

3) Racemose
raceme   spike   spadix   corymb
simple

panicle
compound

simple umbel   compound umbel

4) Capitulum

**Fig. 12 Types of inflorescence (in each diagram
larger spheres denote older flowers)**

Barks

Barks are procured by stripping from the trunk or branches of the appropriate tree or bush and are thus obtained in relatively narrow strips. Strictly, the bark consists of all tissues outside the active cambium layer. During the drying process unequal contractions of the different layers cause the dried barks to assume different shapes. (These and the terms used to describe the bark surface are illustrated in Fig. 13.)

Where possible the bark should be snapped so that its *fracture* can be assessed. This is a key feature in its identification.

Underground structures

These are used by plants most often as storage organs, carrying fluid and nutrients to keep the plant alive during lean spells. They exhibit a variety of forms. Being often swollen they are frequently sliced and cut into small pieces to facilitate drying; some are also scraped to remove the outer dark cork and to give a lighter product.

They include the following:

> *Roots*: these have no buds, scale leaves or leaf scars and have a central core of woody xylem tissue.
>
> *Rhizomes* and *stolons*: underground stems (stolons are those which 'run' along under the ground putting up new shoots at intervals); they possess buds and scale leaves and scars; they have a central pith surrounded by woody xylem tissue.
>
> *Bulbs*: fleshy underground compressed leaves and stem (see Fig. 14).
>
> *Corms*: fleshy underground compressed stems with scale leaves attached (see Fig. 14).

Fruits

Fruits are the organs of plants containing the seed. They are often specialized to assist seed dispersal. They arise from the ovary and sometimes other parts of the plant. The main classes of fruit are illustrated (see Fig. 15).

Bark shapes

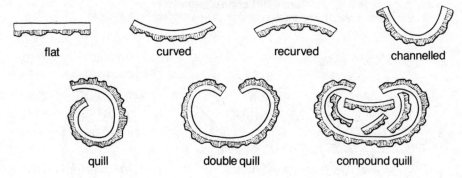

flat   curved   recurved   channelled

quill   double quill   compound quill

Bark surfaces

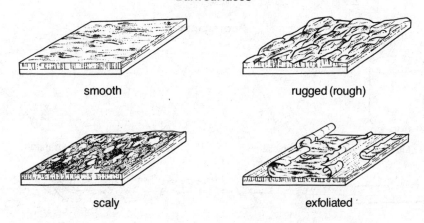

smooth   rugged (rough)

scaly   exfoliated

Bark fractures
(when the bark is snapped across the gain)

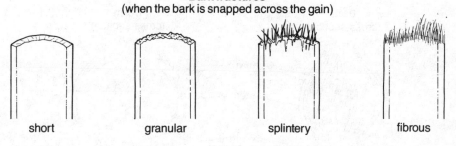

short   granular   splintery   fibrous

Fig. 13 Barks

Root – Direction of growth
(determined by orientation of shoots and rootlets to main axis)

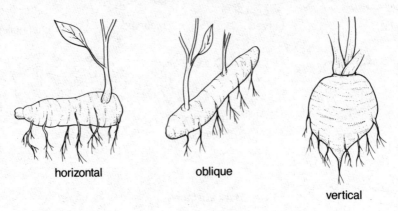

horizontal   oblique

vertical

Root shapes

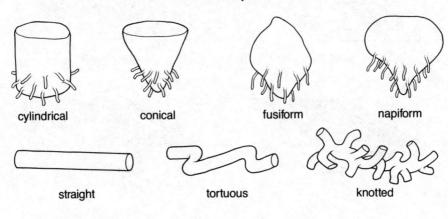

cylindrical   conical   fusiform   napiform

straight   tortuous   knotted

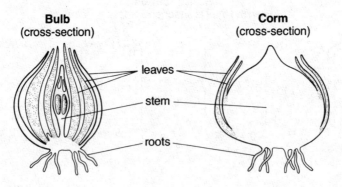

Bulb
(cross-section)

Corm
(cross-section)

leaves

stem

roots

Fig. 14 Roots

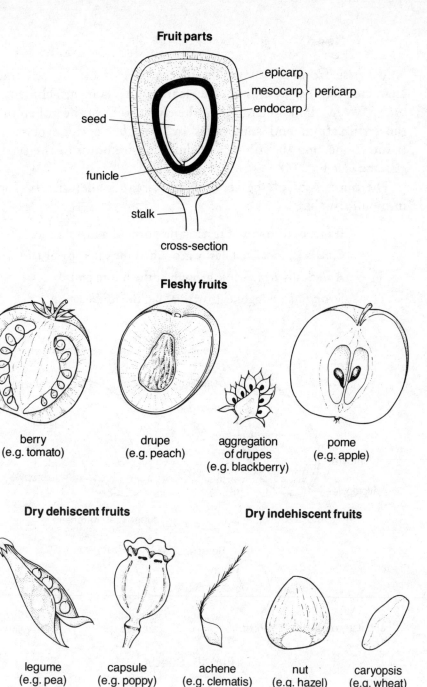

Fruit parts

epicarp ⎫
mesocarp ⎬ pericarp
endocarp ⎭

seed

funicle

stalk

cross-section

Fleshy fruits

berry
(e.g. tomato)

drupe
(e.g. peach)

aggregation
of drupes
(e.g. blackberry)

pome
(e.g. apple)

Dry dehiscent fruits   **Dry indehiscent fruits**

legume
(e.g. pea)

capsule
(e.g. poppy)

achene
(e.g. clematis)

nut
(e.g. hazel)

caryopsis
(e.g. wheat)

Fig. 15 Fruits

Seeds

Seeds arise from the ovules in the carpels of the flower and are characterized by a *hilum*, the scar from their attachment, the *micropyle*, a small hole marking the entry point of the pollen tube at the fertilization, and sometimes by a *raphe*, a ridge of vascular tissue connecting the hilum and the opposite point of the seed, the *chalaza* (see Fig. 16).

The outer coat of the seed, or testa, can sometimes be formed into outgrowths:

Wing: outgrowth of testa in the form of a membrane.

Caruncle: localized fleshy growth at the micropylar end.

Aril: fleshy or hairlike growth at the hilum end.

Strophiole: winglike growth along the raphe.

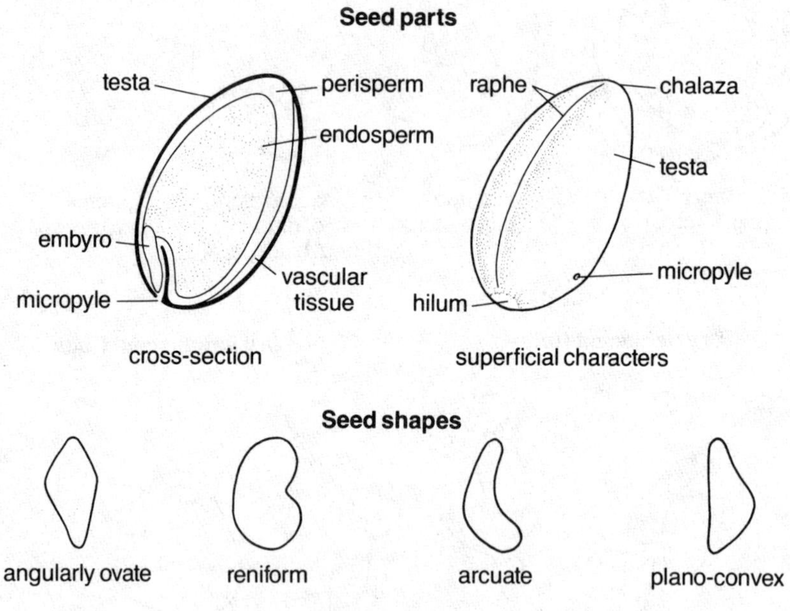
Seed parts
testa
perisperm
endosperm
embyro
micropyle
vascular tissue
cross-section
raphe
chalaza
testa
micropyle
hilum
superficial characters
Seed shapes
angularly ovate
reniform
arcuate
plano-convex

Fig. 16 Seeds

Pharmacy

Introduction

This section is designed to introduce the principles of remedy preparation and application. How a herb is dispensed will radically affect its action, and will also be important in determining the most practical way of handling and using it on a day-to-day basis.[2]

The preparation of remedies for administration is a subject that has been intensively investigated and recorded through the ages. In modern times, when we are used to seeing only a small selection of medicinal preparations like capsules, tablets and ointments, it might be surprising to discover the enormous range of preparations regularly supplied in earlier times. The traditional pharmacist was a highly skilled technician, making to order an amazing selection of applications for both internal and especially external use. For those who wish to explore the full potential for herbal remedies today, it will be very useful to look again at some of the range, and if possible try out a few preparations apart from the most basic.

The external preparations will repay particular attention as the legal position regarding their applications is likely to be easier.

Many of the preparations and instructions follow the standards set by official pharmacopoeias, such as the *United States Pharmacopoeia (USP)*, the *British Pharmacopoeia (BP)*, the *British Pharmaceutical Codex (BPC)* and *Martindale The Extra Pharmacopoeia*. These standards derive in turn from earlier established practices, but once entered in an official pharmacopoeia become a formal convention. In many cases, however, we can adapt the procedures to suit modern needs and techniques.

The universal unit of measurement in modern pharmacy is the metric one and this is used throughout this text. One advantage of using metric is the easy conversion of units of weight and volume for most purposes, e.g. one litre of water (l) weighs one kilogram (kg), one millilitre (ml) or cubic centimetre (cc) weighs one gram (g). To be precise these equivalences are for pure water at 4°C, but in practice they hold for aqueous solutions and those in alcohol at room temperature as well.

List of metric weights equivalents:

1 ml (millilitre) = 0.035 fl. oz. (Imperial) = 0.034 fl. oz. (USA)
1 l (litre) = 1.76 pt, or 0.26 gal. (Imp.) = 2.11 pt, or 0.22 gal. (USA)

1 fl. oz. (fluid ounce): (Imp.) = 28.41 ml; (USA) = 29.56 ml
1 pt (pint): (Imp.) = 0.57 l; (USA) = 0.47 l
1 gal. (gallon): (Imp.) = 4.54 l; (USA) = 3.78 l

1 g (gram) = 15.432 grains
100 g = 3.527 oz.
1 kg (kilogram) = 2.204 lb, or 35.27 oz.

1 grain = 65 mg
1 oz. (ounce) = 28.35 g
1 lb (pound) = 454 g, or 0.454 kg

Obtaining the Crude Drug

The processes of preparation begin with obtaining suitable raw material. The first priority is to ensure this is of good quality (see 'Herb Recognition and Quality Control', on pp. 348–64). For those collecting their own specimens, or able to control harvesting, the following guidelines are suggested for obtaining the best material to start with.

Harvesting

'*Herb*' (aerial parts, including leaves and flowering tops): ideally collected just before the flowers open, in the morning after any dew has dried.

Flowers: ideally collected on dry days, preferably at midday.

Seeds: generally collected in dry weather when fully mature.

Bark: generally collected in dormant seasons, either early spring or late autumn.

Underground parts: generally collected in the autumn, winter or early spring while the plant sap is low. Perennial plants are harvested after at least two years, biennials in the season after their first year's growth. Annual roots are collected just before flowering.

Drying

A few preparations rely on the use of the fresh herb, but the vast majority use dried specimens. The aim of drying is to ensure adequate storage life as well as to reduce bulk, thus concentrating the remedy, all without unduly damaging the plant's constituents. A well-dried specimen should retain most of its natural colour and aroma, indicating that little more than water has been lost.

Natural drying is best accomplished out of direct sunlight, which damages several plant constituents, but with adequate ventilation and not during damp weather. An open barn is ideal.

Artificial drying is conducted at its simplest by strewing the herb material on to netting trays in a chamber whose temperature is raised by dry heat to between 25–40°C (approx. 80–100°F) for leaf and flower material, and to between 40–60°C (approx. 100–140°F) for root, bark and woody material. Again adequate ventilation is necessary. These temperatures are adjusted to suit individual samples, so as to ensure brisk drying (to reduce enzymatic deterioration) without scorching or other damage. In commercial operations vacuum-drying, de-humidifying and freeze-drying are options, and these provide a better-quality product.

Storage

The aims of storage are to protect the plant material from moisture, light, oxidation and pests. The storage environment should be dry and cool, ideally never warmer than 15°C (59°F). The container should be sufficiently porous to avoid condensation (avoid glass and plastic) but not so much as to allow excessive oxidation. Heavy brown paper is ideal for moderate quantities, although some external protection may have to be provided to reduce pest attack.

Herbs stored well will last a long time but not indefinitely. As a guide herbs should be stored for one year, although barks and root material have a longer life.

Basic Processes

There are a number of processes common to most preparation techniques.

COMMINUTION

Breaking down herb samples to suitable size used to be the hardest work of all the processes of preparation, entailing hours of labour with the pestle and mortar, usually by young apprentices! Nowadays these implements are little more than picturesque ornaments and cutting, slicing or grinding is done by machinery of various types; cutting is done by machines adapted from the tobacco industry, whilst grinding is done with metal-disc or hammer mills. For personal use the kitchen blender will perform many functions quite adequately, although to get the fine powders necessary for some applications a special mill with sieves of varying gauge will be necessary.

EXTRACTION

This is the procedure by which the soluble, and hopefully active, constituents of a crude drug are separated out. The main aim is to obtain a preparation that is reasonably concentrated, optimally active and, where possible, one whose qualities can be predicted and reproduced.

A liquid is chosen which will have the best chance of dissolving the required active ingredients. This liquid is called the *menstruum*, the solid material left after extraction is referred to as the *marc*. Most commonly the former will be either water or a mixture of water and ethyl alcohol. Alcohol is necessary when the extract is to be kept for any length of time or when water-insoluble constituents need to be dissolved. Four strengths of alcohol-in-water are used in the *British Pharmacopoeia*: 45 per cent, 60 per cent, 70 per cent and 90 per cent, depending on the constituents selected as desirable. For the purposes of professional practice in the UK, the majority of herbs, for which extraction in water alone would be sufficient, are extracted in 20–25 per cent alcohol, this being the minimum necessary to sterilize and preserve the extract. For home use, however, simple aqueous extraction (i.e., with water alone) is adequate for most purposes, provided the extract is not stored for long (no more than 24 hours out of a fridge, three to four days if refrigerated). Other menstruums are used in some cases, notably acetic acid (e.g. vinegar), glycerol (or glycerine), ether and seed oils.

There are four main procedures used in extraction: infusion and decoction (in which the menstruum is usually hot water), and maceration and percolation (in which the menstruum is usually a cold alcohol/water mixture).

Infusion

This process is chosen when the active principles of the crude drug are readily soluble in water and easily obtained from the tissues. In practical terms it is appropriate for leaves, flowers and non-woody stems, but not for woody material, bark or root (except if finely powdered).

369 Pharmacy

The technique is to steep the material in hot water for a certain period and then to strain off the liquid. Where the extraction of mucilage is a priority, it is better to steep the herb in its equivalent weight of cold water for 15 minutes before adding the rest of the hot menstruum. To reduce loss of volatile constituents it is essential to cover the infusion while steeping, and in fact an ideal container is a wide-necked Thermos, or vacuum flask (this has the twin benefits of retaining all volatile constituents and keeping the temperature up, so increasing extraction performance and sterilization). Traditional quantities are 1 ounce of dried herb steeped in 1 pint of water (30 g to 500 ml). This may have to be adjusted if the herb is particularly bulky.

Steeping time is generally taken as between 15 minutes and 2 hours, although the use of the Thermos flask will allow longer infusion times (even overnight). The liquid is then strained off: it is usually unnecessary to press the marc for more liquid although this may be done if desired, or if the marc is particularly bulky. The extract should be used quickly: in many cases it is best taken while still hot anyway (use of the Thermos flask will allow the dose to be decanted off as required when the medicine is used domestically).

Decoction

This process is used when the active principles are soluble in water but the drug is woody or otherwise slow to relinquish its constituents. It involves boiling the material for some time. Traditionally around 30 g material was boiled with 700–850 ml water until it was reduced, so that around 500 ml water could be decanted off. This entailed boiling for at least 10–15 minutes. While this was certainly the most commonly used technique in pre-urban herbalism, and remains so in Chinese herbalism, for example, its relative inconvenience makes it less popular in modern times. It is still, however, the only way of extracting tough material with water and will continue to have a part to play for that reason. It is possible to avoid the problems of steaming cauldrons, and the obvious loss of volatile constituents they involve, by using electric slow-cookers or crock-pots instead. These are designed to cook food at temperatures a little less than boiling point and the lids are so placed as to form a liquid seal from the condensation. Using them for decoctions (when preparation times are of course extended to 6–8 hours) will lead to a very high-quality extract, rich in volatile constituents. This latter quality is likely to be very important for that action of some Western remedies like the aromatic roots of valerian, elecampane and angelica. It is worth stating, however, that traditional claims for many remedies, and certainly for most Chinese herbs, come from their use as decoctions. Given that different extraction techniques will leave a different profile of plant constituents in the final product we must be prepared to see slightly different actions as well.

Maceration

This is a process by which the herb is steeped in the menstruum at room temperature. By definition, therefore, the menstruum needs to prevent fermentation and deterioration during the process, and in most cases an alcohol/water mixture is used, although vinegar is occasionally used as well. The plant material is generally cut or powdered and left in the menstruum, with daily agitation, for many days (often around two weeks). At the end of this time the liquid is drained off and then the wet marc is pressed to extract as much as possible of that remaining. The proportion of liquid to herb is usually carefully defined (often 1 part of herb to 5 parts of liquid, as in the 1:5 tincture), so that the final product is carefully standardized. This means that it is inappropriate to add fresh menstruum to make up the quantity (this would dilute the extract at a variable rate), so that it makes sense to get as much liquid out of the marc as possible. Hand-squeezing is much less efficient than a wine-press, and this can be bettered by the use of hydraulic presses in commercial outfits. The final preparation will have a long shelf-life and will usually be more concentrated than the infusion or decoction, so that a smaller quantity is necessary in any dosage. This explains the popularity of tinctures among professional practitioners in the UK.

Percolation

Probably the most efficient means of extraction, percolation involves letting the menstruum trickle down through a mass of herb that has been finely ground and placed in a columnar 'percolator'. The ground herb is pre-moistened for several hours in a fraction of the menstruum to allow the particles to swell before the wet mass is passed through a coarse sieve and lightly packed in the chamber, with a wad of gauze below and filter paper above. The drainage at the bottom is closed and sufficient menstruum is added to cover the powder completely: the vessel is covered and maceration is allowed for around 24 hours. The drainage is opened and fluid is allowed through at the rate of 10–30 drops per minute, the rest of the menstruum being added at the top as required; the process is carried on until three-quarters of the fluid intended has been collected or until the herb is exhausted. The powder is then pressed and the fluid added to the percolate, this being topped up to the final quantity with fresh menstruum. It is possible to obtain very concentrated extracts by re-percolating fresh herb with the first extract up to several times, and concentrations of even 1 : 1 (herb to percolate) may be obtained in this way.

Expression

The process of forcibly separating fluid from solids, used of course in the processes of maceration and percolation to obtain the rest of the fluid from the marc. The term is most often used, however, to refer to the pressing of fresh plant material to obtain the juice (succus or green extract). Homoeopathic mother tinctures are made from expressed extracts of fresh plant material to which alcohol is added as a preservative. Some immediate preserving is essential as decomposition proceeds rapidly, although freezing or chilling will be sufficient. It is possible to obtain a reasonable succus with suitably sappy material by using a domestic liquidizer and pressing the resultant substance through fine-mesh material.

Distillation

Used to selectively extract one liquid fraction from another, either from an already extracted fluid or from a macerating mixture, and used in pharmacy mainly for extracting volatile oil fractions from aqueous mixtures (and of course, for the same purpose in perfumery). Crude distillation techniques are easy to apply, as variants on the widely used alcohol-extraction methods. However, for any accurate extraction, either fractional distillation or, for volatile oils from aqueous solutions (the usual requirement), steam distillation will need to be invoked.

Making Mixtures

In practice it is usually necessary to mix together two or more ingredients to make a liquid prescription. When it is simply a number of herbs in an infusion or decoction then few complications will arise. However, it is often the case that other types of blending will be needed and problems may arise with varying degrees of immiscibility. It is thus desirable to explore basic principles in making a mixture (or mistura).

The mixture of two miscible liquids, or of a liquid with a solid that is soluble in it, will lead to stable, true solutions; when the blends are of two immiscible liquids, of liquids that react with each other to form precipitates, or of a liquid with a solid that does not dissolve in it, then some form of 'dispersion' is required. Two main types of dispersion are *colloids* and *suspensions*, the former having finer particles and different physical properties from the latter. When there is a solid fine enough to be diffused through the solution by shaking, then suspension is effectively achieved in this way. In other cases, specific agents will need to be added to disperse one component in the other. The main examples of the process are as follows:

Mucilages

These are suspensions employing in most cases acacia or tragacanth gums in sufficient quantity to increase the viscosity of the liquid

373 Pharmacy

and thus suspend insoluble solid material. Acacia gum is a finer material that may in certain circumstances increase the likelihood of fine solid particles caking. Gum tragacanth is more viscous and is able to suspend heavier solids. Often a 1:1 blend of the two powders is used, called 'Compound Tragacanth' powder. The principle of preparation is to mix the solids with the powdered gum in a mortar before adding the liquid in small portions at a time to form a smooth cream. The amount of gum to add depends on the type used: acacia alone at 0.5–1 g per 100 ml of liquid, tragacanth at half that level.

If two liquids are to be blended that would form a precipitate when mixed (e.g. tinctures of calendula, myrrh, lignum-vitae or hops added to aqueous solutions), a similar process may be adopted to produce a colloid. The gum powders are mixed with the main liquid by degrees to form the smooth cream, and the precipitate-forming liquid is added to the result. Acacia gum is probably the best for this operation: gelatine is used in some solid or semi-solid preparations.

Emulsions

These are mixtures of immiscible liquids (usually oily liquids with water: milk is a common example of such an emulsion; waxes, resins and volatile oils are frequent variants on the oily phase). If the two liquids are mixed together simply and shaken, they will emulsify briefly before separating. Adding a third ingredient will allow the formation of a more stable emulsion. The choice will depend in part on the relative proportions of the two liquids: when the aqueous portion is the major one the mixture is referred to as an oil-in-water (o/w) emulsion; the opposite is termed a water-in-oil (w/o) emulsion. The emulsifying agent in herbal preparations will usually be one of three main groups.

> *Carbohydrates*: acacia gum, agar-agar, Irish moss and the mucilages of seeds like psyllium are examples – they are used for o/w emulsions.
>
> *Proteins*: gelatine, egg yolk and casein are examples used also for o/w emulsions.

Complex alcohols and fats: wool fat (lanolin), cholesterol, beeswax and spermaceti are frequent examples used for w/o emulsions (the latter, derived from sperm whales, is no longer used).

There are wide variations in the details of the emulsion-preparing process, and some are described in pharmacopoeias. However, the essential feature of most is that a primary emulsion is prepared first, this being a concentrated mixture of the emulsion. In o/w emulsions the oily phase is usually blended with the emulsifying agent first, before a little of the aqueous liquid is added to make a smooth cream. This primary emulsion is then diluted with the rest of the aqueous liquid. In w/o emulsions the process is reversed.

Some Specific Processes

We now turn to consider specific preparations for medicinal use. We shall divide them into two groups, for internal and external use.

INTERNAL USE: LIQUIDS

Elixirs

Sweetened preparations, in which tinctures, fluid extracts and other constituents are mixed with a sugar/water mixture, often in the proportions of 1 part of sugar to 2 of water. They were primarily designed to give medicines to young children.

Fluid (liquid) extracts

An extract of a drug in fluid so that one part by volume of the preparation is equivalent to one part by weight of the original drug; in other words it is a highly concentrated preparation. The advantage is clear: a litre of fluid extract takes up much less space than a kilogram of most dried herbs and is instantly prescribable in small doses. The disadvantage comes in considering the processes usually applied. Many commercial extracts used to start out as tinctures of the herb in some form of industrial spirit: this was evaporated off to leave a residue in the vessel which was then reconstituted with the desired amount of alcohol. The result was often a preparation devoid of appreciable volatile oils, which thus rarely had the aroma of the original herb and probably did not have the pharmacological effect of the constituents either (although traditional decoctions probably had similar drawbacks). Moreover, the preparation was often caramelized in the evaporation process, thereby imparting a characteristic taste to all such extracts, and probably pointing to further damage to other plant constituents. Far more efficient an extraction process is repeated percolation, described earlier; this is however more labour-intensive and such extracts are rarely obtained commercially.

Glycerins

Using glycerin as a solvent and preservative is particularly useful for remedies containing a lot of phlobotannins (see 'Tannins', on pp. 282–6) as it can dissolve them. It generally has a solvent action midway between alcohol and water, and this also applies to its preservative qualities: at least 30 per cent of glycerin is necessary for preservation of plant material, and even 50 per cent may not always be sufficient to prevent bacterial contamination. Glycerin tastes sweet and this can help in treating children.

Linctuses

These are thickened solutions designed to be taken for throat problems, the idea being to form a film of solution over the membranes to exert soothing, healing or antiseptic action locally. Mucilages, emulsions, glycerins and syrups are often used to form the basis of these preparations. They are usually sipped and swallowed slowly after meals.

Mels

Medicines made with honey, this being used both to disguise taste, and as a healing and soothing agent, for burns and throat inflammations.

Spirits

Solutions of volatile substances (such as oil of peppermint) in alcohol.

Syrups

Concentrated sugar solutions, used either alone for flavouring, or as part of an extraction process for preserving. The sugar needs to be dissolved by heating the solution, and should be at levels of at least 70 per cent by weight of the fluid it seeks to preserve. Marshmallow, horehound and wild cherry syrups were widely used for coughs, throat and chest problems in children.

Tinctures

The most popular means of administering herbs among herbal practitioners in the UK. They are preparations of medicinal substances in alcohol, most often the result of macerating or percolating herbs with alcohol/water solutions. The concentration of herb to fluid is generally higher than that in infusions or decoctions, with proportions of 1:3, 1:4, 1:5, 1:8 and 1:10 widely recognized for different preparations. Most herbs used in practice are 1:5. The strength of alcohol in water also varies, depending on the type of constituent that needs to be extracted, with 25 per cent alcohol used for most simple extractions (with an extraction most closely comparable to infusions), and 45 per cent, 60 per cent, 70 per cent and 90 per cent used where volatile oils, alkaloids and resins (all largely insoluble in water) are to be extracted. The techniques used have been surveyed above, when discussing maceration and percolation, and specific details of the individual preparations for the different Western herbs are listed in the materia medica section. It is possible to prepare tinctures by diluting fluid extracts, and most commercial 'tinctures' are unfortunately obtained in this way.

Although theoretically legitimate, the quality of the product is far inferior to that of the tinctures prepared by direct maceration or percolation, and they should be avoided.

Vinegars

These are extracts made with acetic acid. The preparation dissolves some alkaloidal constituents well, and the vinegar gives extra expectorant, diuretic and diaphoretic properties. The extract may be obtained by maceration or percolation in the cold. Because of the taste honey is often added as well (the mixture is then referred to as an oxymel).

Wines

In former times wines were the most readily available alcohol/water solvents and were often used to prepare an early form of tincture. The main problem with them was their variable and usually low alcohol content, which, especially after maceration or percolation, was often insufficient to preserve the final preparation fully. For this reason, if wines are to be used they must be of the fortified variety. It is possible to obtain wines by fermenting herbal infusions, but these are unlikely to be strong enough to give an adequate dosage of the herb without risking intoxication, and in any case there is almost certainly alteration of some plant components, especially the glycosides, during fermentation.

INTERNAL USE: SOLIDS

Capsules

The use of gelatine capsules has largely superseded the tablets, pills and other solid preparations so familiar in the past. They may even be prepared on the small scale with capsule-filling machines, or blanks may be filled by hand, and they do provide a convenient way of administering herbal remedies, especially where the taste is a problem, or where what is desired is to provide a mucilaginous, astringent or other direct action on the gut wall. Capsulated preparations seem to have an advantage in the following cases: when giving cayenne for circulatory stimulation, when providing urinary antiseptics, when administering slippery elm powder as a protection against acid damage in the stomach, and for bulk laxatives like psyllium seed or flaxseed (linseed). They are inappropriate where the taste is important, as in the bitter effect. Herbal material will need to be powdered before being put in capsules: a kitchen blender or liquidizer will do the job adequately. As most capsules are still made with gelatine, this may be a problem for vegans or macrobiotics. At this point, enteric and slow-release capsule shells are not readily available, so we cannot take advantage of their resistance to gastric breakdown to deliver their contents directly lower down the gut.

Lozenges

These are traditionally made by cutting out and drying a paste made with acacia-gum mucilage and powdered sugar. They are designed to be sucked as soothing agents for throat problems.

Pastilles

These are softer versions of lozenges using a heated mixture of gelatine and glycerin in water as a base (a ratio of 1:2:2 respectively) instead of acacia mucilage.

Pills

A traditional means of dispensing medicines based on binding the medicinal agent with an adhesive or absorbent excipient and sufficient fluid to form a malleable paste. This is rolled out and cut into balls for drying and probably coating. The techniques involved are highly skilled and practical, and special equipment is also required. However, as there is in any case a reduced demand for pills today, this must be classed as a dying craft in developed countries.

Powders

It used to be quite common to have powders dispensed, to be taken dispersed with a little water, but this practice grew up mainly for inorganic or mineral medicines: it is not generally a suitable way to provide herbal material, which deteriorates quickly when stored as powder and is difficult to disperse in water.

Solid extracts

These are the residues obtained by drying the fluid extract completely. They are generally supplied in the block form or powdered. As all volatile constituents will be lost and many others altered by the process, only a very few herbs are likely to be particularly effective in this form. One of the notable examples of these is liquorice, which in powdered form is most effective mixed with other herbs in capsules.

Tablets

Like pills, the production of compressed tablets is a complicated process, requiring special equipment and a complex formulation of binders, lubricants, disintegrating agents, and so on. Unlike pills, tablets are widely produced commercially, and the technology has developed apace. It is not generally practicable to make tablets on a small-scale basis, but commercial houses in the UK will produce them to special order if sufficient are requested. Tablets are generally designed to be chewed before swallowing, so they are not suitable for strong-tasting ingredients.

EXTERNAL USE: LIQUIDS

Baths

Using immersion in water at various temperatures is an ancient European traditional approach to healing. The cold, tepid and hot baths beloved of the Romans have survived as techniques to the present day in Europe, although they are very much in decline in the UK. The aim is to influence and provoke circulatory activity and renewal (although the terminology arose long before blood circulation was understood), and the revival in use of the treatment bears witness to its effects. Hot baths are just higher than body temperature at 38–43°C (approx. 100–110°F), tepid baths are at 29–35°C (85–95°F), whilst cold baths commence at 29°C (85°F) to be lowered to 15°C (60°F) with ice. Adding herbs or volatile oils to baths has been a common variation, with the particular benefit of allowing inhalation of the volatile components in the steam. One common application of the bath is the mustard bath, used to bathe feet or hands affected by arthritic trouble, or as a means of stimulating circulation generally throughout the system. Mustard powder is added at up to 1 per cent by weight to warm (not too hot) water and the part bathed in it till cool. A notable proponent of the dual benefits of bathing and herbs has been the German, Father Sebastian Kneipp (1821–97), who started a tradition still maintained in the Kneipp spa at Bad Wörishofen in the Bavarian Alps. In another context, there has also been the work of the French herbalist Maurice Messegué, who has popularized an approach using hand and foot baths instead of internal applications. Both these and other similar approaches may be of interest to the prospective unregistered herbalist practising in an unsympathetic legislative climate, as their use is likely to bypass any legal strictures on prescribing medicines.

Douches

Aqueous solutions directed against the body or into a body cavity to cleanse or disinfect. The vaginal douche is the most frequently used: infusions of astringent or antiseptic herbs may be prepared and applied deep into the vagina whilst the patient is lying supine via a bulb syringe or similar applicator, for vaginal and cervical infections and inflammations. Douches can also be used for the nasal cavity although this is rarely done nowadays.

Ear-drops

These are applied to conditions of the external ear canal, to help clear obstructions (warm olive oil is sufficient for most cases), to treat inflammation or infection of the canal or eardrum, or to influence the middle ear by diffusion across the eardrum. They are mostly oil- or alcohol/water-based preparations, and in any case should be prepared with due regard to the possibility of bacterial

381 Pharmacy

contamination. Garlic and mullein flowers are particularly highly regarded remedies for application by this route, especially where it is necessary to affect middle-ear problems: they are usually applied steeped in oil. Glycerin should be avoided in ear-drops.

Enemas

Liquids applied via the rectum, either to allow absorption of medicine into the body to avoid so-called 'first-pass' liver metabolism, in which case small quantities only need to be introduced (see also 'Suppositories', below), or to apply nutrients in extremely cachexic conditions, or most frequently to provoke bowel evacuation. The liquid should be at body temperature and applied with douche can, bowel syringe or similar apparatus. Care must be taken to avoid introducing air into the bowel, and cleanliness must be observed scrupulously. Total quantities to promote evacuation should be between 500 ml and 1 l in the adult.

Eye-drops

Usually aqueous solutions are applied directly to the surface of the eye to treat conjunctival and corneal infections, and problems of the eyelids. Great care must be taken to ensure sterility of the fluid as bacteria introduced to the eye surfaces can occasionally lead to serious trouble. To ensure sterility any herbal solution must be boiled for at least 15 minutes in its final container (or added to a sterilized container after boiling). Any water added to the preparation must also be sterilized. Decoctions of eyebright, fennel seed, agrimony and liquorice root, made at standard strengths and possibly diluted 1:1 with water, may be used with great benefit for a number of eye problems.

Gargles

Preparations in water or alcohol/water solution to be used for throat problems. They are usually antiseptic, soothing and/or healing. Many gargles are meant not to be swallowed, but in practice herbal gargles may be swallowed after gargling to obtain a secondary, systemic effect. Effective gargles can be made with tinctures of sage, myrrh, calendula and echinacea, these ideally combined with fluid extract of liquorice or other mucilaginous ingredients. Honey is another effective ingredient.

Inhalants (*or* vapours)

Volatile components may be inhaled either from a pad applied to the nose and mouth, or from liniments or ointments applied to the skin under the nose or on the chest, or most effectively with steam from hot water. They allow deep and accurate penetration of medicinal agents throughout the whole respiratory system, including the sinuses and middle ear; they will clear catarrhal congestion, soothe irritable mucous membranes, and reduce some hypersensitivity reactions. The simplest steaming bowl of water can form an effective inhalant with a few drops of volatile oil or simple dried herbs applied.

Liniments (*and* embrocations)

Liquid or semi-liquid preparations usually prepared in oily or alcoholic solution (embrocations refer to the former) and designed to have rubefacient or analgesic properties. They are rubbed into usually unbroken skin. Examples include liniments of mustard and capsicum, used to stimulate circulation, and liniment of arnica for analgesic and healing properties. In some cases the preparations involve emulsification with soap.

Lotions

The name given to non-oily liquids applied externally and generally not rubbed in. They are applied to the body surface or any external orifice.

EXTERNAL USE: SEMI-SOLIDS

Creams

Semi-solid emulsions of oil in water or water in oil that are readily absorbed by the skin. They may have various remedies dissolved in either the oil or water fraction. Creams are generally softer than

383 Pharmacy

ointments and are more complex in their formulation. For this reason they were not common in pharmacies of the past, but they are very prominent today, in part because of the advances in technology, in part because of their popularity for the cosmetic industry. Their preparation requires a degree of technological sophistication (and the willingness to use modern emulsifying and preserving ingredients) and is barely practicable on the personal scale.

Jellies

Semi-solid suspensions or colloids made from gums, pectin or gelatine. They allow non-oily preparations to be applied to mucous membranes (like the vagina and rectum) and to open or discharging wounds or lesions. They are the most effective way of applying a strongly astringent treatment, especially if gum tragacanth is used as the gelling/suspending agent (it contains its own high level of tannins). Infusions, juices or tinctures may be used for the fluid part, the latter being recommended where the jelly is to be kept for any period and where the antiseptic action of myrrh or calendula is to be incorporated; tinctures may however lead to smarting and in this case fresh infusions will need to be prepared. The technique is to add powdered gum tragacanth slowly to the liquid being agitated in a food blender or liquidizer, to the point when the mixture thickens sufficiently. Soothing astringent preparations made with comfrey or witch hazel are ideal for irritated wounds, slow-healing leg ulcers, or haemorrhoids; tinctures of myrrh and calendula may be added for treatment of vaginal infections or cervical problems.

Ointments (*or* unguents)

Semi-solid solutions of various preparations in non-aqueous bases that are not absorbed easily into the skin and are therefore used to provide a protective or remedial film over the skin. Being immiscible with water or skin secretions, ointments effectively form an occlusive layer over the skin, preventing evaporation (sweat forms only part of a large loss of fluid from the skin by transpiration). The result is similar to that seen when occlusive dressings are applied: the skin becomes waterlogged (hydrated). This permits easier absorption of water-soluble materials that might be contained in the ointment, and where this is an important consideration, the base should be chosen to be able to carry an appreciable aqueous component. Some bases also penetrate to a degree themselves, with vegetable oils and animal fats being the most likely to do so. It is considerations such as these which determine the choice of base.

The fatty or oily bases (including the paraffins, vegetable oils and animal fats) form clearly occlusive applications, but are greasy, difficult to remove and easily stain clothing. These effects may be alleviated with the use of absorptive bases (such as wool fat, or lanolin) which can absorb a degree of aqueous fluid, emulsifying bases (such as waxes, whether natural, like beeswax, or synthetic), or a few water-soluble bases like polyethylene glycol. These components are blended together in a range of official and unofficial formulae.

Pastes

It is often necessary to incorporate powdered material into ointment bases, especially to provide bulk, absorptive and protective healing benefits (as for example when applying to a dressing or bandage). When the solid component is substantial the preparation is called a paste. It is prepared by blending with the ointment or colloid base in the cold, using a stiff spatula on a tile or glass surface, working small amounts of the solid into small amounts of base, bringing all the portions together at the end.

Pessaries

These are solid preparations, suitable for vaginal insertion and made in a similar way to suppositories (see below).

Plasters

Unlike the modern item, traditional plasters were impregnated dressings applied over the skin where a long-term and concentrated medication was required. The plaster mass was a waxy, rubbery, resinous or other base, incorporating medical agents and spread on to fabric of some description. It was often designed to convey rubefacient, analgesic or protective effects. A plaster can be made quite easily with a 1:1 mixture of lanolin and beeswax melted together, to which is added a herbal tincture or essential oil.

Poultices

Hot soaked masses of material prepared in a fabric bag and applied to the skin while still hot. Poultices have particular ability to draw wounds and infections and to soothe, heal and astringe. A simple poultice may be prepared by putting powdered or chopped herbal material into a small pouch of muslin or similar fabric, pouring enough boiling water on just to soak the material in a shallow dish, working the moisture through the herb until hot enough to be bearable, and applying to the affected area until cold. Linseed, comfrey, marshmallow and cabbage leaf are frequently used in poultice form in traditional practice.

Powders

Fine powders, often based on zinc oxide, magnesium carbonate, or sterilized starch, kaolin or talc, designed to be dusted on to open wounds or broken skin as absorbent and healing agents, or to skin where chafing might occur. Sterility is an obvious requirement for open wounds and any naturally extracted material will need baking on open trays at 150°C (302°F) for at least an hour. This will remove all volatile ingredients (these may be added afterwards in the form of volatile oils, although only small quantities can be used and the oils need to be mixed in the form of a fine spray), but the technique is still applicable to finely milled astringent (especially tannin-rich) herbs, whether these are blended with excipients or not. One example is powdered witch hazel bark, which may for example be inhaled as a snuff for nasal inflammation or polyps. The dose inhaled should be small to prevent the herb reaching the rest of the respiratory system: a portion enough to cover a typed vowel on a page will usually be sufficient. The same or similar powders may be dusted over varicose or other external ulcers or slow-healing wounds.

Snuffs

See powders.

Suppositories

Solid preparations suitable for rectal insertion, generally consisting of a solution or suspension of active agents in a solid base designed to melt at body temperature. Two main types of base are cocoa butter and gelatine-glycerin mixes. The former is most immediately applicable where dry herbal preparations are to be added, the latter will be better able to absorb a certain amount of fluid. To make suppositories, moulds will be required, these being either traditional polished metal, or disposable plastic. Cocoa butter is melted gently in a water bath (avoiding condensation) portions of it are mixed with powders on warmed slabs, and the mixture added back to the container. The final mixture, which needs to be stirred constantly, is added quickly to the moulds, allowing a little overflow. The moulds are then cooled and excess cocoa butter trimmed off. The suppositories can be taken out (unless in disposable moulds) and kept at temperatures below 27°C (80°F). Certain oils and liquids may be added at the last moment before pouring, using beeswax (up to 5 per cent) where necessary to keep the melting point from being lowered too much.

Although gelatine-glycerin mixes are capable of holding more fluid, the use of glycerin in these versions will lead to drying of the mucosal membranes, and this may provoke inflammation if used frequently.

8 Remedies

Introduction

The remainder of this text is given over to discussing several herbal remedies in some detail.

The list is smaller than is usual in herb books and is made up only of herbs of which the author has personal experience in clinical practice.

There are a number of reasons for such a decision. In the first place there is already a considerable literature on herbal remedies, both of the popular and more technical sort. It is possible quickly to collect information about a great many remedies from many parts of the world from a simple perusal of the bookshelves. It seems unnecessary to add more of the same.

On the other hand, there is a singular dearth of accounts of herbal remedies based on actual clinical experience. The majority of texts available is actually very derivative, many writers in the field not having professional training or even being practising herbalists at all. The accounts of each remedy are usually rather shallow, often little more than lists of symptoms, as if herbs were simply gentle versions of conventional drugs. Where scientific information is inserted it also usually has little relevance to clinical experience of the action of the herb.

What is needed is a broad-based account of the herb as a partner in treatment, combining personal experience of its effect with a presentation of available research literature. In Britain at least, conditions for such an enterprise have not been good until recently: the profession has only just been revitalized after a long period of desperately keeping the torch alight against a powerful scientific climate of disapproval. The new generation has understandably waited for a decade or so of practical experience before feeling confident enough to go into print.

The most notable accomplishment to date has been the production of the first volume of the *Compendium* of the *British Herbal Pharmacopoeia* in 1990, in which a highly disciplined review of the clinical and research evidence is made by experienced practitioners and scientists. This is the text most recommended for hard information about herbs in the British tradition.

There still remains another goal: to present, as fully as possible, the *remedies as herbal remedies*, that is, in a way that stays true to their real qualities. The preceding text has attempted to provide a medical framework against which to assess such qualities. The following attempts to apply the clinical detail.

Simples vs. formulae

Many traditions, notably those of the Far East, have a strong written tradition of using mixtures of herbs, or formulae, rather than individual herbs (simples) on their own. There are even those who suggest that it only makes sense to use such formulae, built up over centuries to provide due balance and effect, rather than to use single remedies.

This author disagrees with that view. Firstly, most formulae that come down from earlier traditions were designed to deal with earlier illnesses, in ways discussed at several points in previous chapters. Secondly, and this is a more fundamental point, it is difficult to learn about the qualities of herbal remedies if they are always in mixtures with others. In personal experience of teaching the subject, it has been found that basic principles are much more easily absorbed if the novice starts with individual plants and gets early feedback from them.

All the better herbal remedies are already complex enough characters, as the following text may illustrate. They will have ample effects on their own, and, if used as suggested, these will often be very speedy. The process of learning will be very much faster if each herb is introduced as an individual.

Then of course it will be possible to learn more about the art of mixing herbs anew, such as inspired the construction of many original formulae in the first place. Professional herbalists in Britain in fact rarely use set formulae. Each patient will get a mixture of simples, uniquely tailored to his or her own needs. This can only be done if the qualities of each individual remedy are understood.

The policy adopted here is to provide herbal *archetypes*, a basic palette of remedies. Most other herbal remedies will be better understood in the light of the characteristics of those picked. Absorbing these archetypal qualities will thus help the reader make sense of the almost infinite diversity of medicinal plants around the world. It will even be possible, with a smattering of information on the use, quality and constituents of a plant, to predict its likely action.

John Parkinson

Throughout the following text references will sometimes be drawn from the appropriate pages of one of the most useful old herbals in the English language. *Theatrum botanicum*, written in 1640 by John Parkinson, is a rich source of information about the actual uses of herbal remedies of the day (unlike the more personalized accounts of some of his contemporaries). His comments, apart from confirming the pedigree of the traditional use of the herbs, are often beautifully phrased, and show how apt the English of the period was in describing human experience.

How to use these herbs

This book is not intended as a substitute for proper training in the practice of herbal medicine. There are options for such further education* and no one should use any of the herbs as recommended here without careful consideration of the implications.

Reference is frequently made to the treatment of medical conditions that would need to be assessed by experts, to exclude the possibility of dangerous deterioration, damage or even worse.

*Particularly recommended is the full professional training course offered as a requirement for membership of the National Institute of Medical Herbalists in Britain, by the School of Herbal Medicine (Phytotherapy), at Bodle Street Green, Hailsham, Sussex. The same school offers a one-year lay-person's course by correspondence.

Nevertheless, all the remedies chosen are on general sale in Britain, and with the exception of one or two have no questions of toxicity hanging over them. Most are freely recommended in popular books and journals for general use. Moreover, herbal medicine has primarily been the medicine of the people, used around the world by many millions without textbooks. This information should be useful to the lay-person.

If the reader is medically untrained, then the information provided here may be taken as theoretical background. At the end of this section is an index of symptoms (see 'Clinical Index') in which each is given a brief assessment and direction to appropriate passages in this and the previous sections. This will help guide such a reader to those conditions safe to treat.

CAUTION: *Many of the symptoms listed here are part of broader syndromes of varying severity. Looking up symptoms out of context can be misleading or even alarming. Before looking up treatment for a symptom it is important to put it into some sort of context: make sure that the rest of the discussion of the treatment of that symptom is appropriate to your case.*

Reference should also be made to the passage earlier in this book: 'How to Use Herbs Safely', on pp. 254–5.

In choosing which herbs to use other material already discussed in this book will also be applicable, and the reader who has come to this section first may find some of the conclusions presented difficult to apply unless these are also scanned.

Dosage is given for each herb. This is usually a broad range. Start at the lowest dose if uncertain, working up the more clear you are about your objective. For children under ten or elderly people over 85 give half the dose, for those under the age of two years give a quarter.

393 Introduction

A note about the references

The academic information available about herbs is very patchy. Some remedies are well documented, others have hardly figured in research papers at all. Most of the references available are for matters chemical rather than clinical: those cited here have therefore been the subject of considerable selection.

Those references provided with full titles have been personally read; those without have not, but have been referred to as significant in other accounts. A good list of non-titled references is now available in a recent revision of *Potters Cyclopaedia*.[1]

Finally, some references are asterisked. This denotes that they are review papers, and thus are particularly recommended. Not only will they provide a full account of the research to date, but they will be a good source of further references (usually very much more than is cited here).

Warming Remedies

These remedies were classified as warm and hot in temperament, and might now be seen as vasodilators or circulatory stimulants. Their application has been already discussed at some length in Part I (notably in 'The Temperaments of Plant Remedies', on pp. 174–82 and in the chapter 'Therapeutics' as a whole). Their use has changed dramatically in the last century and it may thus be useful to compare their former application with the one most likely today. The main difference in practice is in the dosage prescribed.

Heroic treatment for acute conditions

The warming remedies were originally used primarily to relieve conditions arising when external pathogenic influences, particularly those classed as 'cold' and 'wind', assaulted the body. The primary symptom of this attack was fever and the required treatment was therefore short-term and heroic, stimulating sweat production (as *diaphoretics*) and supporting the heat-generating defence.

This point is worth emphasizing: the remedies that follow were used primarily for acute conditions, with symptoms that in modern times might appear too threatening for herbal treatment. It certainly demands considerable clinical experience and confidence to use these remedies in the way designed for them. Moreover, traditional indications will not be encountered very often: in modern times the major infectious diseases have been largely eliminated and have been replaced by more insidious and more surely debilitating conditions (such as the all-pervasive 'viral' infection). These latter-day conditions are less obvious indications for warming strategies. In fact, the most likely opportunity to use them will be in the first diseases of childhood, provided, of course, the child can be persuaded to take them, and in that case the dose will have to be scaled down. Fortunately, as we shall see, most of the remedies have supplementary uses and as has already been done in Europe, may be adapted to several frequently encountered modern conditions. This latter use does not have to suffer the cautions that attend the more heroic application.

The main caution to be observed is to ensure, when using the heroic dosage, that the condition really is an acute one. If there are deeper disturbances, there is a real risk that in stirring up the active defences the body's reserves might be threatened (the traditional Chinese view was that in 'opening the surface' and letting perspiration flow, one might actually be draining off precious 'fluids' necessary to maintain the integrity of the organism). In other words *one is strongly advised not to use these remedies as diaphoretics in fever management if the constitution is not robust.*

We may summarize the contra-indications and cautions as follows:

1 One should not use these remedies in any heroic dose if there is:

   (a) a feeling of cold and sensitivity to cold following debility;
   (b) fever resulting from debilitated conditions;
   (c) night sweats;
   (d) haemorrhage.

2 Any sign of weakness in the constitution will at least demand that the appropriate tonifying remedies be added to the prescription (see 'Tonics and Hormonal Remedies', on pp. 505–41).

3 The use of these remedies in any heroic form must be subject to constant review (every 1–2 hours) and withdrawn as soon as the effect is achieved.

Circulatory stimulants for chronic conditions

Following Thomson's espousal of heating remedies as primary agents of therapy (see 'Thomson and the four elements', on pp. 154–8), they have played an important part in the Anglo-American tradition. The requirements for them have shifted gradually in the intervening periods, as febrile infections have diminished, and cardiovascular and other degenerative diseases have escalated. The heroic use of heating remedies has given way to the gentle use of vasodilators and circulatory stimulants. Dosages have dropped and remedies have come to take on qualities barely understood in previous generations. (This will be obvious from looking at the properties of the remedies described in the following section.)

Nevertheless, it is useful to keep fundamental principles in mind when applying these new strategies. It will still be better to use these remedies in ways compatible with the old guidelines. It is one thing to identify a symptom (e.g. poor circulation to the hands and feet) that seems to need warming remedies; it is better, however, to take into account whether such remedies are really indicated. A review of the following traditional cautions will be advisable.

The main indications for circulatory active remedies are symptoms best described as 'cold' (see the chapter 'Traditional Pathology'). They can arise in two ways:

1 through the effects of environmental cold, chronic hunger and deprivation of the body, producing feelings of cold, especially in the abdomen, diarrhoea, other abdominal pains, lack of thirst, poor appetite, pale and cyanosed complexion, pale body of tongue with white coating, and deep, tense or slow pulses;

2 through debilitating illness, with such symptoms as fatigue, spontaneous sweating, shivering, feeling cold, abdominal distension, depressed reproductive functions, and frail or depressed pulses.

While heating remedies will correct these disturbances, they should not be used uncritically: any undue circulatory stimulation will tend to exhaust the body. The following guidelines should therefore be heeded:

the more debilitated the constitution the less aggressively heating should be the prescription;

heating remedies should not be used in 'hot' conditions (see the chapter 'Traditional Pathology') most especially if these

397 Warming Remedies

arise out of a debilitated condition (the only exception would be the discrete use of peripheral vasodilators for short periods);

if circulatory stimulants are being used and a febrile infection (e.g. a cold or flu) develops while on treatment, then peripheral vasodilators must be applied, preferably in heavier doses (moving towards the heroic level);

the dosage of heating remedies should be carefully controlled in hot weather.

Peripheral Vasodilators

These remedies might be classified as 'hot in the first degree' in Galenic terms (see 'The Temperaments of Plant Remedies', on pp. 174–82).

They used to be, and may still be, used as diaphoretics in fever management but have taken on new roles in modern times, applied particularly to circulatory diseases and as part of a broader strategy to 'relax' or 'open up' the peripheral circulation, perhaps in consort with more vigorous circulatory stimulants discussed later.

YARROW

Achillea millefolium L.
Family: Compositae
Synonyms: milfoil, thousand-leaf, nosebleed, staunch-
grass, soldier's woundwort, sanguinary, bloodwort.

Description: a perennial creeping herb, with tough, erect, furrowed, woolly stems, 10–60 cm in height. The leaves are 5–15 cm in length, lanceolate, 2–3 times pinnate. The basal leaves are long and stalked, the upper short and sessile. The flowerheads are numerous, white or pink, 4–6 mm in diameter, in dense terminal corymbs; the involucre is ovoid, with rigid, oblong and blunt bracts; 5–6 florets in each head. Fruit: achenes 2 mm. Characteristic odour; taste slightly bitter.

Habitat: common in pastures, grassy banks, hedgerows, waysides, waste places, especially in dry sunny conditions. Throughout the British Isles and Europe and North America, Australia, New Zealand and Asia.

Parts used: the herb, collected while flowering; many traditions specify the flowers.

Cultivation: may be grown from seed or from cuttings of the creeping rhizome in any soil in a sunny spot; it is likely to spread.

Harvesting: the plant flowers between June and October.

Preparation: the herb should be dried in gentle heat or in cold circulating air as quickly as possible; to prepare make an infusion, for internal use, or put in a bath for bathing; a tincture can be made at 1:5 in 25 per cent alcohol.

Dosage: 1–4 g dried flowers three times a day.

Constituents: volatile oil (incl. cineol, pinene, azulene, eugenol, thujone, camphor, achillin, sabinene, camphene); bitter constituents (incl. ivain); cyanogenic glycosides; salicylates; asparagin; flavonoids (incl. luteolin, apigenin, kaempferol, quercitrin); glyco-alkaloid (achilleine); tannins; aconitic and isovalerianic acids; fluorescent substance; hydroxycoumarins; resins.

Pharmacology: cineol has antiseptic and expectorant properties; azulene reduces inflammation and stimulates the formation of granulation tissue (in wound healing); achilleine has experimentally reduced clotting time without toxic side-effects, and decoction of the whole herb has the same effect *in vitro* and *in vivo*; the bitter action can be expected to stimulate digestion and the tannins to have an astringent effect on the exterior or internal (gut) surfaces of the body; diuretic, expectorant and digestive stimulant action can readily be explained by volatile oil content; the cyanogenic glycosides and isovalerianic acid have sedative action; asparagin is a potent diuretic.

Toxicology: the presence of a fluorescent substance accounts for the occasional case of photosensitivity after consuming the plant in quantity.

References:
*Chandler, R. F. *et al.* (1982) 'Ethnobotany and phytochemistry of yarrow, *Achillea millefolium*, Compositae', in *Economic Botany*, New York, 36 (2), pp. 203–23

Anderson, L. A. and Phillipson, J. D. (1984) 'Herbal remedies used in sedative and antirheumatic preparations: part 2', in *Pharm. J.*, 28 July, pp. 111–15

Autore, G., Capasso, F. and Mascolo, N. (1987) 'Biological screening of Italian medicinal plants for anti-inflammatory activity', in *Phytother. Res.*, 1, 1, pp. 28–31

Benigni, R., Capra, C. and Cattorini, P. E. (1962) *Piante medicinali: chimica farmacologia e terapia*, Inverni & Della Beffa, Milan, pp. 1–3

British Herbal Pharmacopoeia (1983)

Falk, A. J. *et al*. (1974) 'The constituents of the essential oil from *Achillea millefolium* L.', in *Lloydia*, Cincinnati, 37, pp. 598–602

Gessner, O., and Orzechowski, G. (1974) *Gift- und Arzneipflanzen von Mitteleuropa*, Carl Winter Universitätsverlag, Heidelberg

Leung, A. Y. (1980) *Encyclopedia of Common Natural Ingredients Used in Food, Drugs, and Cosmetics*, John Wiley, New York, pp. 326–28

Madaus, G. (1938) *Lehrbuch der biologischen Heilmittel*, Part I, Heilpflanzen, Leipzig

Martindale The Extra Pharmacopoeia (1982), 28th edition

Schneider, E. (1963) *Nütze der Heilkräftigen Pflanzen*, Saatkorn-Verlag, Hamburg

Temperament: warm.

Taste: aromatic bitter; acrid.

Action: astringent; peripheral vasodilator; diaphoretic; digestive stimulant; antispasmodic; menstrual regulator.

Applications: in traditional usage yarrow was most widely regarded as a wound herb, 'for Dioscorides saith that his Achillea sodereth or closeth bleeding wounds and preserveth them from inflammations, and it stayeth the flux of blood in women being applied in a pessary, and the powder of the dryed herbe taken with Comfrey or Plantaine water doth also stay inward bleedings' (Parkinson). Similar considerations led to its use for catarrhal conditions of the mucous membranes, for enteritis and diarrhoea. These healing properties were often vital in earlier martial times and yarrow's botanical name properly thus refers to Achilles.

Second in importance was its application as a digestive stimulant, to improve appetite, to settle digestion, for gastritis and dyspeptic conditions ('for them that cannot reteine meate in their stomack', according to Parkinson), and to stimulate bile flow and liver function. These actions can readily be explained on the basis of yarrow's bitter and volatile oil constituents.

In more recent European usage, yarrow's antispasmodic properties are highlighted in its use for intestinal colic, stomach and other cramps, nervous dyspepsia, palpitations, painful periods, asthma and convulsions, especially in children. These qualities are reminiscent of chamomile, to which yarrow is pharmacologically close.

Yet further experience points to an effect on the peripheral circulation, in its middle-European use for haemorrhoids and varicose veins, for lowering moderately high blood pressure, and in its physiomedical reputation as a diffusive vasostimulant (used to open up peripheral circulation when constructing a prescription). Some of these actions can be explained as a local flavonoid effect, but there is no doubt a general influence on the vasculature, possibly largely mediated by the volatile oil. The most obvious effect is seen when yarrow is given by hot infusion during fever, for at this point it becomes notably diaphoretic, increasing perspiration and effectively cooling the temperature of the body (it does not have this effect in non-febrile states and may even help to increase body temperature if it is low – thus fulfilling its role as a remedy 'hot in the first degree' (see 'The Temperaments of Plant Remedies', on pp. 174–82).

One of yarrow's constituents, achilleine, was isolated and used as a quinine substitute at the turn of the century for intermittent fevers especially, and this simply emphasizes the potential that yarrow has for fever management. When some of its other activities are taken into account it is easy to see how applicable it really is: its digestive tonic activity will help the digestion cope with potentially toxic food material and 'redirect heat' to the process (see 'Bitter', on pp. 190–91); the relaxant effect will reduce the tendency to fits and convulsions, especially in the very young, and will generally calm and soothe; the astringent effect will be helpful in gastro-enteric infections or when diarrhoea is a major source of debility.

In brief, yarrow may be used as the central ingredient in any fever-management programme, helping to reduce the unpleasant symptoms of the process, keeping the body temperature from rising too high (its effect in hot infusion is quite quick, so it can to a large extent be taken on demand), helping after the crisis to resolve the post-febrile state more effectively, while having a minimal suppressant effect on the course of the fever.

Finally, there is a strong tradition for using yarrow in gynaecological conditions, particularly for heavy and painful menstrual bleeding. The evidence of steroidal constituents may help to explain this activity.

HAWTHORN

Crataegus oxyacantha Thuill. and *C. monogyna* Jacq.
Family: Rosaceae
Synonyms: mayflower, whitethorn, quickset, maybush.

Description: a deciduous shrubby tree of the hedgerows with smooth thorny shoots; the leaves are 3-lobed and stipulate; there are small white or pink flowers in corymbs, each with 5 petals, short triangular sepals, prominent stamens arranged around the nectary and carpels; the haw berry is red with white mealy flesh and a large stone; there are botanical differences between the two species but they hybridize freely and in any case there seems little medical difference between them.

Habitat: in hedgerows and copses throughout Britain and all temperate regions of the northern hemisphere.

Parts used: the flowers, fruit and leaves; on balance the flowers with leaves are probably slightly preferable.

Cultivation: rarely necessary in Britain, but will grow from seed if the 18-month germination time is taken into account; alternatively hardwood cuttings may be taken; most hawthorn in Europe was planted by humans.

Harvesting: the flowers are ready for collecting in late spring to early summer, the berries in the autumn.

Preparation: the flowers will be most suited to infusion, the berries to decoction; tinctures of 1:5 in 25 per cent alcohol will suit both.

Dosage: 0.25–1 g flowers, fruit or leaves three times a day.

Constituents: flavonoid glycosides (incl. rutin and quercitrin); 'crataegus lactone' (mixture of triterpenes incl. ursol and sitosterines); saponins; coumarin; cyanogenic glycosides; trimethylamine (in the young flowers); condensed tannins.

Pharmacology: the flavonoid fraction of this plant is vasodilatory, as also is the condensed tannin (phlobaphene) fraction; these not only dilate the peripheral circulation significantly, but they have a specific action on the coronary circulation (phlobaphene potentiating the action of caffeine and adrenaline in this, and also increasing the amplitude of the heartbeat); the cyanogenic glycosides are sedative and increase the parasympathetic (vagal) tone of the heart, so slowing it down (there is an additional anti-cholinesterase action exhibited by the whole plant that probably contributes to this latter action); in addition the trimethylamine stimulates the pulse rate slightly, and has a peripheral vasoconstrictor effect. The combination of these properties helps to account for the paradoxical and valuable effect of exerting a sympathetic action on the coronary circulation and a parasympathetic action on the myocardial muscle. The results include a rise in oxygen consumption and energy metabolism of the heart and a sensitization to cardioactive glycosides (leading to a possible diminution of their dose). The sedative effects of the cyanogenic glycosides combine with the vasodilatory effects to lower high blood pressure, but in another paradoxical effect the cardiotonic activity actually helps to raise low blood pressure. Early clinical research showed clearly that the fruit reduced hypertension in cases caused by both arteriosclerosis and chronic nephritis, and clinical trials with the flowers showed significant improvements in heart patients, especially in cases of mitral stenosis and ageing heart. Other clinical observations include: a decrease in elevated blood levels of pyruvic and lactic acids; normalization of prolonged systole; prevention of ECG changes due to hypoxia. Finally, it has a favourable effect in cardiac arrhythmias, especially extrasystoles and paroxysmal tachycardia.

References:

Braun, H. (1974) *Heilpflanzen-Lexicon für Ärzte und Apotheker*, 2nd edition, Gustav Fischer Verlag, Stuttgart

Fasshauer (1951) *Deutsche Medizinische Wochenschrift*, Stuttgart, 76, p. 211

Gessner, O. and Orzechowski, G. (1974) *Gift- und Arzneipflanzen von Mitteleuropa*, Carl Winter Universitätsverlag, Heidelberg

Graham, J. (1939) *BMJ*, 22 Nov.

Han, F. *et al.* (1960) *Arzneimittel-Forschung*, Aulendorf, Germany, 10, p. 825

Hoffman, F. (1961) *Pharmaceutica Acta Helvetiae*, Solothurn, Switzerland, p. 36

Osol, A. *et al.* (1955) *The Dispensatory of the United States of America*, 25th edition

Starfinger, W. (1969) *Acta Phytotherapeutica*, Oct.

Weiss, R. F. (1974) *Lehrbuch der Phytotherapie*, 2nd edition, Hippokrates-Verlag, Stuttgart

Temperament: warm.

Action: coronary and peripheral vasodilator; bradycardic effect on the myocardium; relaxant.

Applications: the range of different actions on the function of the heart demonstrated in the pharmacology are well reflected in the clinical indications for hawthorn, indications that make it a very useful heart remedy.

Among professional practitioners its primary application is for treating patients with angina or a history of coronary troubles: here its ability to dilate the coronary circulation and to stabilize heart muscle contractility really comes into its own. The stabilizing action also makes the remedy applicable for palpitations, tachycardia, ectopic beats and other arrhythmias. Such use is wholly inappropriate for those not medically experienced, and even among these care is always advisable when other heart-drug treatment is being provided, but evidence suggests that the main concern lies with concurrent administration of digitalis drugs; there appears to be less risk of interaction with beta-blockers. The action of hawthorn is largely cumulative and very gentle, so low doses taken over a long period are the norm.

Hawthorn has almost as strong a reputation for treating peripheral circulatory diseases, particularly those associated with arteriosclerosis, such as intermittent claudication, hypertension and senile dementia, but also those linked with hypersensitivity conditions like arteritis and Raynaud's disease.

In other areas hawthorn demonstrates its relaxant properties with tranquillizing effects: it is a visceral relaxant, suitable for controlling diarrhoea, colic and other intestinal spasms. This action supports hawthorn's use in cases like palpitations, angina and hypertension.

LIMEFLOWERS

Tilia platyphyllos Scop. and *T. cordata* Mill.
Family: Tiliaceae
Synonyms: lindenflowers, *T. europoea* L.

Description: an imposing tree of a largely tropical family, the lime, or linden, is recognized by its large, broadly ovate leaves and the graceful arching of its branches. There is a difference in leaf size between the two species but there are no known differences in therapeutic activity. The leaves are dark green above and light below, with sharp-toothed margins, acuminate at the tip and cordate at the base, and with long stalks. The flowers are in cymes, in groups of 4–10, pendulous, yellow-white, and include 5 sepals and petals and many prominent stamens; their long stalks arise from the centre of large pale-green bracts. The fruit is about 8 mm crosswise, and pale yellow-green. The flowers are delightfully scented.

Habitat: as a specimen tree or in avenues in parks and large gardens, and wild in woods and thickets in sunny positions throughout the temperate world.

Parts used: the flowers with bracts.

Harvesting: collection is during flowering time in June.

Preparation: the flowers should be dried quickly but very carefully (temperature not exceeding 27°C – or approx. 80°F) as they spoil easily; an infusion is readily made, or a tincture at 1:5 in 25 per cent alcohol.

Dosage: 1–4 g flowers or their equivalent three times per day.

Constituents: volatile oil (incl. farnesol); saponins; flavonoids; condensed tannins; mucilage; oestrogenic substances.

Pharmacology: clinically, the effect of limeflowers on the blood vessels is seen to be a synergic effect of the saponins with flavonoids (there is an interest in some saponins for their potential in this area – as seen in the effect of horse chestnut on the veins); experimental work with the remedy has supported its antispasmodic and relaxant action, and demonstrated an oestrogenic effect.

References:
Benigni, R., Capra, C. and Cattorini, P. E. (1962) *Piante medicinali: chimica farmacologia e terapia*, Inverni & Della Beffa, Milan, pp. 1606–14
British Pharmacopoeial Codex (1949)

Duquénois, P. A. (1977) 'Rétrospective sur les hydrolats de tilleul, narcisse, bourrache et primevère', in *Q. J. Crude Drug Res.*, 15, pp. 203–11

Martindale The Extra Pharmacopoeia (1982), 28th edition.

Temperament: warm.

Action: peripheral vasodilator; diaphoretic, with restorative effect on blood-vessel walls; relaxant; diuretic.

Applications: this plant is widely used on the continent for its gentle sedative effects, most valuable to induce a restful sleep, especially in children, and to relax a tense nervous system and musculature.

It is also an anticatarrhal remedy and, being a diaphoretic, is much used for feverish colds and other respiratory infections, earning a place as a useful fever herb in general. It has been used as a specific in Germany for influenza in children.

These effects provide a fascinating background to the postulated action of limeflowers on the circulatory system. There is a persistent reputation for it helping with cases of arteriosclerosis (like the horse chestnut, that shares a similar saponin). Modern practice has also seen its potential in the treatment of other disorders of the vasculature: varicose veins, phlebitis, migraine and auto-immunological attacks on the vessel walls, such as arteritis. It has long been used in England and France as a remedy for migraines and other headaches, cases where a 'soothing' effect on the vessel walls would be reinforced by a background relaxation and spasmolytic effect. The vasodilatory action will also reduce any constrictory tone in peripheral vessels.

MA HUANG

Ephedra sinica Stapf., *E. equisetina* Bge., *E. intermedia* Shrenk and C. A. Meyer
Family: Ephedraceae

Description: the dried young stems of perennial herbs, *E. sinica* comes in stems up to 30 cm long and 2 mm in diameter, grey-green, and slightly rough. Short (4 mm) leaves arise out of nodes about 3–6 cm apart. In cross-section the young stem exhibits 6–10 bundles of fibres. *E. equisetina* has woody stems that are much branched; the gap between the nodes is only 1–1.25 cm, the apex of the leaves is shorter than *E. sinica* and is not recurved, and the leaves tend to be dark in colour. The actual stems can be found very much longer in commerce. *E. intermedia* has rough and greenish-yellow stems about 30–40 cm long, branched, with 2.5–6 cm between each node. The leaf apex is short but sharply acute and often fissured at the base. There are always 8 bundles in transverse section. All samples of *Ephedra* are dry and brittle, with little odour and a slightly bitter taste.

Habitat: native of northern China and Inner Mongolia.

Preparation: decoction.

Dosage: 1–5 g per day.

Constituents: protoalkaloids, notably l-ephedrine; d-ephedrine; pseudo-ephedrine; morephedrine; l-methylephedrine (not less than 1.25 per cent of alkaloids calculated as ephedrine).

Pharmacology: notable among the protoalkaloids (these are alkaloids without the heterocyclic ring structure) are l- and d-ephedrine. The former has a pronounced α-adrenergic action, constricting most blood vessels, constricting sphincters in the digestive tract and relaxing visceral musculature otherwise, dilating the pupils, increasing blood-sugar levels and contracting the musculature of the reproductive system. This represents the first stage of epinephrine-sympathetic arousal and is potentially hypertensive. This effect is largely in the whole plant, however, eclipsed by the action of pseudoephedrine, which is essentially β-adrenergic. This means that blood supply to the skeletal muscle and periphery is increased, the bronchial airways are dilated, there is relaxation of the gut and reproductive musculature. With no doubt the contribution of other constituents, this means that the whole herb does not have the same hypertensive effects as the isolated ephedrine; nevertheless, it is inadvisable to use it in cases of hypertension, especially with coronary thrombosis, or with monoamine oxidase inhibitor (MAOI) antidepressants.

References:
British Pharmacopoeial Codex (1949), pp. 318–19
Martindale The Extra Pharmacopoeia (1967), 25th edition, p. 58
Roi, J. (1955) 'Traité des plantes médicinales chinoises', in *Encyclopédie de Biologie*, 47, p. 51

Temperament: warm.

Taste: acrid, a little bitter.

Action: opens up the surface; diaphoretic; dilates the airways and relieves bronchial spasms; diuretic.

Applications: the principal action of Ma Huang is in treating febrile congested catarrhal conditions of the respiratory system. It is thus indicated for the symptoms of flu, at the stage where the patient is feeling chilly and is shivering, and when sweating has not broken out yet (that is, when the body temperature is high but is still rising). Headaches and diffuse pains around the body accompanying these conditions are additional indications for the use of this remedy. Its effect in such cases is to provide a considerable perspiration and to provide a feeling of warmth, this accompanying a real fall in actual body temperature.

Its virtues are also evident in dealing with asthmatic symptoms: breathlessness and a feeling of constriction in the chest. It may be applied generally to associated conditions of hypersensitivity in the airways, such as allergic rhinitis (including hay fever and ragweed sensitivity), where the symptoms accord. Given their common origin, even wider hypersensitivities such as urticaria and atopic eczema may be helped with Ma Huang.

The warming quality of this remedy dominates all its other effects. It is reflected in its effect as a cardiac and circulatory stimulant, in its role dispersing catarrhal congestion, and as a diaphoretic in fevers. Closely associated with the above is the action of Ma Huang on fluid accumulations in the body. Whether through its diaphoretic or diuretic effects, it acts to relieve symptoms of oedema. The total combination means, for example, that as far as the lungs are concerned, the remedy is applicable to bronchial congestive conditions as well as to asthmatic drying of the airways, and that it is ideal for bronchial asthma.

Circulatory Stimulants

The following remedies have a more obvious warming effect after consumption, most marked if they are applied when a person is feeling cold, or suffering from the effects of the cold.

Their use has been widely discussed in this volume. They are progressively contra-indicated as vital reserves are depleted.

ANGELICA

Angelica archangelica L.
Family: Umbelliferae
Synonym: garden angelica.

Description: a large member of the parsley family, this biennial plant in its first year appears as a rosette of large bipinnate leaves on long stout hollow stalks, much dilated at the base; the double subdivision of the leaves means that the foliage appears as a mass of bright-green serrated leaflets. In the second year, a hollow fluted stem arises, reaching up to 2 m in some cases, surmounted by a series of umbels of small greenish-white flowers, succeeded by pale-yellow oblong fruits with membranous edges, flattened on one side and convex on the other, this latter bearing three prominent ribs. The roots are long, spindle-shaped and fleshy, with many descending rootlets, the whole often achieving great bulk. The whole plant has a strong pleasant aroma that most helps to differentiate it from other members of the family.

Habitat: possibly originally a native of the Levant that spread to northern latitudes and entered Europe from the north. It has been widely cultivated for its candied stems and is found most often as a naturalized escape. It prefers moist places, ravines, woods and coastal regions. It is also found as an escape in the USA, but a wild form, *Angelica atropurpuea*, is common there and may be used in the same way.

Parts used: the root, leaf and seeds.

Cultivation: the seeds should be sown as soon as they are ripe, as they quickly lose their ability to germinate; the young seedlings can be transplanted as soon as they are large enough for their first year's growth, and then again for their second, when they will need a spacing of 1 m between plants; they prefer moist, deep and rich soil.

Harvesting: the roots should be dug up either in the autumn of the first year or, for larger but possibly less robust specimens, in the summer of the second year before the flowering stem dies down; the leaves at the end of the first year, the seeds when ripe in the second year.

Preparation: the root should be chopped into medium-sized pieces and dried as efficiently as possible; preparation of root and seed is by decoction, and of leaf by infusion; or a tincture of the root may be made at 1:5 in 45 per cent alcohol.

Dosage: 1–2 g dried root or seed, 2–5 g of leaf, three times a day.

Constituents: volatile oil (incl. phellandrene); angelic acid; fluorescent (therefore photosensitizing) bitter furanocoumarins (angelicin, osthol, osthenol, marmesinin, apterin); in the root notably: tannin and resin.

Pharmacology: phellandrene, the major component of the volatile oil, has a stimulating action on the nervous system; the furanocoumarins (found incidentally mostly in those plants growing in the open, rather than in enclosed woody areas) have insecticidal properties that work by UV-activated destruction of insect DNA: this photosensitivity can be transferred to humans if large amounts of angelica are consumed and the patient exposed to bright sunlight, or in some cases on skin contact with the fresh sap of the plant. The bitterness of the furanocoumarins accounts for digestive stimulating effects, but there is so far little pharmacological information on the circulatory stimulating components; whether some of the activities noted for constituents of *Angelica dahurica* apply to this remedy is an interesting point.

References:

Beck, R., Dietz, U. and Schimmer, O. (1980) *Planta Medica*, Stuttgart, 40 (1), pp. 68–76

Braun, H. (1974) *Heilpflanzen-Lexicon für Ärtze und Apotheker*, 2nd edition, Gustav Fischer Verlag, Stuttgart

Charbonnier, J. and Molho, D. (1982) *Planta Medica*, Stuttgart, 44 (3), pp. 162–5

Escher, S. *et al.* (1979) *Helvetica Chimica Acta*, Basel, Switzerland, 62/7, pp. 2061–72

Kimura, Y. *et al.* (1982) *Planta Medica*, 45 (3), pp. 183–7

Kozawa, M. *et al.* (1981) *Shoyakugaku Zasshi*, Kyoto, 35 (2), pp. 90–5

Lemmich, J. *et al.* (1983) *ibid.*, 22 (2), pp. 553–6

Lemmich, J. and Thastrup, O. (1983) *Phytochemistry*, 22 (9), pp. 2035–8

Temperament: hot.

Taste: aromatic acrid; bitter.

Action: warming digestive tonic; relaxing expectorant; antispasmodic and carminative; diuretic.

Applications: Parkinson summed up the traditional European view of angelica when he stated, 'it resisteth poison by defending the heart, the blood and the spirits, and giveth heate and comfort to them'. There was generally a view that angelica was a prime tonifying agent, with almost supernatural (hence its common and especially botanical name) ability to protect against an often morbid and cold environment.

Its warming benefit is most often felt on the digestive tract, 'to warme and comfort a cold or old stomack', having, even more than cinnamon (see below), a generous blend of the digestive stimulant but cooling effect of its bitter constitutents and the warming acrid principle. The bitter effect allows it to stimulate gastric and pancreatic secretions, and 'openeth the obstructions of the Liver and Spleene', allowing the plant to be of particular use in stimulating appetite and digestion in convalescence or debility.

Secondly, it is carminative, the volatile oil acting like that of fennel, dill and the like to soothe intestinal overactivity, colic or flatulence and to reduce pain and spasms in enteric infections. The combination of these activities in practice makes it of immense value in a great variety of digestive ailments.

Warming also produces diaphoresis, and angelica can be considered a useful fever remedy, to provide a more substantive stimulating effect than yarrow.

The action on the lungs is that of a moderately relaxing expectorant formerly used in all manner of lung infections and even chronic bronchitis. It is seen as essentially strengthening the lung in debility.

Angelica was also used as a diuretic and to encourage a normal menstruation.

It is difficult to quantify adequately the potential of angelica today. It has indeed been neglected in some quarters, probably due to the passing of the debilitating infectious disease in modern times. Yet it is clear that it still has great value. It can certainly be relied upon whenever there is infection, particularly when febrile or subfebrile and involving the digestive system and lungs. For various reasons the remedy was seen principally as a protection against 'contagion'. Whether angelica belongs to a former age when confrontations with toxins were more vigorous, when it could be relied upon to support and strengthen an embattled body, or whether it still has an application in the greyer areas of today's conflicts with pathogenic forces is a very valid question. However, there is no doubt that it still has an important application in its other major role, as a warming restorative in debilitating diseases and through convalescence. There is probably no better convalescent remedy in the Western materia medica.

CINNAMON

Cinnamomum verum J. S. Presl
Family: Lauraceae
Synonyms: Ceylon cinnamon, *C. zeylanicum* Garc. ex. Blume.
NOTE: In the UK there are two varieties of cinnamon widely used. The other species, *Cinnamomum cassia*, or Chinese cinnamon, is a less fragrant and aromatic product called 'cinnamon' in the USA and 'cassia' in the UK. It is the primary form of the remedy used in China, where it is applied for much the same purposes as given below.

Description: a 10 m high tree with alternate long elliptical leaves with densely hairy panicles of creamy-white flowers giving way to clusters of globular drupes. The bark is dried from 5–6-year-old trees, curling as it does into quills (generally single), the exterior surface a pale, earthy-brown colour, the interior surface lighter red-brown and finely granular; the fracture is short and granular in the outer part, but fibrous in the inner part. The odour is fragrant, the taste sweet and aromatic.

Habitat: Sri Lanka, but cultivated throughout the Tropics.

Parts used: the dried inner bark.

Preparation: decoction.

Dosage: 1–5 g daily.

Constituents: essential oil (incl. cinnamaldehyde 60–70 per cent – forming cinnamic acid – eugenol, methyleugenol, phellandrene, cinnamyl acetate), coumarins, condensed tannins.

Pharmacology: cinnamaldehyde has experimental sedative, hypothermic and antipyretic activity. Extracts of the remedy have *in vitro* antifungal and antibacterial activity, and the essential oil has antiviral activity, is a circulatory stimulant and vasodilator, stimulates digestive secretions, and is antispasmodic.

References:
British Herbal Pharmacopoeia (1983)
Leung, A. Y. (1980) *Encyclopedia of Common Natural Ingredients Used in Food, Drugs, and Cosmetics*, John Wiley, New York

Temperament: hot.

Taste: acrid; sweet.

Action: warms the interior; relieves pain; carminative and astringent.

Contra-indication: pregnancy.

Applications: this remedy is applied specifically to conditions with such symptoms as feeling cold, poor circulation to the extremities, oedema, diarrhoea and loss of appetite.

It is also used as a warming tonifying remedy in general conditions of exhaustion, and especially in prolonged illness, with pallor and loss of vitality.

It can be considered as rather more warming than angelica, and can be used like it for chest infections (an effective remedy for the onset of chesty colds is a tea of powdered cinnamon mixed with fresh ginger).

The presence of tannins helps to account for the use of the remedy as a symptomatic treatment for diarrhoea. This action is combined, however, with a wider tonifying effect on the digestion, gently stimulating digestive secretions, and encouraging effective peristaltic movements (most notably by reducing griping and flatus – the carminative action). This balance of beneficial actions on the digestive tract has made cinnamon a favourite traditional remedy for problems in the area.

The other major folk application of cinnamon was as a supportive heating remedy in the management of fever conditions. It has always been a favourite remedy for use in convalescence from illnesses as well. It is one of those most useful remedies that stimulates both digestion and circulation.

It has appreciable uterine stimulating properties and has been used to help in difficulties after childbirth. This accounts for its contra-indication of pregnancy.

GARLIC

Allium sativum L.
Family: Liliaceae

Description: a familiar item: garlic 'heads' are the compound bulb divided into component corms or 'cloves', each of which is completely autonomous with its own roots.

Habitat: a native of central Asia, but now grown throughout the world in warm climes as a crop, especially in southern Europe.

Parts used: the bulb.

Cultivation: propagation is by seed or more usually by splitting the bulb into cloves and planting these out 10 cm apart in rows 30 cm apart. The ground should be very well manured, and well dug as, unlike onions, garlic does not naturally push itself out of the ground as it grows. Garlic should be in the warmest and sunniest spot available.

Harvesting: the bulbs are collected in late summer when the leaves have died down, and are then hung to dry.

Preparation: well-dried garlic keeps satisfactorily in cool conditions until the following spring when it begins to sprout. The simplest and most effective way to take it is simply to swallow it fresh, chopped into pieces. This technique will, of course, lead to strong-smelling breath and possibly stomach reactions: to avoid these the deodorized capsules, or 'perles', are available. These are likely to have reduced antiseptic effects, but may well be sufficient for some of the other effects of garlic, as long as the dosage is sufficient.

Dosage: for long-term treatment, 3–8 garlic perles may be taken daily, or one clove cut to last through the day; for intensive use, 2–6 good-sized cloves may be taken daily for up to 3–4 days.

Constituents: volatile oil (containing alliin: when the plant's tissues are crushed this comes in contact with an enzyme called alliinase that converts it to allicin, which then forms the odorous volatile diallyl disulphide); hormone-type substances; glucokinins; germanium; mucilage.

Pharmacology: considerable research work has been done on garlic, providing support to almost all the clinical claims made below. Unlike most other plants the work has largely been done with the whole remedy so it can be incorporated into the main text. However, we, know that diallyl disulphide is antibacterial, even when diluted to 1:125,000, inhibiting the growth of *Staphylococcus*, *Vibrio cholera*, *Bacillus typhosus*, *B. dysenteriae*, and *B. enteritidis*; it also possesses the acrid properties of the mustard oil glycosides. The mineral germanium, found by Japanese researchers to be present in large quantities, is credited with further vasodilatory properties; the glucokinins appear to lower blood-sugar levels, and possibly improve the pancreatic performance in producing insulin.

References:
*Adetumbi, M. A. and Lau, B. H. S. (1983) '*Allium sativum* (Garlic) – a natural antibiotic', in *Medical Hypotheses*, Lancaster, 12, pp. 227–37
*Ernest, E. (1987) 'Cardiovascular effects of garlic (*Allium sativum*): a review', in *Pharmatherapeutica*, 5, pp. 83–9
*Lau, B. H. S. *et al.* (1983) '*Allium sativum* (Garlic) and atherosclerosis: a review', in *Nut. Res.*, 3, pp. 119–28
Bordia, A. (1981) 'Effect of garlic on blood lipids in patients with coronary heart disease', in *Amer. J. Clin. Nutr.*, 34, pp. 2100–103
Foushee, D. B. *et al.* (1982) 'Garlic as a natural agent for the treatment of hypertension', in *Cytobios*, 34, pp. 145–52
Hikino, H., *et al.* (1986) 'Antihepatotoxic actions of *Allium sativum* bulbs', in *Planta Medica*, 56, Stuttgart, pp. 163–8.
Leung, A. Y. (1980) *Encyclopedia of Common Natural Ingredients Used in Food, Drugs, and Cosmetics*, John Wiley, New York, pp. 176–8
Martindale The Extra Pharmacopoeia (1982), 28th edition

Temperament: hot.

Taste: acrid (when raw); sweet (when cooked).

Action: antipathogenic (especially in the digestive tract and respiratory system); hypocholesterolaemic and hypolipidaemic; reduces clotting of blood platelets; vasodilatory; expectorant; antihistaminic.

Applications: such are the virtues claimed for garlic that it might all be thought too good to be true if most of them were not being independently supported by research.

The protective effects of garlic against infections have long been well known, and in the past it has been used locally for ulcerous sores, to rid the gut of worm infestations, and as a prophylactic against many infectious diseases. It was credited with preventing gangrene and sepsis in the trenches of the First World War, and has been used to this day as a general antibiotic and antiseptic ('Russian penicillin').

Its internal effects are notable in two areas, the gut and the lungs. In the gut, the evidence points to significant inhibition of pathogenic organisms (as listed above), with little such effect on beneficial flora: it has been used effectively in dysentery, typhoid, cholera and in bacterial food poisoning, and it proves a safe and efficient antiworming agent. Its action on the lungs is due to the volatile oil being excreted there (hence the breath odour): in passing through, it effectively sterilizes the alveoli and bronchial tree. It is thus an excellent agent for bronchitic infections, and has also been used for tuberculosis. If crushed in the mouth, garlic sterilizes the whole area, and it is worth considering it in cases of oral thrush, dental infections, throat infections and tonsillitis. It is a superb agent in cases of the common cold. Its antifungal properties have been noted too. The Chinese have reported trials showing a successful application of garlic to cryptococcal meningitis; they have also pointed to garlic's general ability to enhance the body's immune defences – a property that clearly takes garlic a stage on from the conventional antibiotic.

There has also been much investigation into the effects of garlic on the circulation, these revealing new insights obviously not recorded in traditional accounts. For instance, garlic lowers blood-cholesterol levels, so that after a meal with garlic these are lower than after the same meal without: this has obvious implications for a prophylactic regime in atheromatous conditions. The action is supported by the finding that on regular ingestion of garlic there is a reduction in the levels of the clotting precursor fibrinogen in the blood, and also that, along with onion, garlic reduces the clotting activity of blood platelets. Further, garlic is shown to be vasodilatory, thus at least transiently reducing blood pressure through increasing blood perfusion through the tissues (not a contradiction). This is a feature of a 'hot' remedy, and garlic shares many attributes of this type of remedy; one example is the simple reduction in pathological deterioration known to occur when oxygenation is increased to an area (an excellent example is the process of atheroma formation known to follow an effective reduction in oxygen supply to the affected artery walls). It is thus not surprising that in countries where garlic is consumed in quantity, there is significantly less cardiovascular disease.

Garlic's effects on the digestive system are manifold, but essentially involve a general stimulation of secretions and of gut activities. Bile secretion is increased (garlic was a traditional remedy for jaundice), and the result of this and other intestinal secretions seems to be to normalize the chemical environment of the gut, and it is as much this effect as garlic's antipathogenic action that makes life uncomfortable for organisms that should not normally be present, yet encourages the presence of normal symbiotic flora. Certainly, it is one of garlic's most notable effects that the gut is detoxified and cleansed when it is administered in the appropriate way (i.e. after 24 hours of near-fast with a gentle purge if necessary, taking 3–6 cloves over 12 hours). The removal of gut toxins is a most profitable activity in many clinical cases (a connection with the earlier effect: German medical practice points to a connection between sluggish bowel activity and hypertension). Garlic also reduces irregularity in gut motility, enhancing a regular rhythmic peristalsis, which, combined with its detoxifying effect, makes it a useful agent in the treatment of colic and flatulence. There also seems to be some impact on assimilation or availability of some nutrients, and blood levels of thiamin have been shown to be higher when garlic is taken. One cannot ignore the effect of garlic on the endocrine pancreas either: there is an improvement in the ability of the pancreas to produce insulin and glucagon, and garlic is among those agents to be recommended to add to the diet of a diabetic or hypoglycaemic sufferer.

The passage of garlic's volatile components through the lungs provides an excellent opportunity for disinfection to occur; this is coupled with an additional expectorant property, in which garlic loosens viscid mucus and promotes its passage up the mucociliary escalator. These paired effects make garlic appropriate for almost all pulmonary and bronchial infections.

Similar antiseptic action can be seen in other eliminatory passages, notably the urinary tract and the sweat glands (especially when these are active, in hot weather or in febrile conditions), being thus a potential benefit in urinary-tract infections and scrofulous skin diseases.

Garlic has been shown to have direct antitumour activity *in vitro* and circumstantially *in vivo* as well. Apart from all the beneficial effects on the body systems, especially digestion, mentioned here, and the mobilization of body defences, there is a clear possibility that some components of garlic positively inhibit the growth of malignant cells. There is certainly an effect on the inflammatory system, seen in the observation that raw onions and garlic both are likely to alleviate the unpleasant symptoms of hay fever and other allergies when eaten, and they have long been reputed to help insect bites and stings. A direct antihistamine action has been suggested.

GINGER

Zingiber officinale Rosc.
Family: Zingiberaceae

Description: a reed-like plant with sheathed leaves bearing an irregularly yellow-green flower with one purple labium with yellow spots on a terminal spike; bulbous rhizomes are joined in racemose clusters: these are fleshy and succulent when fresh with easily scraped pale skin; when dried they shrink considerably to flattened pieces a few centimetres long with short fracture and fibrous interior, with the transverse surface exhibiting numerous yellow oil cells; the characteristic odour and taste are well known.

Habitat: originally tropical Asia, but cultivated in the Carribean, Africa and, from earliest antiquity, India. It grows well at subtropical temperatures where the rainfall is at least 20 cm per year.

Parts used: the rhizome, fresh or dried.

Preparation: decoction; in Western herbalism, the powdered dried root, or the grated fresh root, is often prepared by infusion, or made up into tinctures (1:1 or 1:3 for dried powder; 1:5 for fresh grated root).

Dosage: 1–9 g daily of the fresh rhizomes; in the Western tradition 0.25–1 g of the dried rhizome is prescribed three times per day, but the dose of the fresh can be much greater.

Constituents: volatile oil (incl. camphene, phellandrene, zingiberine, zingiberol, eucalyptol, citral, borneol, linalol); phenols (gingerol, zingerone, shogaol); resin.

Pharmacology: many of the volatile oil constituents in ginger are the same as in other peripheral vasodilators or circulatory stimulants; this leads to the supposition that it is these constituents that have such properties. In this plant, the acrid principle is supplied particularly by gingerol, an oily liquid made up of a mixture of similar phenols, the more aromatic zingerone, and a breakdown product of gingerol, shogaol. These have local irritant or acrid effects on mucous membranes and it is very possible that the vascular stimulation that follows from taking ginger comes either from direct action on metarterioles or by reflex from sensory receptors at other sites (it is temporarily hypertensive in humans on chewing, not on swallowing). There is certainly adequate explanation here for its effects on the digestive system (shogaol has been implicated as a prime agent in producing the observed anti-emetic effect in humans and experimental animals; gingerol suggested as stimulating gastric secretion and peristalsis; together they are antipyretic, analgesic, antitussive, reduce peristaltic activity, and are antispasmodic). The similarity in structure of the phenols to aspirin has been suggested as an explanation for an observed anticlotting *and* anti-inflammatory action after ginger was consumed (combining inhibition of both thromboxane *and* the prostaglandins. PG_{E_2} and PG_{F_2}). Recent clinical investigation has clearly supported the traditional use of ginger as a protection against motion sickness – it having superior action to dimenhydrinate. At least some of the volatile elements are eliminated from the body through the lungs and this leads to expectorant and possibly antiseptic effects rather similar to those of garlic.

References:

*Suekawa, M. *et al.* (1984) 'Pharmacological studies on ginger. I. Pharmacological actions of pungent constituents, [6]-gingerol and [6]-shogaol', in *J. Pharm. Dyn.*, 7, pp. 836–48

Backon, J. (1986) 'Ginger. Inhibition of thromboxane synthetase and stimulation of prostacyclin: relevance for medicine and psychiatry', in *Medical Hypotheses*, Lancaster, 20, pp. 271–8

British Pharmacopoeia (1988)

Grøntved, A. *et al.* (1988) 'Ginger root against seasickness: a controlled trial on the open sea', in *Acta Otolaryngologica*, Stockholm, 105, pp. 45–9

Kiuchi, F. *et al.* (1982) 'Inhibitors of prostaglandin synthesis from ginger', in *Chem. Pharm. Bull.*, 30 (2), pp. 754–7

Leung, A. Y. (1980) *Encyclopedia of Common Natural Ingredients Used in Food, Drugs, and Cosmetics*, John Wiley, New York, pp. 184–6

Martindale The Extra Pharmacopoeia (1982), 28th edition

Srivastava, K. C. (1984) 'Effects of aqueous extracts of onion, garlic and ginger on platelet aggregation and metabolism of arachidonic acid in the blood vascular system: *in vitro* study', in *Prostaglandins, Leukotrienes and Medicine*, 13, pp. 227–35

Temperament: hot (the fresh less so).

Taste: acrid.

Action: 'diffusive' circulatory stimulant, calms nausea and vomiting, removes catarrh, and settles cold, wet coughs; the fresh rhizome is more peripheral in action, the dried rhizome is more hot and central; the dried especially expels 'cold-wind' conditions.

Applications: this remedy is used widely around the planet as a favourite heating agent. In China, for example, the indications are almost identical with those applied in the West and elsewhere.

They include a primary application to phlegmatic bronchial coughs or bronchitic conditions (with an action roughly comparable to garlic). A very common folk tradition, dating from Roman times in the West, and probably India and China of even earlier eras, is to use it to ward off the common cold, or at least those examples associated with cold and draughts (it probably dilates the blood vessels in the mucosal tissues).

Its action on the digestive functions is reflected in its use to relieve nausea and vomiting, the feeling of cold in the abdomen and the diarrhoea that often follows, and digestive over-reactions to fish and shellfish (classic 'cold' foods).

Following immediately from the above, the remedy is applied to warm generally, for poor circulation to the extremities, and for the treatment of shock. In the North American physiomedical tradition, ginger was seen as a diffusive circulatory stimulant (compared, say, with cayenne), most appropriate for increasing peripheral circulation rather than having a solely central effect. This leads to its use in opening up congested or toxic tissues at the periphery or the skin.

A specific role, often referred to, is in reinstating menstrual flow and correcting dysmenorrhoea, where the pelvic area is subject to congestion. A possible contra-indication, on the other hand, is pregnancy (although this is not so for the culinary use of the plant).

CAYENNE

Capsicum minimum Roxsb., *C. frutescens* L., and *C. anuum* L.
Family: Solanaceae
Synonyms: chilli, red pepper, bird pepper, *C. fastigiatum* Bl.

Description: a member of the nightshade family, along with potatoes, tomatoes, tobacco, datura and henbane, this remedy is available in spice shops as either the familiar red powder, or in the form of dried pods of variable colour and size containing many seeds. It is wise to taste the powder for strength, as adulteration with lead oxide is an occasional practice.

Habitat: originally native of Central America, introduced to Europe and India in the fifteenth century by the Portuguese, and to Africa soon after, from which most British supplies now come.

Parts used: the dried ripe fruits.

Cultivation: by seed in light and well-tilled ground in full sun and heat.

Preparation: an infusion may be made, generally using the remedy to fortify another; a tincture may be made at 1:3 or 1:20 in 60 per cent alcohol.

Dosage: usually limited by taste; an accepted adult dose is 30–120 mg, or 1 g in 570 ml water taken in doses of two tablespoonfuls, or 0.06–0.2 ml of the strong (1:3) tincture, or 0.3–1 ml of the 1:20 tincture, all dosages three times daily.

Constituents: alkaloids (incl. capsaicin); carotenoid pigments (incl. capsanthin, capsorubin); flavonoids; ascorbic acid; volatile oil.

Pharmacology: capsaicin is known to mimic the effect of some of the prostaglandins; a patent US skin cream 'Zostrix' containing capsaicin has been shown to improve healing from postherpetic neuralgia and to reduce pain in diabetic neuropathy – an antisubstance-P activity has been suggested; this supports the claims made for the remedy stimulating circulation, digestive secretions and perspiration; the volatile oil is also likely to be a significant factor.

References:

*Christopher, J. R. (1980) *Capsicum*, Christopher Publications, Springville, Utah

Chad, D. (1988) *Report to American and Canadian Pain Society*, Toronto

Janscó-Gábor, A. and Szolesányi, J. (1976) 'Sensory effects of capsaicin congeners. Part II. Importance of chemical structure and pungency in desensitising activity of capsaicin-type compounds', in *Arzneimittel-Forschung*, Aulendorf, Germany, 26, pp. 33–7

Merck Index (1968), p. 203

National Dispensatory (1887), USA, p. 381

Ramamurthy, S. (1988) *Report to American and Canadian Pain Society*, Toronto

Temperament: hot.

Taste: acrid.

Action: a strong circulatory stimulant and diaphoretic; stimulates gastric secretions; carminative; antiseptic; counter-irritant.

Contra-indications: hypertension, hyperacidity, peptic ulceration.

Applications: T. J. Lyle, in *Physio-Medical Therapeutics, Materia Medica and Pharmacy* (1897), commenced a very long entry on this remedy as follows:

The fruit is a most positive, pungent stimulant. It is an excellent antiseptic and is very nutritious. It is the most powerful and persistent heart stimulant known. It increases arterial force, enlarges its calibre and slightly increases its frequency. Its influence is permanent and reaches every organ through its primary influence upon the circulation.

Cayenne was the key ingredient in the materia medica of Samuel Thomson (with *lobelia*) and later in the physiomedical canon because of its intense ability to bring 'vital heat' to the body. It was not the remedy to use for gentle effects – 'Capsicum by itself is not very diffusive. It is quite local in its influence, but is gradually permeating' – but in a time when crude and heroic treatment was often the only life-saving option, it enabled the early practitioners to develop a good reputation in primary health care and to compare very favourably indeed with the attempts of the early 'Regular' physicians.

The drastic indications are now largely gone: the terminal fever, the savage infectious disease, the exhausted and dying casualty of such events, but cayenne still has a valuable role today.

Added to a prescription it will ensure that the ingredients are propelled vigorously into all tissues against the poorest of circulations or the worst cold conditions. It will bring to cold, congested or cyanotic tissues improved arterial blood supply and toxin removal. Applied externally in the form of ointment or plaster, it will produce an appreciable counter-irritant effect, stimulating a significant increase in circulation in the subdermal tissues beneath, so reducing the need for the body to invoke painful and debilitating inflammation.

For the clinically experienced it may be used to provoke a therapeutic fever: by directly raising body temperature it may be taken internally to provoke a subfebrile, catarrhal, congestive condition into a febrile one, so raising the stakes and the body's defensive measures.

A further use, still very relevant in equatorial and tropical regions, is to stimulate stomach-acid production, so increasing the sterilizing capacity of the stomach against potential enteric infections. This makes it potentially troublesome in some gastric conditions of hyperacidity or ulceration. It is generally unwise to take it in severe hypertension and in those cases where reactions to a disease are already too violent or hyperactive.

Aromatic Digestives

These remedies seem to act on the assimilation and circulation of food material from the digestive tract. They are particularly indicated for symptoms such as gastric congestion, nausea, vomiting or belching, diarrhoea, loss of appetite and fatigue, these especially when associated with increased salivation, an insipid taste in the mouth, and a white, slippery or sticky and thickened tongue coating. Such symptoms have been classified as 'cold-dampness' affecting the digestion (see 'Cold-dampness', on pp. 138–9).

These remedies were also traditionally used to treat the effects of rapid cooling of an overheated body by cold bathing, cold drinks, etc., with symptoms including fever, diarrhoea, constant perspiration, headache, shivering and vomiting.

They are heating and relatively strong-acting, and so lead to exhaustion if given for too long. Although not as stimulating as other 'hot' remedies they need to be treated with caution if vital reserves are depleted.

FENNEL

Foeniculum vulgare L., var. *vulgare* (Mill.) Thelung
Family: Umbelliferae
Synonym: bitter fennel.

NOTE: sweet fennel *Foeniculum vulgare* var. *dulce* (Mill.) Thelung is sometimes sold as medicinal fennel: the judgement of many is that it is not as effective.

Description: a short-lived perennial umbelliferous plant with erect branched stems, 60–90 cm high (taller when cultivated); leaves 3–4 times pinnate with very narrow linear segments; rather large umbels of more than 15 rays producing the fruit: these are 4–10 mm long, 1–4 mm wide, oblong, laterally compressed, straight or slightly curved, green-to-yellow brown, with 5 equally prominent ridges; the odour and taste are aromatic and characteristic.

Habitat: indigenous to Europe, but cultivated widely in China, India and Egypt.

Parts used: the fruits.

Preparation: decoction.

Dosage: 1–6 g daily (the usual dosage is 0.3–0.6 g three times daily).

Constituents: volatile oil (mainly anethole, also fenchone, limonene, phellandrene, camphene, pinene); tannins; fixed oil; stigmasterol; coumarins.

Pharmacology: research indicates that naturally present isomers of anethole, dianethole and photoanethole are active oestrogenic agents. Anethole has structural similarity to the catecholamines adrenaline, noradrenaline and dopamine: this may account for some of the sympathomimetic effects of fennel and anise (which also contains large quantities of anethole), such as ephedrine-like bronchodilator action and amphetamine-like facilitation of weight loss. The traditional lactogenic effect may be due to competitive inhibition of dopamine inhibition of prolactin secretion as much as to any direct hormonal activity. The relationship of anethole to psychoactive chemicals like mescaline, asarone and myristicin from nutmeg has been noted and may account for a psychoactive and aphrodisiac tradition for fennel and anise. Alcoholic extracts of the remedy reduce the spasmogenic effect of histamine and acetylcholine on isolated ileal tissue.

References:

Albert-Puleo, M. (1980) 'Fennel and anise as estrogenic agents', in *J. Ethnopharmacol.*, 2 (4), pp. 337–44

Autore, G., Capasso, F. and Mascolo, N. (1987) 'Biological screening of Italian medicinal plants for anti-inflammatory activity', in *Phytother. Res.*, 1, 1, pp. 28–31

Benigni, R., Capra, C. and Cattorini, P. E. (1962) *Piante medicinali: chimica farmacologia e terapia*, Inverni & Della Beffa, Milan, pp. 605–7

British Pharmaceutical Codex (1973)

Forster, H. B. *et al.* (1980) 'Antispasmodic effects of some medicinal plants', in *Planta Medica*, Stuttgart, 40 (4), pp. 303–19

Leung, A. Y. (1980) *Encyclopedia of Common Natural Ingredients Used in Food, Drugs, and Cosmetics*, John Wiley, New York, pp. 169–70

Martindale The Extra Pharmacopoeia (1982), 28th edition

Temperament: warm.

Taste: acrid.

Action: warms and harmonizes digestive functions; powerful carminative; local anti-inflammatory; diuretic; stimulates lactation.

Applications: fennel is applied to conditions of digestive debility, with anorexia, belching, hiccuping or reflux, persistent epigastric pain relieved by warmth or pressure, white slippery coating on the tongue and slow pulse rate. As Parkinson noted, it is used 'to digest the crude flegmaticke qualitie of Fish, and other viscous meats', or to stay 'the hickocke and taketh away that loathing which often happeneth to the stomackes of sicke or fearish persons'.

It has also been used to settle intestinal cramps, colic and flatulence (especially in children and infants – fennel is an ingredient of gripe water for infant colic), and in high doses (9–15 g at once) has been used in Chinese hospitals for more acute conditions like intussusception or intestinal obstruction.

Throughout European tradition, fennel has been highly valued for increasing milk production in both humans ('for Nurses to increase their milke') and other mammals (notably farm animals). A possibly linked quality has it as a remedy for provoking a more complete menstrual flow ('helpeth also to bring downe the courses and to clense the partes after delivery'), and it may be that hormonal influences are behind the aphrodisiac effects noted in the thirteenth-century herbal *Macer Floridus de Viribus Herbarum*, 'fennel seed drunk with wine stirreth lechery', or again, 'The decoction of fennel drank often will make old men to seem long young. This proveth authors and philosophers, for serpents, when they be young and woolly, wax strong, mighty and young once more, they go and eat often fennel, and so become youthful and mighty.'(!)

There is evidence that fennel was the drug of immortality in the Prometheus legend. It was also known to have diuretic qualities ('provoke Urine and to ease the paines of the Stone and helpe to breake it'), choleric and expectorant properties ('much more helpeth to open the obstructions of the Liver, Spleene and Gall and thereby much conduceth to all the diseases arising from them as the painfull and windie swellings of the Spleene and the yellow jaundies; as also the Goute and Crampes, the seede is of good use in pectorall medicines, and those that helpe the shortnesse of breath, and wheezing by obstructions of the Lungs'). All these properties are made use of by modern herbalists (for example, using fennel oil in steam inhalations for bronchial conditions).

Modern practice also has fennel decoction as a useful eyebath, in which application its anti-inflammatory properties are most appropriate, or, as Parkinson puts it 'as also to be dropped into the eyes to clense them from all enormities risen therein'.

CARDAMOM

Amomum cardamomum L.
Family: Zingiberaceae
Synonyms: *A. compactum* (Soland. ex) Maton., round
   cardamom, Bai Dou Kou

Description: the familiar brown aromatic seeds in pale yellow to green fibrous capsules.

Habitat: Indonesia, India and south-east Asia.

Parts used: the seeds.

Preparation: decocted briefly, or powdered in pills.

Dosage: 1–6 g daily.

Constituents: essential oil (incl. borneol, camphor, pinene, humulene, caryophyllene, carvone, eucalyptole, terpinene, sabinene).

Temperament: warm.

Taste: acrid; bitter.

Action: broad warming stimulant to digestion.

Applications: a strong warming remedy for congestive digestion with abdominal pain and distension, diarrhoea, nausea and vomiting, and loss of appetite.

It is a valuable strategy in cases where poor digestion and assimilation appear to be at the root of a chronic debility. It is less stimulating than some in this category and there is thus less risk of putting too many demands on a weakened constitution.

It is also traditionally used for difficulties during pregnancy, such as nausea and vomiting, vertigo, headaches, aversion to eating, tiredness and threatened miscarriage.

Cooling Remedies

These are remedies of a general cooling action, used against conditions originally classified as resulting from internal 'heat' (see 'Heat', on pp. 137–8), with such traditional signs as serious fever, a feeling of heat, flushed complexion, swelling of the affected parts (i.e. inflammation), neuromuscular tension and pain.

Cooling remedies always reduce vital activity, and are applied only to mitigate excessive vitality. They should be avoided in any case of subdued vital signs and in debility, and particular care should be taken not to prescribe them in cases where apparent vitality occurs against a background of severe debility (as sometimes occurs in fatigue syndrome or terminal illness).

Many of the former indications for cooling remedies – violent fevers, haemorrhaging, delirium, pathological thirst and acute diabetes – were emergency conditions requiring desperate measures. They are barely encountered in modern herbal practice or any medical context outside acute hospital wards. The remedies that were applied to these problems are thus less appropriate to modern needs, at least until they have demonstrated new properties at lower doses.

Attention here will instead focus on two groups of cooling remedies that have particular application to problems of modern developed society. They are on the whole less drastic in their effects and more likely to have positive restorative properties as well.

They may be subdivided into further groups: the bitters and the relaxants.

Bitters

These remedies have been discussed at some length in the chapters 'Therapeutics', and 'Traditional Pharmacology'.

They are a powerful strategy for the treatment of a number of inflammatory and digestive disorders, acting in brief to switch on the engine of digestion where this is failing and thus appearing to 'earth' hyperactivities in some other areas.

In former times they were seen to be specifically effective against 'damp-heat' syndromes (see 'Damp-heat', on pp. 139–40), marked by the presence of thick, opaque sputum, diarrhoea or constipation, nausea and vomiting, scanty dark urine, thirst but little drinking, sore watery inflamed eyes and/or malodorous yellow vaginal discharge, with thick yellow coating of the tongue. If these syndromes are actually present in the modern era, then they will be firm indications for bitters prescription. Their most common application nowadays will be for less clear-cut symptoms.

Bitters may be considered for treatment of the following:

> biliary disorders, including gall-bladder disease and even some cases of high cholesterol levels;
>
> many liver conditions (they were a prime strategy in the treatment of jaundice), notably those marked by low-grade disability, such as an intolerance of greasy foods and alcohol, previous exposure to undue levels of alcohol, recreational drugs and many prescribed drugs;
>
> loss of appetite, poor digestion, poor breakdown of food in the gut, liability to food intolerances;
>
> reactive hypoglycaemia (low blood sugar), as part of dietary control of late-onset diabetes;
>
> any other clinical condition *linked to* any of the above, but notably chronic inflammatory diseases of the skin, joints, vascular system and bowel, migrainous headaches and fevers.

Bitters are universally classed as tonics and may thus also be applied where any of the above conditions appear to be contributory factors in cases of fatigue or debility.

The bitters are to be considered as counter-weights to the aromatic digestive remedies. Both were seen to move 'damp' conditions, the first 'damp-heat', the second 'cold-damp'. 'Damp', as has been stated already (see 'Dampness', on pp. 138–40 and the Appendix), was seen to uniquely affect the digestive and assimilative systems (or *Spleen* in Chinese medicine), and the bitters and aromatic digestives can be seen as alternatives for such digestive disorders, depending on whether the prevailing condition requires cooling or heating respectively.

It follows that bitters should not be used where there are clear symptoms of 'cold': depressed circulation or metabolic rate, pallor, copious urination, etc., or chronic respiratory congestion, arthritis, or other symptoms linked to 'cold-damp'.

Clinical experience shows that bitters work quickly. The response time from the taste buds through to gastrin secretion is measured in fractions of a second, and the subjective experience, if the right button has been pressed, so to speak, is sometimes apparent in minutes. Certainly, most conditions for which bitters might be prescribed should respond in some way within hours or a day or so at most. The obverse to this is also sometimes found: bitters prescriptions may have more dramatic results in the short term than they do in the long term. Ideally, they should be seen as doing a specific job, as a prelude to other treatment to be established if the effect of the bitters wears off, or in repeated short treatments rather than one continuous long regime.

The stimulating laxatives are also bracketed in with the bitters. They share this essential property but of course add the effect of stimulating bowel activity (see 'Anthraquinones', on pp. 288–90). In practice their temperament means that they too are most useful in the syndromes outlined above.

The link between bitter and stimulating laxative is most obvious in the function of bile (see 'Removal', on pp. 95–117). Bile is a natural laxative and also interacts closely with bowel function and bowel disease on a wider basis. It is certain that bitters alone can act to promote bowel movement in certain conditions, possibly by changing bile flow. It is equally clear that the anthraquinone laxatives are sometimes useful in correcting 'toxic' conditions linked with liver-bile as well as with bowel disorder. A gentle combination remedy like yellow dock, discussed here, can have a very wide application indeed.

DANDELION

Taraxacum officinale Weber
Family: Compositae
Synonyms: *T. dens-leonis* Desf., *pissenlit*, lion's tooth, fairy clock.

Description: a very well-known plant that is however confused with a number of similar plants such as the hawkweed, hawkbits and cat's-ears. The dandelion arises as a rosette of leaves in a variety of shapes, from almost entirely lanceolate, to deeply pinnatifid with 3–6 often backward-pointing triangular lobes likened to lion's teeth (dandelion is *dent-de-lion* in French). From the centre of the rosette arises a single hollow stem, yielding white sap on cutting, and terminating in a yellow capitulate flowerhead made up of 200 or more yellow ligulate bisexual florets, each giving way in turn to the familiar floating pappus with seed: it is the globular mass of these pappi that comprise the 'fairy clock' so beloved of children. The long taproot issues from a short rhizome: all the under-ground parts are covered by a dark-brown bark, but are almost white inside, and like the stem, produce a bitter-tasting white milky sap.

Habitat: originates in central Asia and prefers moist soils, in pastures, meadows, lawns, waysides and waste places up to the snowline and into the Arctic regions, mostly in the northern hemisphere, but now in most parts of the world.

Parts used: the roots and leaves.

Cultivation: propagation of the plants is easily achieved by either sowing the seed or dividing the roots; the cultivated vegetable form obtained in vegetable seed catalogues is not as medicinally active as the wild plant; the plant will quickly spread and will need its flowers picking before seeding to contain it.

Harvesting: the root should be collected no earlier than the second year after sowing, and the later the better; for most purposes the root should be picked in early spring rather than the usual autumn because of the improved bitterness of that time (due to the plant using up the slightly sweet and starchy inulin during the winter months). The leaves are picked in the spring or early summer.

Preparation: the roots are cut into long pieces (do not cut up too fine, as there is a risk of losing sap on drying) and dried by gentle heat; they can be chopped further before use and prepared by decoction; the leaves are prepared by infusion. Both roots and leaves can be made into a tincture at 1:5 in 25 per cent alcohol.

431 Cooling Remedies

Dosage: 2–8 g dried root, 4–10 g dried leaves three times a day.

Constituents: bitter glycosides (incl. taraxacin, lactupicrin, lactucin); waxy substances (incl. lactucerol, taraxerin); triterpenoids (incl. taraxasterol, taraxerol, faradiol, arnidiol); tannins; volatile oil; inulin; potassium salts – 4.25 per cent.

Pharmacology: bitter cholagogue action has been demonstrated for dandelion experimentally; in work on the leaves researchers have found a pronounced diuretic effect, improved by the fact that the potassium content is so high (3 times that usual for plant tissues) that the normal potassium loss of diuresis is more than replaced, leading to a net increase in potassium levels after the use of dandelion leaf for diuresis.

References:

Autore, G., Capasso, F. and Mascolo, N. (1987) 'Biological screening of Italian medicinal plants for anti-inflammatory activity', in *Phytother. Res.* 1, 1, pp. 28–31

Benigni, R., Capra, C. and Cattorini, P. E. (1964) *Piante medicinali: chimica farmacologia e terapia*, Inverni & Della Beffa, Milan, pp. 1593–9

Gessner, O. and Orzechowski, G. (1974) *Gift- und Arzneipflanzen von Mitteleuropa*, Carl Winter Universitätsverlag, Heidelberg

Leung, A. Y. (1980) *Encyclopedia of Common Natural Ingredients Used in Food, Drugs, and Cosmetics*, John Wiley, New York, pp. 154–5

Martindale The Extra Pharmacopoeia (1977), 26th edition

Osol, A. *et al.* (1955) *The Dispensatory of the United States of America*, 25th edition

Racz-Kotilla, E. *et al.* (1974) 'The action of *Taraxacum officinale* extracts on the body weight and diuresis of laboratory animals', in *Planta Medica*, Stuttgart, 26, pp. 212–17

Temperament: cool.

Taste: bitter.

Action: digestive and hepatic tonic; cholagogue; diuretic; laxative; detoxifier.

Applications: dandelion is one of the cornerstones of herbal treatment in many cultural traditions, certainly seen as such by the medical herbalist in the UK.

The great herbal archivist of the seventeenth century, John Parkinson, sums up dandelion's effect in his first lines of description: 'by the bitternesse doth more open and clense, and is therefore very effectuall for the obstructions of the liver, gall and spleene, and the diseases that arise from them, as the jaundise and the hypochondriacall passion . . .' (It is worth noting the humoral connection in the last indication.) This standard bitter cholagogue effect is augmented in the eyes of most herbalists by a specific restorative effect on the liver, making dandelion an effective and safe foundation for many modern prescriptions, given the particular strains on the organ imposed in the present day. Dandelion is seen not only to help the liver in its self-cleansing role, but to encourage it in its capacity for renewal and repair. It may be used without hindrance for most liver disorders or diseases, even active hepatitis (where some hepatics ought to be applied with caution) and so also gall-bladder inflammation and gallstones (for which problems it has been particularly recommended).

Parkinson moves straight on from extolling the hepatic virtues of dandelion to say:

it wonderfully openeth the uritorie parts, causing abundance of urine, not onely in children whose meseraical veines are not sufficiently strong to containe the quantitie of urine produced in the night, but that then without restraint or keeping it backe they water their beds, but in those of old age also upon the stopping or yeelding small quantitie of urine; . . . it also powerfully clenseth apostumes and inward ulcers in the uritorie passages, and by the drying and temperate qualitie doth afterwards heale them . . .

It has, in fact, been demonstrated that dandelion does have powerful diuretic properties, although large quantities of leaves are needed for the most dramatic effects. The French word for dandelion, *pissenlit*, (literally 'piss-in-bed') provides a graphic reminder about the risks of taking it last thing at night, but this does not invalidate Parkinson's recommendation that it be applied to cases of enuresis in children: it is simply a case of giving diuretics earlier in the day so helping to readjust the system's diurnal rhythm. The leaves are a most appropriate treatment in cardiac and hepatogenous oedema (dropsy and ascites respectively), and for water retention from any cause. The high level of potassium is particularly useful when digitalis heart drugs are being prescribed as these will provoke irritability of the heart muscle when potassium levels are low. It is thus interesting to note that dandelion has been an almost constant accompaniment to foxglove or lily-of-the-valley in traditional herbal treatments for dropsy (a symptom produced, of course, by left-heart failure).

With these two main recommendations it is easy to appreciate that dandelion also has a reputation for treating stones, as it effectively dilutes both the bile and urine, thus reducing the propensity for crystal and stone deposition in each and even allowing a certain amount of redissolving to occur. In short, dandelion can be seen as improving both the liver and kidney functions.

Similar remedy: In Chinese medicine a dandelion is also used, *Taraxacum mongolicum* Hand.-Mazz. (as well as other species), called *Pu Gong Ying*. It is most likely that the character of the plant will be very similar to dandelion and many of the popular usages are similar. In Chinese terms the plant is seen as having cooling and cleansing effects, and it is much used in toxic, inflamed and chronically infected conditions, those classified as 'damp-heat' problems in particular. This accords with the qualities adduced to dandelion above, given the detoxifying roles of liver and kidney (and Parkinson's assertion of it 'clensing the malignant humours'), and the cooling and drying properties of all bitters. There is a tradition for using *Pu Gong Ying* as a stimulant to lactation that is not recorded in Europe.

GENTIAN

Gentiana lutea L.
Family: Gentianaceae
Synonym: yellow gentian.

Description: a perennial herb with a single stem up to 120 cm high with glabrous grey-green opposite leaves cupped around whorls of golden star-shaped flowers; the large taproot, when dried and cut, forms whole or split cylindrical pieces, externally yellow-brown to brown, longitudinally wrinkled, with short and hard fracture showing a transverse surface red-yellow in colour with a dark cambium ring inside a wide bark. The taste is initially sweet then bitter.

Habitat: at high altitudes (over 600 m) in lime-rich soil in central and southern Europe.

Parts used: the rhizome and roots.

Cultivation: propagation is by splitting crowns or sowing seeds, planting into deep loamy soil in full sun.

Harvesting: in autumn in the second or third year, before the plant is mature enough to flower.

Preparation: decoction or tincture at 1:5 in 45 per cent alcohol.

Dosage: 0.5–2 g three times per day.

Constituents: bitter glycosides (incl. gentiopicrin, gentiopicroside, amaropanin, amarogentin and amaroswerin: gentiin and gentiamarin are formed from gentiopicrin on drying); alkaloids (incl. gentianine); flavonoids (incl. gentisin).

Pharmacology: amarogentin is used as a bitter standard (it is able to be tasted at concentrations of 1:50,000); gentianine has anti-inflammatory activity.

References:
British Pharmacopoeia (1988)
British Pharmacopoeial Codex (1973)
European Pharmacopoeia, vol. 1, p. 295
Leung, A. Y. (1980) *Encyclopedia of Common Natural Ingredients Used in Food, Drugs, and Cosmetics*, John Wiley, New York
Hänsel, R. and Steinegger, E. (1988) *Lehrbuch der Pharmakognosie und Phytopharmazie*, Springer-Verlag, Berlin, pp. 594–9
Martindale The Extra Pharmacopoeia, (1989) 29th edition

Temperament: cold.

Taste: bitter.

Action: pronounced bitter digestive stimulant; anti-inflammatory.

Applications: the archetypal bitter remedy, sure-safe and without side-effects, is to be used as a foundation for any prescription seeking to use the cooling, drying and digestive stimulant effects of the bitter principle.

The anti-inflammatory effect, highlighted by the action of one of

435   Cooling Remedies

gentian's constituents, is of course an extension of the bitter effect, and incidentally points to one of its most frequent modern indications.

Similar remedies: chicory (*Cichorium intybus*); centaury (*Erythraea centaurium*).

WORMWOOD

Artemisia absinthium L.
Family: Compositae
Synonym: absinthe.

Description: an aromatic perennial plant with erect stems up to 1 m tall, very tough, but dying back each autumn; the whole plant is greyish-white and covered with fine down. The leaves are almost orbicular in general outline, but much cut into long and oblong lobes: the lower leaves are tripinnate, the upper bipinnate or entire. The flowerheads are numerous and arranged in dense racemose panicles: each head is drooping, nearly hemispherical, yellow, with multiple tubular florets surrounded by grey-green bracts, the outer linear, the inner broad. The taste of the leaves is intensely bitter, with a characteristic odour.

Habitat: on roadsides and waste places over the greater part of Europe, eastern North America, and central Asia, having been naturalized from earlier cultivated crops in most places. Truly indigenous to maritime areas of Britain and Europe.

Parts used: the whole herb, gathered when the plant is in flower.

Cultivation: propagated by dividing the roots in autumn or by sowing seeds at the same time and transferring the young plants to a sunny position.

Harvesting: the herb flowers in August and September; the leaves and flowers should be stripped off the stem.

Preparation: infusion or by making a tincture at 1:5 in 45 per cent alcohol.

Dosage: 1–2 g of the dried herb is the therapeutic dose; it is such a strong bitter, however, that a powerful effect may be had simply by tasting the tincture or strong infusion.

Constituents: essential oil (incl. thujone, thujol, isovaleric acid); bitter sesquiterpenes (incl. caryophyllene and cadinene); bitter sesquiterpene lactones (incl. germacranolides (e.g. costunolide, ridentin, novanin, balchanolide), guaianolides or 'azulenes' (e.g. artabsin, absinthin, anabsinthin, arborescin, globicin) and santanolides (e.g. santonin and artemisin)); triterpenoids (farnesol); terpenoids (incl. artemisia ketone, santolinyl and lavendulyl skeletons); flavonoids (a great number); hydroxycoumarins (incl. hernianin, scopoletin and scoparone); polyacetylenes; tannins; resin; silica.

Pharmacology: this plant is notable for the large number of powerful ingredients it contains, making it something of a single-handed pharmacy of bitters. Most of the sesquiterpenes, flavonoids and essential oil constituents have classic bitter effects (see 'Bitter Principles', on pp. 321–7), but many have other actions as well. For example, the germacranolide group of sesquiterpene lactones are significantly antitumour in effect; the azulenes are anti-inflammatory; santonin is a strong vermifuge; absinthin and anabsinthin are insecticidal. The essential oil is carminative, but the thujone and thujol in isolation are simulating to smooth muscle and also antiseptic; the polyacetylenes, present at least in the fresh plant, are antiseptic; the tannins and resin give an astringent action; the silica promotes connective tissue repair.

Toxicology: the essential oil when extracted is called absinthe and was used as the basis of a potent liqueur in France much favoured by the more degenerate for its narcotic and hallucinogenic properties (Van Gogh was a notable consumer): it has been illegal for many years because it was discovered to severely damage the central nervous system; therapeutic use of the whole plant is most unlikely to provide enough absinthe to cause concern (there are certainly no worries about consuming that other popular drink based on wormwood: vermouth) but, nevertheless, it would be advisable to restrict its use in long-term prescriptions and to use gentian if only a simple bitter effect is required. The plant has some abortifacient properties and must not be used in pregnancy.

References:
Gonzales, A. G. *et al.* (1978) *Planta Medica*, Stuttgart, 33, p. 356
Hartwell, J. L. (1967–71) *Lloydia*, Cincinnati, 30, pp. 379 *et seq.*

Temperament: warm.

Taste: bitter, acrid.

Action: bitter digestive stimulant; antiparasitic; uterine stimulant.

Contra-indication: pregnancy.

Applications: this is a powerful remedy with a paradoxical temperament. Although one of the bitterest plants commonly used, it also has acrid constituents that effectively raise its 'temperature', so that Dioscorides called it a heating and drying remedy. Parkinson elaborated by pointing out, 'the astringent quality therein, is stronger than the bitter: but by reason of the sharpnesse it partaketh more of heate than of cold, so the temperature thereof, is hot in the first degree, and dry in the third'.

There are certainly particular qualities in this remedy which make it more than just a powerful bitter digestive stimulant. It is an antiparasitic, much used, as its name suggests, for the treatment of intestinal worms. In large doses it is quite cathartic, and at these levels, the action of the constituents in killing parasites and incidentally checking bacterial populations, is quite appreciable. Killing endoparasites always involves some risk as by necessity a relatively toxic material needs to be applied (although the best vermifuge remedies utilize the different metabolism in parasites compared with the host), and in practice antiworming treatment needs to be approached with care, and only by those with experience of the procedures. It is certainly possible, however, to use the dosages recommended above for other gastrointestinal infections, and it is a tendency to get such infections (say, linked with inadequate stomach secretions and thus sterilization of food, a general indication for bitters) that is one of the main indications for wormwood. The acrid principle probably increases gastric-acid secretion even over and above the bitter effect.

There are intestinal antispasmodic and astringent effects allowing wormwood to be used for colic conditions, and the plant is also used to quieten the uterus in spasmodic dysmenorrhoea. Although contra-indicated in pregnancy it has been used to relieve the pain of childbirth (another role that should not be utilized except by experienced personnel).

Throughout tradition, wormwood has been used to treat tumours and other severe chronic inflammatory conditions. There is some evidence of anti-inflammatory and antitumour activity in some of its constituents, especially the sesquiterpene lactones.

438   Remedies

Related remedies: many members of the Artemisia genus are used in medicine around the world. The mugwort (*A. vulgaris* L.) is a less bitter version used principally for its stimulating effect on the uterus, which improves congested menstruation and brings it on if tardy (it is also an abortifacient, as are all members of the genus). The southernwood or lad's love (*A. abrotanum* L.) is another more aromatic bitter with similar properties.

The moxa used in acupuncture is made up of *Artemisia argyi*, *A. vulgaris*, *A. lagocephala*, and/or *A. selengensis*.

GOLDEN SEAL

Hydrastis canadensis L.
Family: Ranunculaceae
Synonym: yellow root.

Description: a small perennial plant with a thick, knotty rootstock sending up a hairy stem about 30 cm high, with two palmate 5-lobed, serrate leaves near the top; the stem is topped by a small solitary apetalous flower whose greenish-white sepals fall away when the flower opens; the fruit resembles a raspberry and consists of fused, two-seeded drupes. The dried rhizomes are obtained in pieces about 2–5 cm long and 4–10 mm thick, yellow-brown in colour, twisted in shape, longitudinally wrinkled, and circled by scale leaf scars; the surface is covered with numerous brittle curved roots sometimes broken to leave yellow root scars; the fracture is brittle and the cut surface dark yellow; it exhibits a thick bark and a ring of 10–20 yellow wood bundles, surrounding a large pith. The odour is distinctive, the taste bitter.

Habitat: rich, shady woodland and damp ground in eastern North America, although rare in many areas due to overcollection.

Parts used: the rhizome and roots.

Cultivation: similar conditions to ginseng are ideal, with deep, rich loam in a partially shaded situation; propagation is by divided rootstocks in the autumn, these planted out about 20 cm apart.

Harvesting: autumn in the third year of growth.

Preparation: decoction or by making a tincture at 1 : 10 in 60 per cent alcohol.

Dosage: 0.5–2 g three times a day.

Constituents: alkaloids (incl. berberine, hydrastine and canadine); volatile oil; resin.

Pharmacology: berberine is a bitter alkaloid with antibacterial and anti-protozoal effects down to dilutions of 1:6000, and is a sedative to the CNS; hydrastine is a stimulant to the autonomic nervous system and appears to exert astringent effects on mucosal surfaces throughout the interior of the body – both these alkaloids are present in large quantities in golden seal and will therefore contribute significantly to its action; canadine is bitter and sedative.

References:

Benigni, R., Capra, C. and Cattorini, P. E. (1964) *Piante medicinali: chimica farmacologia e terapia*, Inverni & Della Beffa, Milan, pp. 731–8

British Pharmaceutical Codex (1949)

Genest, K. and Hughes, D. W. (1969) 'Natural products in Canadian pharmaceuticals. IV. *Hydrastis canadensis*', in *Planta Medica*, Stuttgart, 4, 2, pp. 41–5

Hänsel, R. and Steinegger, E. (1988) *Lehrbuch der Pharmakognosie und Phytopharmazie*, Springer-Verlag, Berlin, p. 525

Leung, A. Y. (1980) *Encyclopedia of Common Natural Ingredients Used in Food, Drugs, and Cosmetics*, John Wiley, New York

Martindale The Extra Pharmacopoiea (1977), 26th edition, p. 2018

Merck Index (1960) 7th edition, p. 528

Shideman, F. E. (1950) 'A review of the pharmacology and therapeutics of *Hydrastis* and its alkaloids, hydrastine, berberine and canadine', in *Bull. Nat. Form. Comm.*, XVIII, pp. 1–2 and 3–19

Temperament: cold.

Taste: bitter.

Action: bitter digestive stimulant; cholagogue; astringent and healing to the gut wall and other mucous membranes; laxative; stimulating adjunct to remedies for the lungs, reproductive tract and kidneys.

Contra-indications: pregnancy and hypertension.

Applications: this remedy achieved great popularity in North America from the middle of the nineteenth century after settlers had learnt about its use from native Americans, and almost 150 tons of the root were being collected in 1905. It was most popular as a tonic remedy assisting digestion and liver function, as an eyebath, and as a local application to infected wounds and ulcers and inflamed skin conditions.

The physiomedicalists regarded it as 'the king of tonics to the mucous membranes', used especially for the treatment of inflammations of the gut wall (perhaps marked by reactive diarrhoea), gastric ulceration and mouth and gum disorders. They further considered it as having a general influence on the venous system, implying a systemic action of the same type, applying it to phlebitis and varicosities.

It was considered a strong bitter digestive stimulant and cholagogue, finding much use in jaundice and liver diseases and dyspeptic conditions: the modern medical herbalist still sees dyspepsia with hepatic symptoms as the main indication for using golden seal.

It is both gently laxative (like the stimulating laxatives making use of the bile connection) yet astringent: as a result, it can be used to contain cases of diarrhoea (especially when associated with infection/inflammation of the upper gut wall, see above), but will also provoke a more healthy bowel movement in cases of constipation.

Its astringent and healing properties have made it a popular douche for the treatment of vaginal problems and its gynaecological reputation is augmented by its systemic use for uterine spasm, heavy menstrual bleeding and post-partum haemorrhage.

In physiomedical tradition it achieved a prime reputation as a valuable adjunct to many treatments, particularly in dealing with toxic, inflammatory and congestive conditions of the lungs, kidneys and reproductive tract. There was often a feeling that, provided other indications were in order, the addition of golden seal to a prescription that was failing to make an impact in such conditions would make all the difference.

Similar remedies: barberry bark (*Berberis vulgaris*); golden thread (*Coptis chinensis*); phellodendron (*Phellodendron amurense*).

MILK THISTLE

Silybum marianum (L.) Gaertn.
Family: Compositae
Synonym: *Carduus marianus.*

Description: a low thistle with purple solitary flowers.

Habitat: Europe, especially close to the Mediterranean.

Parts used: the seeds.

Preparation: decoction or by tincture 1:5 in 25 per cent alcohol.

Dosage: 2–4 g three times a day.

Constituents: flavolignans (collectively referred to as 'silymarin', incl. silybin, silychristin, silydianin); bitter principle; polyacetylenes.

Pharmacology: a number of investigations have shown an effect of the remedy in protecting against the effect of liver poisons, such as carbon tetrachloride, and notably the death-cap mushroom (*Amanita phalloides*); it has also been shown to be effective in the treatment of hepatitis and cirrhosis.

References:
Benda, I. and Zenz, W. (1973) *Wiener Medizinische Wochenschrift*, Vienna, 123, p. 512
Devault, R. L. and Rosenbrook, W. (1973) *J. Antibio.*, 26, p. 532
Hruby, K. *et al.* (1983) *Hum. Toxicol.*, 2 (2), p. 183
Poser, G. (1971) *Arzneimittel-Forschung*, Aulendorf, Germany, 21, p. 1209
Qiu, S. J. *et al.* (1981) *Chin. J. Cardiol*, 9, p. 61
Tuchweber, B. *et al.* (1973) *J. Med.*, 4, p. 327

Temperament: neutral.

Taste: bland; slightly bitter.

Action: protects the liver; digestive tonic; galactogogue.

Applications: after being used widely in Europe as a digestive tonic and as a stimulant to milk flow in nursing mothers this plant has been given a powerful new identity as the result of considerable research, particularly in Germany. It is now a popular remedy for a full range of real or perceived liver disorders.

This is an unusual case where a remedy has been introduced into the dispensary of professional medical herbalists as a result of modern research. However, the plant had been widely used in a way that is at least compatible with its new guise, and many of the tasks which it is called on to do are peculiarly modern. It finds a place in many prescriptions where burdens on the liver are seen to be a dominant feature in the condition treated, especially in the aftermath of a drug-abuse problem, alcoholism or long-term treatment by conventional medicinal drugs (see also 'The liver' in Part I, on pp. 84–5).

It has advantages in that it is not particularly bitter. It can therefore be used in cases where bitter herbs are contra-indicated, or as a buffer to their effect. Its action is essentially gentle, and protective as much as assertive. It has been recommended as an emergency treatment for consumption of liver poisons, notably death-cap mushrooms (in which its effects are said to be dramatic), but its main use is for longer-term treatment of chronic toxic syndromes. It has a valuable potential role in liver 'detox' regimes.

A further potential benefit is hinted at by research that suggests an effect in lowering fat levels in the blood. As the liver is the organ most involved in affecting such levels after the effects of diet and exercise are taken into account, then the connection may not be too tenuous.

Similar remedy: artichoke (*Cynara scolymus*).

YELLOW DOCK

Rumex crispus L.
Family: Polygonaceae
Synonyms: curled dock, narrow-leafed dock.

Description: there are several species of dock, not all sharing the same properties, so attention to identification is important; this plant has narrow leaves, usually wavy or curled at the edges, very variable in size, diminishing higher up the stem till they become mere bracts; the flowers are numerous and small, greenish turning red, in dense whorls or panicles; the roots are thick and deeply rooting, having a clear-yellow colour when scraped. When dried and cut they have a grey-brown cork, yellowish

443   Cooling Remedies

cortex and pale, radially split wood; treatment with aqueous alkali rapidly turns the fragments intense dark red.

Habitat: in arable farmland, on roadsides, ditches and waste places throughout the civilized world.

Parts used: the root.

Cultivation: very easy if desired, but it spreads quickly and is not a welcome addition to the garden.

Harvesting: any time from late summer, after the fruit is ripe.

Preparation: the root is cleaned and chopped into small pieces while fresh; it can be prepared by decoction or made into a tincture at 1:5 in 25 per cent alcohol.

Dosage: 1–4 g root three times a day.

Constituents: anthraquinone glycosides (incl. emodin, chrysaphenol); tannins; volatile oil.

Temperament: cool.

Taste: bitter.

Action: mild laxative and cholagogue.

Applications: this can best be seen as a mild version of cascara or rhubarb, having the same bitter and choleretic properties, but less laxative action.

In modern clinical practice yellow dock is most used as an alterative or blood-cleansing remedy, applicable to the treatment of systemic toxic states of any sort where the main trouble is seen to lie in what might be termed the 'bile–bowel' axis. In other words, if there is a skin disease, or arthritic or other toxic degenerative condition, and there is the suggestion that liver and bowel dysfunction is implicated, then yellow dock is the remedy of choice, provided of course that its cold temperament is otherwise indicated. It is often seen as a useful companion for dandelion root.

It is significantly astringent too, and has found much use as a wound dressing and mouthwash; its particular strength is for slow-healing ulcers. It is also unusually rich in iron.

CASCARA SAGRADA

Rhamnus purshiana D.C.
Family: Rhamnaceae
Synonyms: cascara, Californian buckthorn.

Description: a shrub or tree up to 130 m high from which the bark is collected; this is obtained in single quills, channelled or nearly flat pieces; the outer surface is smooth, purple-to-brown cork bearing scattered lenticels, occasional patches of white lichen and small pieces of moss and liverwort; inner surface yellow to black, longitudinally striated and faintly corrugated transversely; fracture short, fibrous on the inner surface, exhibiting narrow cork, yellow-grey cortex showing groups of sclerenchymatous cells, brown phloem traversed by medullary rays; taste bitter and persistent, odour characteristic.

Habitat: Pacific coast of North America; increasingly cultivated, especially in British Columbia, as native stocks are depleted.

Parts used: the bark.

Preparation: the bark is collected through the summer and then must be stored for a year before use; it may then be prepared by decoction or by making a tincture at 1:5 in 25 per cent alcohol.

Dosage: 1–5 g bark in one dose before bed.

Constituents: anthraquinone glycosides (incl. emodin, chrysophanic acid, aloe-emodin, cascarosides A, B, C and D – these after storage for a year: certain more griping constituents such as franguloside are broken down in this process); tannins; volatile oil.

Pharmacology: it has been demonstrated that the combined purgative action of the anthraquinones in cascara is greater than the sum of their individual actions (this demonstrating the synergic principles common to many plant remedies); like all anthraquinone remedies (see 'Anthraquinones', on pp. 288–90) it works 8–14 hours after administration by stimulating the intestinal musculature, probably via a prostaglandin mediation.

References:
*Fairburn, J. W. (ed.) (1976) 'The anthraquinone laxatives', in *Pharmacology*, 14, Suppl. 1, pp. 7–101
British Herbal Pharmacopoeia (1983)
British Pharmacopoeial Codex (1973)
European Pharmacopoeia (1971)

Fairburn, J. W. *et al.* (1977) *J. Pharm. Sci.*, 66, pp. 1300–3

Temperament: cold.

Taste: bitter.

Action: stimulating laxative; cholagogue and bitter digestive stimulant; antiparasitic.

Applications: this is to be recommended as possibly the most gentle but effective stimulating laxative available, able to procure a sure bowel movement without undue griping (although in any such prescription the addition of carminatives like dill, fennel, etc., is to be recommended). It is indicated whenever atonic constipation or sluggish bowel is interfering with health or recovery, either as a short-term treatment to move accumulations, or as part of a longer-term management of chronic atonicity. It must be emphasized that indiscrimate use of laxatives alone is harmful to the process of encouraging bowel tone, and such usually self-administered treatment should be actively discouraged. An acceptable formula for the re-education of bowel function, to be taken daily for many weeks, but effective in even the most debilitated bowel, is as follows:

> cascara sagrada: 1 part
> chamomile: 2 parts
> psyllium seeds: 4 parts

The whole is powdered and taken in doses of 1 teaspoonful 3 times per day before meals, as a powder with water or made up into capsules.

Like all anthraquinone remedies, cascara should not be used for constipation arising from bowel tension.

The laxative effect of cascara is usefully augmented by a pronounced bitter stimulating effect, particularly active in promoting liver function and bile secretion. This is often a most appropriate activity given the intensely close relationship between bile and bowel functions (it is a property shared with yellow dock above).

Cascara may also be used like its close European cousin, alder buckthorn or frangula bark (*R. frangula* L.) as a local antiseptic, applied to the scalp for lice and scabies, as a mouthwash for gum, throat and mouth infections, and even in toothpastes for protection against dental caries. This property of course helps in its action on the gut and adds gut toxicities in general to its indications.

Similar remedies: rhubarb (*Rheum officinale*); senna pods (*Cassia* spp.).

Relaxants

These are remedies that are used to reduce the symptoms of tension in the body. The components of this tension are both psychological and neuromuscular and the best herbs in this class appear to work broadly across both areas.

The word 'relaxant' is not widely used in herbal texts. The remedies that reduce mental and psychological tension have been called 'tranquillizers' or 'sedatives'; those that reduce neuromuscular tension have been termed 'antispasmodics' or 'spasmolytics'. Each is a specific term and as it is true that any one remedy can be said to have one quality more than others, it is also the case that most of those widely used share all of them.

A relaxant can be used as a short- to medium-term measure to reduce the effects on the body of either external stresses or internal anxieties. The ideal is to use them as a management strategy in developing other stress-reduction measures rather than as a long-term solution. Apart from any other factor it is likely that any benefits wear off after a time.

The more sedative a remedy – and this review excludes notable sedatives – the nearer the remedy comes to depressing vital functions. The obvious example of a plant sedative is the opium poppy, and its negative properties are well known.

These remedies are all classed as 'cooling' in this review. This is in a slightly different sense than that otherwise used, but refers to their role in reducing (vital) activity, and even depressing it. They should in fact be used with increasing care if illness or stress has already drained the body.

Some cases of tension actually originate from depression of the nervous or metabolic functions (for example, many cases of tension follow clinical depression, and menopausal or premenstrual tensions often signify an underlying exhaustion). In such cases relaxants need to be used very sparingly and, most importantly, should be fortified by a 'tonic' or restorative regime.

CHAMOMILE

1: *Matricaria recutita* L., 2: *Anthemis nobilis* L.
2: Roman chamomile, true chamomile, *Chamaemelum nobile* L., double chamomile.
Family: Compositae
Synonyms: 1: German chamomile, wild chamomile, *Chamomilla recutita*, M. *chamomilla*

Description: 1: an annual of erect stem up to 60 cm high, with few wispy 2- to 3-pinnate leaves, and terminal peduncles supporting single flowerheads; the receptacle is raised and hollow; implanted on it are yellow tubular florets without membranous bracts; these are surrounded by one row of white ligulate florets, often bent downwards and easily lost on drying; odour strong and characteristic, taste bitter and aromatic.
2: a perennial plant of generally lowly growth with denser foliage but otherwise similar appearance; the receptacle is solid throughout, the white florets less vulnerable.

Habitat: found in fields and many other places throughout southern England, Europe, Russia and introduced throughout North America; they prefer cultivated ground.

Parts used: the flowerheads, ideally a few days before opening.

Cultivation: 1 is grown easily from seed, sown in light to loamy soil in a sunny position; once established it is self-sowing although it suffers from competition by other plants and the site will need clearing of perennial weeds. The same is true for 2, which is slower in growth: sowing should be into seed trays with the small young plants transplanted to well-cleared beds and carefully nurtured in the first few months.

Harvesting: the flowerheads are plucked at intervals throughout the summer.

Preparation: an infusion of the flowers, or a tincture made at 1:5 in 45 per cent alcohol.

Dosage: 1–4 g three times per day.

Constituents: 1: volatile oil (incl. proazulenes, bisabolol, farnesine, terpenes such as pinene, anthemal, spiroether, angelic and tiglic acids); flavonoids (incl. anthemidin and luteolin); bitter glycoside (anthemic acid); coumarin; malic acid; tannins.
2: volatile oil (with similar constituents as above but no spiroether); sesquiterpene lactone (nobilin); flavonoids (incl. patuletin, quercitrin, luteolin, apigenin); acetylenic salicylic derivative; cyanogenic glycoside; bitter glycoside (anthemic acid); coumarins (incl. scopolin); valerianic acid; tannins.

Pharmacology: although botanically distinct there is sufficient overlap in the constituents and pharmacology of the two chamomiles to justify their overlap in clinical use: the azulenes and bisabolol are anti-inflammatory and antispasmodic, reducing histamine-induced reactions such as anaphylaxis and hay fever, allergic asthma and eczema – they also are shown to speed up the healing of peptic ulcers; the flavonoids (especially anthemidin) are also antispasmodic; spiroether is more strongly antispasmodic than papaverine; valerianic acid is sedative, as are the cyanogenic glycosides; heteroglycan polysaccharides have been shown to have significant immunostimulating properties; the whole plants are antispasmodic *in vitro*, inhibiting contractions provoked by histamine, acetylcholine and bradykinin; they are also anti-inflammatory; the bitter effect is noticeable and will be apparent in the action of the remedy.

References:
1: *Carle, R. and Isaac, O. (1987) 'Die Kamille – Wirkung und Wirksamkeit', in *Zeitschrift für Phytotherapie*, Stuttgart, 8, pp. 67–77
Achterrath-Tuckerman, U. *et al.* (1980) 'Pharmacological investigations with compounds of chamomile. V. Investigations on the spasmolytic effect of compounds of chamomile', in *Planta Medica*, Stuttgart, 39, pp. 38–50
British Pharmacopoeia (1988)
European Pharmacopoeia (1985)
Glowania, H. J. *et al.* (1987) 'The effect of chamomile on wound healing – a controlled clinical-experimental double-blind trial', in *Zeitschrift für Hautkranheithen*, Berlin, 62, (17), pp. 1262–71
Isaac, O. (1979) 'Pharmacological investigations with compounds of

Chamomile. I. On the pharmacology of (-)-α-bisabolol and bisabolol oxides', in *Planta Medica*, 35, pp. 118–24

Jakovlev, V. *et al.* (1979) 'Pharmacological investigations with compounds of chamomile. II. New investigations on the anti-phlogistic effects of (-)-α-bisabolol and bisabolol oxides', in *Planta Medica*, 35, pp. 125–40

(1983) 'Pharmacological investigations with compounds of chamomile. VI. Investigations on the antiphlogistic effects of chamazulene and matricine', in *Planta Medica*, 49, pp. 67–73

Leung, A. Y. (1980) *Encyclopedia of Common Natural Ingredients Used in Food, Drugs, and Cosmetics*, John Wiley, New York, pp. 110–12

Martindale The Extra Pharmacopoeia (1982), 28th edition

Szelenyi, I. *et al.* (1979) 'Pharmacological investigations with compounds of chamomile. III. Experimental studies of the ulcerprotective effect of chamomile', in *Planta Medica*, 35, pp. 218–27

Wagner, H. *et al.* (1985) 'Immunstimulierend wirkende Polysaccharide (Heteroglykane) aus hoheren Pflanzen', in *Arzneimittel-Forschung*, Aulendorf, Germany, 35, (II), 7, pp. 1069–75

2: Benigni, R., Capra, C. and Cattorini, P. E. (1962) *Piante medicinali: chimica farmacologia e terapia*, Inverni & Della Buffa, Milan. pp. 187–9

British Pharmacopoeia (1988)

Leung, A. Y. (1980) *Encyclopedia of Common Natural Ingredients*, pp. 110–12

Martindale The Extra Pharmacopoeia (1989), 29th edition

Melegari, M. *et al.* (1988) 'Chemical characteristics and pharmacological properties of the essential oils of *Anthemis nobilis*', in *Fitoterapia*, Milan, LIX, 6, pp. 449–55

Morelli, I. *et al.* (1983) 'Selected medicinal plants', *FAO Plant Production and Protection Paper 53/1*, FAO, Rome, pp. 36–9

Action: anti-inflammatory; visceral and general relaxant; bitter; uterine relaxant; peripheral vasodilator.

Applications: Chamomile has been used from the earliest times for convulsions, ague, nervous tension and insomnia. It may be used for anxiety states, spasmodic or colicky pain, vertigo, and notably for children's problems, governed as these commonly are by nervous excitability or tension. Chamomile proves itself again and again as the parents' standby when tension, sleeplessness or pain compounds upon itself to affect their offspring, as it allows sleep or rest to intervene on many occasions where the explosive vitality of the child threatens to dangerously exhaust its small constitution. Chamomile is both effective and very gentle, acting without depression, after-effects or habituation.

The remedy has a particular orientation towards the digestive tract, being used specifically in modern clinical practice for dyspeptic conditions with a nervous component. On the one hand, it relaxes the gut wall, slowing or regulating peristaltic movements, relieving colic, nervous or irritable hyperactivity, diarrhoea and spastic colon: the volatile oil is also carminative, reducing flatulence. On the other hand chamomile is an appreciable bitter stimulant, maintaining adequate digestion, bile flow and pancreatic action, so never allowing digestive depression to occur.

Traditionally chamomile has been used as a local healing poultice for ulcers, skin inflammations and slow-healing wounds, as a mouthwash or eyebath, or in steam inhalations for catarrh and inflamed respiratory mucous membranes. These uses have been strongly supported by modern investigations showing constituents of the oil having anti-inflammatory effects.

The generic name of one of the chamomiles, *Matricaria*, deriving from matrix, meaning mother or womb, underlines the early prominence given to the plant for problems of the female reproductive system. It has been successfully used in a number of problems, including vomiting in pregnancy, menopausal symptoms, painful periods, mastitis, amenorrhoea due to psychological problems (e.g. anorexia nervosa, for which the plant is also indicated), and hysterical symptoms in their strict medical sense. It seems that chamomile will be helpful wherever hormonal problems, uterine tension and nervous tension coincide.

Chamomile has many constituents in common with yarrow, this supporting its use in fever management. It obviously has particular place for fevers in children, and where convulsions, undue tension, digestive irritability and associated symptoms are significant.

LEMON BALM

Melissa officinalis L.
Family: Labiatae
Synonyms: honeyplant, bee balm.

Description: this slightly mint-like plant is well known for its unmistakable lemony scent; the leaves are petiolate, decussate, ovate, dentate, and arise from erect square stems, branching little at first, but much more at flowering. The small white flowers grow in cymes of 3–5 in the upper-leaf axils: they are typically labiate, i.e. 2-lipped, with 4 curved stamens and a 5-toothed calyx. The roots do not 'creep' in stolons like other mints.

Habitat: native to southern, eastern and central Europe, from the Caucasus on to Iran, it is found naturalized throughout the world.

Parts used: the herb, just before flowering.

Cultivation: very easily grown from seed or root cuttings, or by taking the many plants that arise naturally around any specimen; it quickly establishes itself and spreads.

Harvesting: flowering time is between June and October: the afternoon is the best time of day to collect.

Preparation: the herb should be dried as briskly as possible, but gently, to preserve the volatile oils; prepared by infusion, or making a tincture at 1:5 in in 45 per cent alcohol.

Dosage: 1–4 g three times per day.

Constituents: volatile oil (incl. monoterpenes: citral, citronellal, geraniol, etc.); tannins; bitter.

Pharmacology: the volatile oils have been closely investigated in Germany where the plant is the main ingredient of a popular medicine known as 'Melissengeist'. Analysis of ingredients showed that many of the monoterpenes had central nervous calming activities, notably citronellal, but also citral, limonene, linalol and geraniol. All were also found to have appreciable antiseptic activity. Their antispasmodic nature was significant: some spasmolytic action was seen at concentrations as low as that seen with papaverine. Even more interesting was the effect demonstrated with what the Germans refer to as psychological-autonomic problems, such as those accompanied by symptoms of excitability, restlessness, headaches and palpitations: a clear clinical improvement was observed in double-blind clinical trials. In animal autopsy, inhaled molecules were actually found to have concentrated in the hippocampus of the limbic system.

References:

Becker, H. and Förster, W. (1984) 'Biologie, Chemie und Pharmakologie pflanzlicher Sedativa', in *Zeitschrift für Phytotherapie*, Stuttgart, 5, pp. 817–23

Forster, H. B., Niklas, H. and Lutz, S. (1980) in *Planta Medica*, Stuttgart, 40, 4, p. 309

Herrmann, E. C. and Kucera, L. S (1967) *Proc. Soc. Exp. Biol. Med.*, 124, p. 865

Holm, E. *et al.* (1974) *Die Heilkunst*, 87, pp. 70–75

Martindale The Extra Pharmacopoeia (1967), 25th edition, p. 858

Wagner, H. and Sprinkmeyer, L.(1973) *Deutsche Apotheker Zeitung*, Stuttgart, 113, pp. 1159–66

Arzneimittel-Forschung, Aulendorf, Germany, 23, pp. 749–55

Action: relaxant; antispasmodic; carminative; diaphoretic.

Applications: this plant has many of the properties of chamomile, being a useful relaxant and digestive remedy. If anything, its action is more cerebrally directed, and it should be considered one of the best central nervous relaxants.

Lemon balm is an effective peripheral vasodilator and diaphoretic useful in the management of those fevers with a tension component. It is an excellent and very safe children's remedy.

VALERIAN

Valeriana officinalis L.
Family: Valerianaceae
Synonyms: garden heliotrope, all-heal, fragrant valerian.

Description: a perennial herb, 60–120 cm high, with one or more fluted stems, supporting especially near the base, pinnate leaves with 9–21 lanceolate segments 2–8 cm long, with a few coarse teeth and a few hairs underneath. The leaves are more infrequent and opposite higher up the stem. There is a short rootstock, giving off a tuft of creeping runners. The stems terminate in broad corymbs of numerous flowers, white tinged with pink, funnel-shaped, with 5 unequal lobes. The dried roots are obtained 2–15 cm long, 1–2 mm wide, longitudinally wrinkled and brittle; the rhizome is upright, more or less truncate, 2–4 cm long and 1–2 cm wide, dark brown, upper portion having a circular stem and leaf scars, the whole often cut into 3 or 4 pieces. The odour is aromatic and pungent (only when the roots, etc. are dried); the taste bitter and camphoraceous.

Habitat: in moist situations, on the banks of streams or ditches and damp areas over the whole of Europe and Russian Asia to the Arctic Circle (becoming an alpine plant in the north); it is a common plant in Britain and is naturalized in the eastern USA.

Parts used: the roots and rhizomes.

Cultivation: will grow from seed in most soils, though it prefers a moist position in a light soil; once established it is prolifically self-sowing.

Harvesting: the roots are dug up in autumn.

Preparation: the roots can be both dry and fresh: the latter state apparently provides the most effective remedy, as drying largely destroys the valepotriates. To preserve the fresh root adequately, pure glycerin should be used: maceration of the roots can be carried out with a kitchen blender, and the whole allowed to stand for several days before being pressed off. Alternatively prepare a decoction of the dried roots or make them into a tincture at 1:5 in 25 per cent alcohol.

Dosage: 1–4 g three times per day.

Constituents: volatile oil (incl. valerianic acid, isovalerianic acid, borneol, pinene, camphene, methyl-2-pyrrole ketone, assorted sesquiterpenes); epoxy iridoid esters ('valepotriates'); volatile alkaloids (valerianine, chatarinine); resin; gum.

Pharmacology: the presence or otherwise of valepotriates in any sample of valerian is a subject of much vexation among phytochemists; they have certainly been shown to have considerable tranquillizing powers, reducing anxiety and aggression and counteracting the effects of ethanol; valerianic and isovalerianic acid are also sedative and antispasmodic; methyl-2-pyrrole ketone is a sedative and potentiates anaesthetics (as does the sesquiterpene fraction as a whole); from the whole root a water-soluble fraction reduces blood pressure, has some cardiotonic properties, and is antispasmodic *in vitro*. An effect in prolonging the activity in the brain of γ-aminobutyric acid, an inhibitory neurotransmitter, extends its similarity to diazepams.

References:
*Houghton, P. J. (1988) 'The biological activity of valerian and related plants', in *J. Ethnopharmacol.*, 22, pp. 121–42
Blackie and Ritchie (1939) *Pharm. J.*, 142, p. 299
Braekon, R. von *et al.* (1972) *Arzneimittel-Forschung*, 22, Aulendorf, Germany
British Pharmacopoeia (1988)
Chauffard, F. and Leathwood, P. D.(1985) 'Aqueous extract of valerian

reduces latency to fall asleep in man', in *Planta Medica*, Stuttgart, pp. 144–8

Eickstedt, K. W. *et al.* (1969) *Arzneimittel-Forschung*, 19, pp. 319 and 995

Jurcic, K., Schaette, R. and Wagner, H. (1980) 'Comparative studies on the sedative action of Valeriana extracts, valepotriates and their degradation products', in *Planta Medica*, 38, pp. 358–65

Leathwood, P. D. *et al.* (1982) 'Aqueous extract of valerian root (*Valeriana officinalis* L.) improves sleep quality in man', in *Pharmacol. Biochem. and Behav.*, 17, pp. 65–71

Leung, A. Y. (1980) *Encyclopedia of Common Natural Ingredients Used in Food, Drugs, and Cosmetics*, John Wiley, New York, pp. 317–19

Martindale The Extra Pharmacopoeia (1982), 28th edition

Riedel, E. *et al.* (1982) 'Inhibition of γ-aminobutyric acid catabolism by valerenic acid derivatives', in *Planta Medica*, 46, pp. 219–20

Temperament: Cool.

Taste: bitter; sweet; acrid.

Action: tranquillizer; antispasmodic; expectorant; diuretic.

Applications: in conventional medicine, the distinction is made between the sedative, which produces drowsiness and a reduction in sensitivity, and the tranquillizer, which in theory reduces sensitivity without interfering with activity and co-ordination (and which for example could be taken while driving). In fact, the distinction is a difficult one to sustain, and even the diazepams, the market leaders among conventional tranquillizers, have sedative actions. It is worth checking claims therefore that valerian is a natural tranquillizer.

On the one hand, it is used to help induce sleep, in those unable to settle down to it; however, this is not a very strong activity and appears to be more an enabling activity, reducing some of the distracting 'noise' in the central nervous system. Again it is occasionally likely to produce a sedation in certain individuals, but this seems more of an idiosyncratic reaction than a standard pharmacological one. It is, in fact, not difficult to agree with clinical research that suggests valerian is the nearest thing to a genuine tranquillizer available. This supports its main applications in modern times to any state of tension, irritability or spasm, where these are disturbing the patient and interfering with recovery.

There are antispasmodic characteristics as well, adding to the application of valerian to states of visceral tension, such as nervous bowel, dyspepsia, cramp, migraine and other vasospasms and similar disorders.

In earlier times, however, it is clear that these potential uses for valerian were not considered important. Old texts emphasize valerian's diuretic and expectorant properties, and the very name of the plant itself is thought to derive from a Latin word meaning 'heal-all'. This highlights the changes that can occur in a remedy when it is adapted to suit modern conditions. It also emphasizes the point that valerian is not just another suppressive agent.

Similar remedy: passionflower (*Passiflora incarnata*).

PEPPERMINT

Mentha x piperita L.
Family: Labiatae

Description: a hybrid of the spearmint, M. *spicata* and M. *viridis*: there are two varieties, black mint, M. *piperita* var. *vulgaris* Sole, and white mint, M. *piperita* var. *officinalis* Sole; the former has purplish stems and leaves; a low, spreading-branched perennial herb with erect or running purplish quadrangular stems, from 15–60 cm high; leaves stalked, ovate and toothed, 2–10 cm long, the upper ones smaller; the lilac or reddish-purple flowers all in axillary whorls, mostly shorter than the leafstalks, the last pair of leaves rarely with flowers; the odour and taste is mentholated.

Habitat: cultivated throughout temperate zones around the world.

Parts used: the leaves.

Preparation: infusion; decocting will lead to loss of the volatile oil; in Western herbal medicine tinctures are made at 1 : 5 in 45 per cent alcohol.

Dosage: 3–10 g daily.

Constituents: volatile oil (incl. variable quantities of menthol, pulegone, menthalone, piperitone, cineole, menthonone, limonene, α-pinene, phellandrene); tannins; flavonoids (incl. rutin, menthoside); bitter principle.

Pharmacology: menthol is a monocyclic monohydric terpene alcohol occurring in its isolated form as solid crystals; its physical properties impart a noticeable cooling effect to the skin (vasoconstriction, later followed by a pronounced vasodilation and rubefacient effect) and mucous membranes, this accompanied by a slight local anaesthetic action (due at least in part to an excitation of cold receptors); it is also a powerful antiseptic (four times the strength of phenol) and antiparasitic (an alcoholic solution of menthol is a local treatment for ringworm or other fungal infestations of the skin); inhaled it has a drying effect on mucous membranes and ingested it has a settling effect on the gastric, intestinal and especially colonic mucosa (a light anaesthetic effect on the gastric mucosa is thought to underlie its anti-emetic action). Whole peppermint has, in fact, more antispasmodic effect on the gut than menthol alone, due no doubt to the action of other constituents, and it has bitter effects in addition (like cholagogue action); it relaxes the gastro-esophageal sphincter, allowing reflux of air and flatus in aerophagy and flatulent dyspepsia; it specifically relieves colonic spasm and bowel irritability and the combination of effects gives it an important action in relieving biliary colic.

References:
Evans, W. C. and Trease, G. E. (1989) *Pharmacognosy*, 13th edition,
    p. 430
Gessner, O. and Orzechowski, G. (1974) *Gift- und Arzneipflanzen von
    Mitteleuropa*, Carl Winter Universitätsverlag, Heidelberg, pp. 296–9
Martindale The Extra Pharmacopoeia (1977), 26th edition, p. 1024
Potterton, D. (1979) *Brit. J. Pharm. Practice*, Sept., p. 35

Temperament: cool.

Taste: acrid.

Action: visceral relaxant; uterine relaxant; cholagogue; hepatic.

Applications: it is used principally to reduce colic, griping and flatulence, to check the spasm of diarrhoea and spastic constipation, and to inhibit vomiting. It is generally relaxant too, so is used in nervous tension, sleeplessness and vertigo ('comfortable for the head and memory' according to Parkinson). It is a notable cholagogue, both because of its bitter effect and because of a specific action of the volatile oil; the effect is to cleanse liver-related toxicities and gall-bladder infections and inflammations.

There is a persistent association with peppermint and generative matters. Parkinson notes, 'It is of especiall use to stay the feminine courses when they come too fast, and also to stay the whites, for which purpose no other herbe is more safe and powerfull' and 'it is good to represse the milke in womens breasts when they are swolne therewith'. It may be used to calm some cases of dysmenorrhoea or painful menstruation.

It also has a traditional reputation as affecting men: 'an especiall remedy for those that have venerous dreames and pollutions in the night, used both inwardly, and the juyce being applied outwardly to the testicles or cods'. On the other hand he also reports: 'Aristotle and other in the ancient times forbade Mints to be used of Soldiers in the time of warre, because they thought it did so much incite to Venery, that it took away, or at least abated their animosity or courage to fight.'

This gentle ambivalence in recommendation is rather in key with the rest of the traditional impression of peppermint, it being classified as 'hot' and 'dry' in Galenic terms, but cooling in common experience.

HOPS

Humulus lupulus L.
Family: Cannabinaceae

Description: a perennial climber with annual stems running to considerable height (up to 6 m) in hedgerow trees and shrubs; the stems twist in a clockwise direction and at intervals give rise to opposite leaves, broadly ovate, more or less cordate at the base, deeply 3–5-lobed and sharply toothed, with a very rough surface; smaller leaves are single-lobed. The flowers are single-sexed: the male flowers in loose panicles in the upper-leaf axils, 5 mm across, yellowish-green; the female are closely stacked cone-like catkins made up of bracts, with the flowers themselves tucked into the bract axils: after fertilization these cones grow around three-fold up to 5 cm long, and change from pale greenish-yellow to yellow-brown and then to brown. The odour of these female 'strobiles' is characteristic and heavy; the taste is bitter.

Habitat: throughout south and east England, locally further north, through Europe and Asia, and as an escape from cultivation elsewhere around the world; naturally found in hedgerows, thickets and open woods.

Parts used: the strobiles; sometimes the oil glands sifted out from these.

Cultivation: plant established plants in a rich well-mulched soil in a sunny position against a hedge or wall with adequate support; it must not be allowed to dry out in a drought, and should be cut hard back to the ground after picking in the autumn.

Harvesting: August to October: long ladders may be needed!

Preparation: drying should be done carefully and thoroughly; the scent will improve when dry, if it is done properly. As the lupulin from the oil glands is very prone to oxidation, the plant does not retain its value after long storage, and should be replaced yearly. If buying hops (e.g. in stores selling it for beer making), some indication of the age of the material is worth inquiring for. The dried herb is best ground somewhat to reduce its great bulk before infusing; otherwise a tincture may be made at $1:5$ in 60 per cent alcohol.

Dosage: 0.5–1 g three times per day.

Constituents: volatile oil (incl. sesquiterpenes such as humulene, and geraniol, linalol, myricin, luparol, luparenol) and bitter-resin complex (including valerianic acid, humulon, lupulon) – the whole constituting 'lupulin'; condensed tannins; oestrogenic substances (100 g hops = 30,000–300,000 IU oestrogen); asparagin; trimethylamine; choline.

Pharmacology: several constituents are likely to have sedative properties: valerianic acid, the resin constituents, and possibly the oestrogenic principles; the resin components, lupulon and humulon are antiseptic, affecting particularly gram-positive bacteria; asparagin is notably diuretic. Work by Caujolle has suggested that the antispasmodic effect is stronger than the sedative, and that it also has antihistamine and anti-oxytocic properties (thus supporting claims for its use in painful menstruation).

Toxicology: chronic exposure to hops by pickers and other workers can produce symptoms of nausea, vomiting, abnormal sweating, somnolence, agitation, fever, bradycardia, mydriasis, and skin reactions such as erythema, conjunctivitis and pustular dermatitis.

References:
Becker, H. and Förster, W. (1984) 'Biologie, Chemie und Pharmakologie pflanzlicher Sedativa', in *Zeitschrift für Phytotherapie*, Stuttgart, 5, pp. 817–23

Benigni, R., Capra, C. and Cattorini, P. E. (1964) *Piante medicinali: chimica farmacologia e terapia*, Inverni & Della Beffa, Milan, pp. 893–907

Caujolle, F. *et al.* (1969) 'Étude de l'action spasmolytique du houblon (*Humulus lupulus*, Cannabinacées)', in *Agressologie*, 10, 5, pp. 405–10

Hänsel, R., Schmidt, H. and Wohlfart, R. (1983) 'The sedative-hypnotic principle of hops. 4. Communication: Pharmacology of 2-methyl-3-buten-2-ol', in *Planta Medica*, Stuttgart, 48, pp. 120–23

Leung, A. Y. (1980) *Encyclopedia of Common Natural Ingredients Used in Food, Drugs, and Cosmetics*, John Wiley, New York, pp. 198–9

Martindale The Extra Pharmacopoeia (1982), 28th edition

Temperament: cold.

Taste: bitter.

Action: sedative; visceral antispasmodic; bitter digestive tonic; local antiseptic and healer.

Applications: the strobiles are most often thought of as a mild sedative, well known in the form of the hop pillow, where the heavy aromatic emanation has been shown to relax, presumably through direct action on the olfactory centres and thus on the central nervous system through the limbic system. Similar effect can be had through more conventional application, so that hops is often used to help with insomnia and restlessness. It has genuinely sedative effects and it is not therefore recommended in depressive conditions.

There is, however, an even more significant property: hops may be used whenever there are signs of visceral tension in the body: it has a particular application to tense bowel states, such as irritable bowel syndrome or any condition of variable bowel performance either from neurogenic causes or as a reaction to local inflammation or irritation (as, for example, diverticulitis or Crohn's disease); it is also useful in nervous dyspepsia, palpitations, nervous coughs and even asthma.

Hops is a notable bitter, and this will round out its effect in any disordered bowel condition, as well as adding to the cooling effect of the whole remedy. Combined with its local antiseptic action, this also makes hops a useful agent for upper-digestive infections. It is possible, however, that the action of hops on the digestion might not suit every individual, and an early review of a hop-containing prescription is advisable.

Hops has an appreciable oestrogenic activity, manifested in the abolition or disturbance of the menstrual cycles of female hop-pickers (getting oil diffused through their skin). This undoubtedly means that it may disturb an unsettled menstrual or other hormonal function, and may contribute to the suspicion that excessive beer-drinking may not after all improve male virility! (Certainly a depressive action on libido in men has been reported with hops.) It may however be used in some cases of amenorrhoea and dysmenorrhoea, where its relaxant, antihistamine and anti-oxytocic effects may be an added bonus.

CRAMP BARK

Viburnum opulus L.
Family: Caprifoliaceae
Synonyms: guelder rose, European cranberry.

Description: a shrub or small tree, the wild form of the common garden cultivar; it bears leaves that are 4–7 cm broad, deeply divided into 3–5 broad pointed lobes, divided in turn into a coarse-toothed margin; they are quite hairless and shiny and on slender leafstalks with 2 or more glands at the top, and fringe-like appendages on the bottom. The flowers are small, white, borne in dense cymes, the outer flowers of which may be considerably larger, yet lacking in any reproductive organs; the fruits are in the form of black-to-red globular drupes. The dried bark is obtained as strips, chips or quills; bark up to 3 mm in thickness, outer surface green-brown and longitudinally wrinkled; few brown lenticels, thicker pieces light grey to brown, finely fissured or scaly; inner surface green-yellow to rusty brown; fracture short; surface showing brown outer bark, greenish phelloderm and yellow inner bark. Odour slight, taste astringent and bitter.

Habitat: in hedgerows and woods over Russian Asia and Europe, including Britain and Ireland; freely naturalized also in the United States, where it is known as European cranberry.

Parts used: the bark of the stem.

Cultivation: cuttings may be taken from the bush by taking off a lateral stem with a heel in the autumn, and striking in sand; the slow-growing plant can then be moved into a position with good loamy soil.

Harvesting: the bark is scraped off young shoots and branches removed from the shrub during flowering in May and June.

Preparation: after drying a decoction can be made or a tincture at 1:5 in 25 per cent alcohol.

Dosage: 1–4 g three times per day.

Constituents: bitter (viburnin); valerianic acid; salicosides; resin; tannins.

Pharmacology: viburnin is antispasmodic on uterine muscle and hypotensive, yet cardiotonic as well; valerianic acid is sedative (see also valerian and hops); the salicosides are anti-inflammatory.

References:
Vlad, L. von *et al.* (1977) *Planta Medica*, Stuttgart, 31, p. 22

Action: smooth and skeletal muscle relaxant.

Applications: cramp bark is used by the herbalist as a specific for relaxing muscle tension. Its name suggests one of its most popular applications; however, it is most appreciated in practice for its ability to control the many forms of visceral tension encountered in modern life. It plays a useful part in the control of nervous bowel, asthma, colicky pain from the gut, gall-bladder or urinary system, migraine, poor circulation following neuromuscular tension and spasm of the arterial musculature, difficulty in swallowing, convulsions in children, spasmodic dysmenorrhoea, and so on. It works more on such smooth muscle than on skeletal tissues, possibly through central relaxant mechanisms as much as directly on the tissues concerned.

Its role is clearly not a restorative one as such, but cramp bark is excellent in the management of a functional disorder, perhaps allowing time for physiological habits to be broken, for normal underlying tone in a structure to be re-established, or simply for relief and rest from a disturbing pattern of reaction. True restoration is more likely to occur under such circumstances.

Related remedy: black haw bark (*Viburnum prunifolium*).

SELF-HEAL

Prunella vulgaris L.
Family: Labiatae
Synonym: heal-all.

Description: a sprawling perennial herb up to 50 cm high but generally smaller, with opposite, petiolate, elliptical or oval leaves with entire or dentate margins; the small bluish-violet flowers are borne in a terminal spike with persistent broad bracts; the individual flowers are bilabiate with finely dentate upper lip and deeply divided paired ciliated lower lip; when dried the spike is a brown colour; the taste is bitter and pungent.

Habitat: throughout the northern hemisphere.

Parts used: the flowering spike.

Preparation: infusion or decoction.

Dosage: 6–15 g three times daily.

Constituents: essential oil (incl. camphor and fenchone); alkaloids; flavonoids; tannins; resin; bitter principle.

Pharmacology: experiments suggest a hypotensive effect.

Temperament: cool.

Taste: sweet; acrid; slightly bitter.

Action: relaxing; anti-inflammatory; lymphatic.

Applications: this is often thought of as a remedy to relieve tension and inflammations in the head, a remedy having both relaxing and restorative properties. It is a traditional internal remedy for eye problems, with such symptoms as conjunctivitis, blepharitis, and other types of inflammation and redness, as well as eye conditions marked by eye tiredness and strain developing through the day.

A wider relaxing effect is seen in its application to such symptoms as headaches and vertigo, and there are apparently modern investigations into a possible hypotensive effect.

The lymphatic properties of the remedy led to its application for lymphadenopathies and similar swellings, glandular fever, mumps, and mastitis. A traditional application to goitre should be treated with scepticism: it looks like but is not a lymphatic enlargement – dietary iodine remains the only real solution.

Diuretics

These remedies are milder alternatives to the purgative remedies that were traditionally used to provoke an urgent expulsion of water in earlier times. By contrast with those rather drastic remedies, the diuretics simply correct disturbances in normal diuresis, being particularly indicated for oliguria (poor urine production) and water retention.

They are generally mild in nature (and often of a bland taste, see 'Bland', on pp. 193–4) and are above all gentle. They may thus be used in a wider range of prescriptions without upsetting other actions. Even so their use should be watched in cases where dehydration might be a possibility (some otherwise inexplicable cases of heat symptoms may be due simply to dehydration, following either inadequate fluid intake, relatively high alcohol consumption, or fluid loss such as perspiration, diarrhoea or vomiting: recent findings suggest that relative dehydration is much more common than was once thought).

Diuretics should be considered particularly applicable to oedematous conditions, especially connected with heart failure and ascites, and also to 'catarrhal' conditions, as these affect the respiratory and digestive functions.

They may also usefully be applied in urinary infections, and as components of prescriptions for scrofulous skin diseases and jaundice, (when such conditions are marked by the description 'damp-heat' in Chinese terms, or liver disturbance in Western terms).

COUCH GRASS

Agropyron repens Beauv.
Family: Graminaceae
Synonyms: *Triticum repens* L., twitch grass, scutch, quick
grass.

Description: a pervasive perennial grass with hollow stems except at the
nodes, with leaves completely ensheathing the stem, and between 4–30 cm
in length. At the top of each sheath, at its junction with the blade, is a
tiny stiff appendage known as the ligule, variably hairy and about 1 mm
in length. The distinguishing feature of the plant is the extensive system
of white-to-yellow rhizomes revealed when the plant is dug up, by which
the plant spreads remorselessly through cultivated land. The dried rhizome occurs in short yellow-brown cylindrical pieces about 2–4 mm in
diameter with a hard smooth longitudinally furrowed surface.

Habitat: in temperate countries almost everywhere where humans have dug
the ground: it is the archetypal weed of cultivation. It is found particularly
on waste land and in abandoned gardens, on roadsides and field margins.

Parts used: the rhizomes.

Cultivation: absolutely not to be considered: the plant requires no help.

Harvesting: the rhizomes are lifted and washed in early spring or late
autumn.

Preparation: drying is little problem; a decoction is made, or else a
tincture at 1 : 5 in 25 per cent alcohol.

Dosage: 1–4 g three times daily.

Constituents: mannitol; mucilage (triticin); inositol; gum; antibiotic substances (formed from agropyrene); glycosides (incl. glucovanilline); saponin; vanillin, silicic acid, potassium and many other minerals (couch
grass is a notable soil 'pirate').

Pharmacology: among the useful components is the sugar mannitol
present in large quantities: this is known as a standard 'osmotic diuretic',
i.e. it is absorbed whole from the gut and excreted largely by the kidney
tubules; its presence in the tubules means that extra water has to be
retained in the tubules to maintain osmotic pressure at the same level. It
is likely that other factors in the plant, e.g. saponin and vanillin, also
have diuretic properties. The silica – present as 30 per cent of the ash
(that is, inorganic residue) – is present in high enough amounts to justify

465 Diuretics

using couch grass for the treatment of slow-healing wounds, and to strengthen the lung and other tissues, and with the antibiotic substances, to limit infections in the urinary tubules and elsewhere.

References:

Bezanger-Beauquesne, L. *et al.* (1981) *Plantes médicinales des régions tempérées*, Maloine Ed., Paris, p. 42

Dadak, V. and Hejtmanek, M. (1959) *Ceskolovenska Mykologie*, Prague, 13, p. 183

Mozes, E. and Racz-Kotilla, E. (1971) *Revista Medicala*, Tirgu-Mures, Romania, 17, p. 82

Taste: mild; sweet.

Action: soothing diuretic; calming pain and spasm in the urinary tract.

Applications: this remedy has a very long tradition of being used for pain in the urinary system, being applied to infections, calculi (stones) and other irritable conditions.

There is in fact support for these actions. Due to the presence of mannitol, a possible immediate effect is to dilute the urine, thus helping to flush out sites of infection and inflammation and so reduce the chance of calculus formation (crystals do not however automatically form in the urine: largely insoluble salts will stay in solution as long as there is no rough surface upon which crystals can deposit or grow – infection or inflammation provides this opportunity and thus in theory is also necessary for crystals to sediment).

Mannitol is thought to have direct soothing action on the mucosa. Silica is also likely to have some healing and tissue-repairing properties. The antibiotic substances would contribute to reducing infections and the saponins and vanillin are thought to further increase urine flow.

The rhizome is considered to be highly nutritious (being very rich in essential minerals); it is taken as a food in convalescence and debility, and is also used, in Germany at least, as a 'cleansing' food, suitable for catarrhal, liver and rheumatic problems.

Similar remedies: corn silk (*Zea mays*); pearl barley (*Hordeum vulgare*).

HORSETAIL

Equisetum arvense L.
Family: Equisetaceae
Synonyms: shavegrass, pewterwort, bottlebrush.

Description: a member of a very primitive family of plants that millions of years ago formed swampy forests that covered the earth and later became our present coal deposits, horsetail is now the most common species in northern temperate climes. In the spring, a spore-bearing shoot rises 15–25 cm, rather like a thin asparagus shoot, covered in scales. After the spore is shed, the stem is replaced by a pale-green brush with erect hollow jointed stems with longitudinal furrows, and with sharply-toothed sheaths covering each joint. From the sheaths of the central stem arise whorls of branches, some of which in turn give off further irregular whorls at their nodes. The whole plant has a fine appearance, and is up to 60 cm in height, in comparison with its relatives that are generally of coarser appearance. When dried the stems are 0.5–3 mm in diameter, bearing 6–19 deep longitudinal grooves. Odour and taste are slight.

Habitat: in waste and moist places throughout temperate regions of the world; prefers non-chalky soil.

Parts used: the sterile brush or herb.

Cultivation: a troublesome weed, spreading as much by its creeping rootstock as by its spores.

Harvesting: the herb is collected during mid- to late summer.

Preparation: drying is non-critical as there are no volatile components present; the plant is best boiled in water for a considerable time (up to 3 hours along with a little sugar) as the best way to mobilize the vast quantities of silica. It will be an advantage to grind the dried herb finely before adding water. An alternative process would be to put the fresh herb with water several times through the juicer. Probably the best preparation is fresh succus, available from some German firms. A tincture may be made at 1:5 in 25 per cent alcohol, but this is unlikely to contain much silica unless made from the fresh herb.

Dosage: 1–4 g dried herb three times daily.

Constituents: saponin (equisetonin); silica; flavonoids; alkaloids (incl. nicotine and palustrine); bitter; phytosterols; many minerals.

Pharmacology: it is the silica which has been credited with most of the healing effects of this remedy, but the saponins and flavonoids are likely to combine to have at least a diuretic effect; evidence of an antirheumatic action and an influence on lipid metabolism (leading to potential benefit for cardiovascular problems) has also been attributed to silica; the juice increases blood clotting, in spite of it containing haemolytic saponins.

Toxicology: although toxic in quantity to cattle, the content of alkaloids is very low and is very unlikely to figure as a problem in therapeutic dosages.

References:
Benigni, R., Capra, C. and Cattorini, P. E. (1962) *Piante medicinali: chimica farmacologia e terapia*, Inverni & Della Beffa, Milan, pp. 333–8
Carlisle, E. M. (1974) *Fed. Proc.*, 33, 6, p. 1758
Franck Bakke, E. L. and Hillestad, B. (1980) *Meddelelser fra Norsle Farma centisle*, Selskap, Oslo, 42, p. 9
Hänsel, R. and Steinegger, E. (1988) *Lehrbuch der Pharmakognosie und Phytopharmazie*, Springer-Verlag, Berlin, pp. 567–8
Hartke, K. and Mutschler, E. (1988) *Schachtelhalmkraut. DAB 9 – Kommentar*, Wissenschaftliche Verlagsesellschaft, Stuttgart
Loeper, J. et al. (1979) *Atherosclerosis*, 33, p. 397
Martindale The Extra Pharmacopoeia (1989), 29th edition
Milne, D. and Schwartz, K. (1972) *Nature*, 239, p. 334
Saint Paul, A. (1980) *Plantes médicinales et phytothérapie*, Angers, France, 14, 2, p. 73
Vernin, J. (1981) *Parfums, cosmétiques et arômes*, Paris, 37, p. 63
Weiss, R. F. (1980) *Lehrbuch der Phytotherapie*, Hippokrates-Verlag, Stuttgart, p. 258

Taste: mild.

Action: astringent and styptic, notably on urinary mucosa; strong diuretic; restorative to damaged pulmonary tissue; supporting inflammatory response; possible detoxifier.

Applications: horsetail has for long had a strong reputation as a healing agent. The most obvious application was as an antihaemorrhagic, used as a poultice to staunch bleeding from wounds. Apart from its clotting promotion mentioned above, it appears to have direct healing action on the connective tissue (a possible silica effect). This impact on external bleeding leads to it being taken when there are signs of internal bleeding, especially from the lungs ('coughing blood') and in the urine. While this connection is not normally justified, in this case the antihaemorrhagic effect does seem to be transferred to systemic action.

The effect on the urinary system is augmented by the pronounced diuretic action of the plant. One study indicated that a 70 per cent increase in urine flow was possible using the remedy, whilst further work suggested that the activity is found in tinctures, thus indicating that the silica is not responsible (a combined action of saponins and flavonoids is suggested as most important). Certainly, the remedy was much used for oedematous conditions and to flush out urinary stones. It is particularly favoured in modern times for the hormonal oedema that marks menopause and some arthritic conditions.

The combination of these properties leads to the major use by modern herbalists of horsetail as a 'urinary astringent', useful for checking infections and damage to the walls of the ureters, bladder and urethra, as well as the prostate in men. It dilutes the urine, possibly increases clotting on site, and may have other healing effects on the mucosa. Even the paradoxical application of horsetail to incontinence and frequency of micturition may be explained, as these symptoms very often arise from irritation of the bladder sphincter or enlargement of the prostate, both conditions which horsetail might benefit.

Other benefits are claimed. Recent research in Russia has apparently indicated that horsetail is effective in removing lead accumulations in the body. If confirmed, this would be an exciting find in these times. It has long been seen as a general 'blood-cleanser', used for rheumatic, arthritic and skin diseases in many traditions.

It has a recognized repairing and healing effect on the lungs and is one of the basic remedies for tuberculosis as well as other cases marked by 'spitting blood'.

Finally, the local astringent and antihaemorrhagic effect explains the application of horsetail to such conditions as bleeding from mouth, nose and vagina, its use to check diarrhoea, dysentery and bleeding from the bowel, and for slow-healing wounds, chilblains and conjunctivitis.

469   Diuretics

UVA URSI

Arctostaphylos uva-ursi Spreng.
Family: Ericaceae
Synonyms: bearberry, mountain cranberry, sandberry, bear grape.

Description: a small evergreen shrub with alternate entire or toothed shiny obovate or oblong leaves up to 25 mm long, arranged in large masses. The long fibrous main root sends out several prostrate or buried stems 10–15 cm high. The flowers are in drooping terminal racemes, small pink-to-white bell-shaped in groups of 4 to 6. The globular bright-red berries, containing several seeds, taste sour and astringent (though liked by bears!). The plant resembles cranberries (though with erect branches and small dots on the undersides of the leaves) and the cowberry (with sepals at the crown of the berry rather than at its base).

Habitat: on dry, heathy or rocky hills, often covering large tracts of ground, extending over the northern hemisphere up to the Arctic Circle.

Parts used: the leaves.

Cultivation: propagation is by layering the shoots or taking cuttings, or by sowing the seeds in the autumn. The plant likes a lime-free soil, and will grow best in a peaty or sandy acid soil. It can be cultivated in a similar way to other members of the heather family.

Harvesting: collected in September or October, only green leaves being selected.

Preparation: dried by exposure to gentle heat; an infusion can be made without any difficulty in any suitable container or a tincture made at 1:5 in 25 per cent alcohol.

Dosage: 1–4 g dried leaves three times per day.

Constituents: glycosides (incl. arbutin, methyl-arbutin and ericolin); tannins (6–7 per cent); flavonoids; resin (ursone).

Pharmacology: the excellent antiseptic effect on the urinary system is brought about by the hydrolysis of arbutin to the antiseptic hydroquinone in alkaline urine; this inhibits growth of *Citobacter*, *Enterobacter*, *Escherichia*, *Klebsiella*, *Proteus*, *Pseudomonas* and *Staphylococcus* (Kedzia), and also by the breakdown of ericolin to a volatile component ericinol. There is thus in fact a delayed-action effect manifesting only at the site of action.

References:

Benigni, R., Capra, C. and Cattorini, P. E. (1964) *Piante medicinali: chimica farmacologia e terapia*, Inverni & Della Beffa, Milan, pp. 1640–48

Frohne, D. von (1970) 'Untersuchungen zur Frage der Harndesinfizierenden Wirkungen von Bärentraubenblatt-Extracten', in *Planta Medica*, Stuttgart, 18, pp. 1–25

Jahodar, L. *et al.* (1978) *Die Pharmazie*, Berlin, 33, p. 536

Kedzia, B. *et al.* (1975) 'Antibacterial action of urine containing arbutine metabolic products', in *Medycyna Doswiadczalna I Mikrobiologia*, Warsaw, 27, pp. 305–14

Leung, A. Y. (1980) *Encyclopedia of Common Natural Ingredients Used in Food, Drugs, and Cosmetics*, John Wiley, New York

Martindale The Extra Pharmacopoeia (1989), 29th edition

Moretti, V. (1977) *Bolletino della Società Italiana della Farmacia Ospedaliera*, Milan, 23, p. 207

Proliac, A. (1980) *Plantes médicinales et phytothérapie*, Angers, France, 24, 3, p. 155

Action: potent and selective urinary antiseptic; astringent effect on lower digestive tract.

Applications: this is a prime remedy for urinary infections such as cystitis, urethritis, prostatitis and similar. It is possibly not appropriate for cases where the kidneys are affected.

The possibility of activity against micro-organisms *Klebsiella* and *Proteus*, among others, adds an intriguing new dimension to a reputation for a benefit in some rheumatic diseases (see 'Autoimmune Disease', on pp. 73–4).

The presence of tannins justifies its use as an astringent for managing diarrhoea and reducing other cases of intestinal irritation.

Similar remedies: Juniper berries (*Juniperus communis*); buchu (*Barosma betulina*).

PARSLEY

Petroselinum crispum Mill.
Family: Umbelliferae
Synonyms: *Carum petroselinum* Benth. and Hook., *P. sativum* Hoffm.

Description: a well-known kitchen herb commonly grown for its curly, pinnate, segmented leaves. The flowers appear in the second year, in the typical umbel form: small yellowish-green flowers in groups of 8–20 and with bracts. Fruit (seed) is ovoid in shape with 5 longitudinal ridges. The root is a rather thick fusiform taproot. The odour is characteristic.

Habitat: a native of eastern Mediterranean countries, now grown and naturalized throughout the world. The naturalized form is found especially in maritime areas, and in limestone and rocky areas otherwise.

Parts used: the whole herb, root and seed.

Cultivation: the plant is grown from seed, sown in rows 45 cm apart, and the seedlings thinned to 15 cm apart. Germination is slow and often patchy: it is helped by pouring over the seeds in the seed trench after sowing boiling water from a kettle – this cracks the outer shell. Parsley enjoys a sunny position in a rich well-dug and limed soil, but will grow in less ideal conditions.

Harvesting: the leaf is collected in early summer, the root in autumn, but the seed will not be ready until the late summer of the second year.

Preparation: the herb can be taken as an infusion, the root and seed as a decoction; alternatively a tincture may be made at 1:5 in 40 per cent alcohol.

Dosage: 1–4 g dried root or leaves or 1–2 g seeds three times daily.

Constituents: volatile oil (containing apiol: 'parsley camphor'); furanocoumarins (incl. bergapten); flavonoids (incl. apiin); large quantities vitamin C, provitamin A, and iron, calcium, phosphorus and manganese.

Pharmacology: the apiol, shared with its close relative celery, is a urinary antiseptic and a stimulant to the womb; it is possible that the furanocoumarin fraction is antispasmodic.

References:
Boni, U. and Patri, G. (1977) 'Prezzemolo', in *Le erbe: scoprire, riconoscere, usare*, Gruppo Editoriale Fabbri, Milan, pp. 494–5
Leung, A. Y. (1980) *Encyclopedia of Common Natural Ingredients Used in Food, Drugs, and Cosmetics*, John Wiley, New York, pp. 257–9

Martindale The Extra Pharmacopoeia (1982), 28th edition
Novak and Mitarb (1965) *Planta Medica*, Stuttgart, 13, p. 226

Action: strong diuretic; carminative and digestive tonic; antispasmodic; uterine stimulant; nutritive.

Contra-indications: the seeds and heavy consumption of the herb are to be avoided in pregnancy.

Applications: long credited as a strong diuretic (according to Galen, 'it provoketh the urine mightily'), parsley (especially the seed) has been used for oedematous conditions and for urinary stones. Like its close relative celery seed it is likely to increase the elimination of uric and other acidic metabolites and so have a particular application for gouty and arthritic conditions.

Parsley has a two-fold action on the gut: on the one hand, it is a sure carminative, effective in allaying flatulence and intestinal colic (and hence its culinary use); on the other hand it has been used in Germany for anorexia and modern research shows it stimulates stomach acid secretions and gastric activity, an action consistent with producing a feeling of hunger. In addition the root of the plant was seen as one of the best cleansers of the 'liver, spleene and belly', used for jaundice and general epigastric disorders.

There are antispasmodic effects, reducing the contractility of smooth muscle, i.e. the muscle of the gut, blood vessels and other internal structures. This property explains the use of parsley for migraines, cramps, asthma, 'weakness of the bladder' (in fact, tension in the bladder muscle) and, of course, dyspepsia and intestinal hyperactivity.

As with many antispasmodics there is a contradictory stimulating effect on the smooth muscle of the womb. So the seed especially is used to bring on suppressed menstruation and help expel the placenta after birth; it is also likely to damage the foetus and must be avoided in pregnancy. It is not likely to be helpful in painful periods. As with some other emmenagogues it promotes milk production and is in general an excellent postnatal remedy, helping as it does the normal involution of the womb.

Parsley is one of the most nutritious vegetables available, being one of the best food supplements for iron-deficiency anaemia and other cases of poor nutrition or deficiency. In this case the fresh leaf is the most effective, preferably freshly picked to optimize its high vitamin C content.

Similar remedy: celery seed (*Apium graveolens*).

Expectorants

The concept of 'catarrh' has a much broader meaning in traditional medicine than it has in modern times, involving disturbances not only in the respiratory functions but also those of the processes of assimilation and elimination. Frequent descriptions of 'catarrh-states' include concepts such as 'dampness', 'congestion' and 'toxicity'.

Specific 'catarrhal' symptoms have been said to include, as expected, mucous congestion, breathlessness and coughing, but also glandular swellings, eczema, weak digestion, nausea, distension (when the upper digestion is involved), cramps, anxiety, tinnitus and even epileptic fits. The diagnosis is confirmed when the symptoms are relieved by provoking an expectoration: in former times *emetic* remedies were applied for more dramatic short-term treatment; in modern conditions these are generally too drastic and more gentle remedies suited to chronic conditions and weakened constitutions are indicated.

Often 'catarrhal' conditions can also be relieved by countering the effects of 'cold-dampness' on the digestive system, using *aromatic digestives*.

Coughing is often, but not always, linked to 'catarrh'. It may also be the result of old age and/or debility (usually producing a classic dryness of the airways), or an inflammatory response to infection or other irritation (such as pollution, earlier lung disease, or, *in extremis*, lung cancer). Such factors will require other remedies and care will need to be taken that any treatment for coughs does not disguise other requirements.

There are three categories of expectorants, of which the last is the one most likely to disguise other troubles:

stimulating and warming expectorants
relaxing expectorants
antitussives

Stimulating and Warming Expectorants

These are remedies with circulatory stimulant properties or stimulating effects on the stomach wall (some in this group are emetic remedies used in sub-emetic dosages). Their prime effect on the lungs seems to be to provoke an expectoration of congested phlegm in the airways, and to dry up excessive catarrhal production.

These remedies are used for 'catarrhal' conditions formerly linked with 'cold' and 'damp' conditions and the pathological influences linked to them (see 'Cold-dampness', on pp. 138–9) with wet and productive cough, thin or clear sputum, painful joints and limbs or swelling.

As well as the one listed here, other warming remedies discussed elsewhere, like ginger, garlic and angelica root are notable warming expectorants. The effect of any stimulating expectorant is in any case likely to be enhanced by combining them with warming remedies. The simultaneous use of diuretic remedies is also often recommended.

Some in this group are gentle enough to be used quite freely but they are often stimulating and heating and even drastic in action, requiring care in their use.

ELECAMPANE

Inula helenium L.
Family: Compositae
Synonyms: scabwort, elfwort, horse-elder.

Description: a large herbaceous perennial consisting of a tuberous branching rootstock of considerable size from which each year arise stiff, robust stems 60–200 cm high. These have at their base elliptical leaves up to 60 cm long on a fleshy stalk, with an acute apex, single hairs on the upper surface and woolly grey hairs underneath. The stem leaves arise alternately, are similar to the basal leaves but smaller and sessile, and with finely toothed margins. The flowerheads are single, at the end of the stem, or in a corymb of 2 or 3. They are 6–8 cm in diameter, with pronounced involucral bracts, broadly ovate and woolly, which support numerous spreading bright-yellow ray florets surrounding a mass of often dark-yellow tubular florets.

Habitat: a native of south-east Europe and west Asia, but found widely in temperate regions over the world as a cultivated escape, including north mid-west USA, and Britain and Ireland; on roadsides or waste places or in old gardens.

Parts used: the roots.

Cultivation: easily cultivated from seed or rootstock, it prefers a moist position, though it will prosper in any good soil.

Harvesting: in the autumn after the stem has died back.

Preparation: the root is chopped while fresh into small pieces; the best aqueous preparation is by infusion in a vacuum flask, the better to extract the volatile oil; this necessitates grinding the root to a coarse powder just before preparation; a tincture may be made at 1:5 in 25 per cent alcohol.

Dosage: 1–4 g dried-root equivalent three times daily.

Constituents: essential oil ('helenin' – solid at room temperature: incl. camphor, alantol, alantoic acid, alantolactone); bitter principles (possibly including sesquiterpene lactone, alantolactone); triterpene saponins (incl. dammaradienol, stigmasterol, friedelin); possible alkaloid; inulin (40 per cent).

Pharmacology: in spite of its mucilaginous quality, this remedy is notable for exhibiting a more stimulating effect on the lungs overall. Two factors are likely to be responsible for this: the essential oil – shown to have a stimulating effect on the mucociliary escalator in a number of other remedies – and the saponins. These exert a stimulating effect on the bronchial structures by reflex from their detergent irritant effect on the stomach wall. The essential oil is additionally antiseptic and is for example active against the tubercle bacillus.

477 Expectorants

References:

Benigni, R., Capra, C. and Cattorini, P. E. (1962) *Piante medicinali: chimica farmacologia e terapia*, Inverni & Della Beffa, Milan, pp. 549–55

British Pharmaceutical Codex (1923 and 1934)

Leung, A. Y. (1980) *Encyclopedia of Common Natural Ingredients Used in Food, Drugs, and Cosmetics*, John Wiley, New York, pp. 162–3

Martindale The Extra Pharmacopoeia (1989), 29th edition

Temperament: warm.

Action: stimulating expectorant; diaphoretic; digestive tonic; relaxant; bacteriostatic.

Applications: due to reflex irritation and other actions, this remedy provokes the mucociliary escalator in the bronchial system to increase the active elimination of mucus from the lung. Coughs are made more productive in congested pulmonary conditions, and because of the camphoraceous nature of the volatile oil there is also reflex stimulation of circulation and respiration. Any harshness, however, is largely mitigated by the soothing effect of the mucilaginous component, so that elecampane is quite safe to use even for the most infirm. In fact, it is an ideal remedy for chronic bronchial conditions of the elderly, but can in general be used for any obstructive pulmonary disease, with its antiseptic effects, warming and diaphoretic effects having valuable back-up benefits.

It is an appreciable relaxant, so is further indicated where there is a nervous component in any coughing.

It may also be considered, like angelica, as a useful warming digestive tonic, this further supporting its role as a remedy for the infirm and convalescent.

Similar remedies: ipecacuanha (*Cephaelis ipecacuanha*); squills (*Urginea maritima*); cudweed (*Gnaphalium uliginosum*); cowslip (*Primula vera*).

Relaxing Expectorants

These are often remedies high in mucilages, occasionally volatile oils (see 'Volatile Oils', on pp. 294–304), that act to reduce spasm and deficient mucus secretion in the airways, either by reflex from the gut or in other ways not established.

These are used for 'catarrhal' conditions linked in the past with the effects of heat and dryness on the lungs, with either copious or scanty thick, yellow, tough expectoration, glandular swellings in the neck, asthmatic tightness in the chest and other visceral spasm.

A range of other linked conditions, such as skin disease, rheumatic inflammatory diseases, and tension conditions like palpitation, may be treated with these remedies if a primary lung problem can be established. It is often useful to add other cooling remedies.

COLTSFOOT

Tussilago farfara L.
Family: Compositae
Synonyms: coughwort, horsehoof, foal's foot.

Description: appears in mid-winter as a hairy flowering stem arising from a network of subterranean rootstocks and creeping stolons: the stems are covered with brown scaly leaves, rise from 5–15 cm, and produce a single flower 15–35 mm in diameter, made up of bright-yellow ligulate florets surrounding a central area of deeper golden tubular yellow disc florets. This all converts to a white downy sphere of wind-borne seedheads at the same time as the characteristic large leaves are appearing, cordate with dentate margins, smooth above with a white down underneath, about 20 cm in diameter. These persevere through the growing season on long stalks. There is no odour, but a most mucilaginous taste.

Habitat: a common invasive weed, especially on heavy clay soils throughout Britain and Europe, North Africa and Asia, and introduced to North America; it is also found in damp areas, river banks and ditches.

Parts used: the leaves and flowers.

Cultivation: rarely desirable, but the rootstock is easily transplanted to any waste site and grown without much assistance. For both medicinal purposes and the goodwill of neighbours and farmers, the flowers should be picked before seeding.

Harvesting: the flowers in early spring, the leaves in late spring.

Preparation: as the leaves are very mucilaginous, the best extraction method is cold infusion, though for sterilization purposes leaving an ordinary hot infusion for a few hours to cool will be satisfactory: the solution will be very mucilaginous. A tincture may be made at 1:5 in 25 per cent alcohol.

Dosage: 0.6–2 g the dried flowers, 2–4 g the dried leaves three times a day.

Constituents: mucilage; bitter glycosides and sesquiterpenes; triterpene saponins (incl. arnidiol, faradiol in the flowers); pyrrolizidine alkaloids; tannins (up to 17 per cent in leaves, very little in flowers); sitosterol; zinc.

Pharmacology: the soothing effect of the mucilages (see 'Gums and Mucilages', on pp. 275–8) is augmented in this remedy by the proven spasmolytic action of the sesquiterpene fraction; their effect on the bronchial system is also broadened, at least in the flowers, by the stimulating expectorant action of the triterpene saponins; the presence of appreciable levels of zinc may account for anti-inflammatory and healing effects, both locally and internally.

Toxicology: the presence of hepatotoxic pyrrolizidine alkaloids (see 'Comfrey', on pp. 544–7) and the finding that when given to rats (at 16 per cent of their diet over a long period) there was an increase in incidence of liver cancer have cast a shadow over coltsfoot's reputation in regulatory circles at least; there can however be little risk in using the remedy in therapeutic doses for the short periods normally applied.

Temperament: neutral.

Taste: bland.

Action: relaxing expectorant particularly effective in reducing non-productive coughs; soothing dry and irritable airways; local healing and soothing remedy.

Applications: this is one of the most established traditional cough remedies, a fact even reflected in its botanical name ('*tussis*' means 'cough'). It demonstrates the virtue of mucilages in reflexly soothing bronchial irritation and increasing bronchial secretions. There must however be other influences as the herb is traditionally used as a smoking herb for asthmatic complaints: this suggests that alkaloidal constituents might be important, but this has not been confirmed. Whatever the basis of its activity, it was seen to be suitable for 'hot, dry cough and for wheesings and shortnesse of breath' (Parkinson): it proves a particular standby for children's coughs, associated as these are with a nervous, spasmodic element.

Coltsfoot is a good local healer and demulcent remedy, notable for badly healing wounds and ulcers; here the mucilage, tannins and zinc probably combine.

COMMON THYME

Thymus vulgaris L.
Family: Labiatae

Description: a perennial low aromatic shrub with much-branched, mostly woody stems forming dense tufts from which arise opposite paired leaves on short stalks, each with two minute leaflets at the base. Each leaf is 6–8 mm long, oblong-lanceolate, 1–2 mm broad, and recurved at the margins, the underside covered with fine hairs. The flowers are arranged in whorls in the axils of the upper leaves, with the typical 2-lipped labiate appearance, pink to lilac in colour. The seed is in the form of ovoid nutlets. The odour is characteristic. There are many subspecies and even species of thyme with variations in smell and appearance: they all have something of the medicinal action of *T. vulgaris*, but the differences may be significant: the standard species should if possible be obtained.

Habitat: an import to many countries from the Mediterranean regions and southern Europe, where it prospers almost anywhere, especially on waste ground.

Parts used: the flowering herb.

Cultivation: grown from seed or from cuttings, suitable for well-drained, lime-rich soil, perhaps in an alpine garden. Established plants should be kept closely cut to avoid their becoming straggly and, in any case, should be replaced by fresh cuttings every few years to maintain vigour. Though able to be grown in northern climes, some winter protection may be necessary.

Harvesting: during flowering, i.e. between May and October.

481   Expectorants

Preparation: drying should be fast, but the temperature should not be too high; storage should be under airtight conditions, as the volatile oils are easily lost; preparation should be by vacuum flask rather than in an open container for the same reason; a tincture may be made at 1:5 in 45 per cent alcohol.

Dosage: 1–4 g dried herb three times daily.

Constituents: volatile oil (incl. thymol 40 per cent, carvacrol, borneol, cymol, linalol); tannins; bitters; flavonoids; triterpenoid saponins.

Pharmacology: the volatile oil is the most notable constituent: thymol is a strong antiseptic agent, twenty times more powerful than the standard, phenol, yet unlike phenol it does not irritate or corrode the mucosa or skin exposed to it; the other components are also antiseptic, relaxing and expectorant: carvacrol stimulates mucosal membranes into secretory activity, while borneol has a camphor effect on the body: it stimulates heart, circulation, respiration, diaphoresis and the central nervous system. The bitters stimulate digestive activity, the saponins are reflex-stimulating expectorants, while the tannins provide an appreciable local astringent effect.

Toxicology: the toxicity of thymol is not significant in therapeutic dosages of thyme; however, it should not be taken in any quantity during pregnancy as it induces contractions in the gravid uterus.

References:

Debelmas, A. M. and Rochat, J. (1967) *Plantes médicinales et phytothérapie*, Angers, France, p. 23

Herrmann, E. C. and Kucera, L. S. (1967) *Proc. Soc. Exp. Biol. Med.*, 124, p. 869

Lemli, J. A. and Van den Broucke, C.O. (1981) *Planta Medica*, 41, p. 129

Litvinenko, V. I. *et al.* (1975) *Planta Medica*, Stuttgart, 27, p. 372

Moyse, H. and Paris, R. R. (1971) *Matière médicale*, Masson, Paris, III, p. 280

Olechnowicz-Stepien, W. *et al.* (1975) *Herba Polonica*, Poznan, Poland, 21, p. 347

Passet, J. (1979) *Parfums, cosmétiques et arômes*, Paris, 28, p. 39

Simeon de Buochberg, M. *et al.* (1976) *Rivista Italiana Essenze, Profumi, Piante Officinali*, Rome, 58, p. 527

Action: relaxing antiseptic expectorant; antispasmodic; carminative and digestive tonic; local antiseptic and astringent.

Applications: the antiseptic qualities of the remedy have attracted interest in modern times. It is antifungal and in quantity is anthelmintic, effective particularly against such intestinal worms as *Necator americanus* and species of *Ascarides* and *Oxyuris*.

Thyme also has a general effect on the bacterial population of the gut, owing to the poor absorption of thymol. Such thymol as is absorbed, however, is responsible for a reasonable antiseptic effect at the lungs and urinary system, at which two places it is excreted from the body: it is thus applied to bronchial (including fungal) and urinary infections. It is also useful locally as a mouthwash and gargle (and is an excellent base for toothpastes) and as a vaginal douche for infections at this site. With the tannin content (of up to 10 per cent) these local effects are potentiated.

The essential oil is the major influence in the antispasmodic action of the herb, manifested as a carminative effect on the digestive tract (along with the tannin effect), relaxing bronchial spasm in asthmatic conditions and nervous coughing. Like many antispasmodics, there is an opposite effect on the womb, and thyme has a tradition for procuring labour and expelling afterbirth: in quantity, it is likely to threaten a pregnancy.

Apart from disinfecting the airways and relaxing bronchial spasm, thyme has a well-recommended expectorant action as well: increasing the fluidity of the mucosal secretions, and promoting their expulsion. Thyme was noted for its ability to 'purge phlegm' and was said to 'cause easy expectorations of tough phlegm' (Parkinson), and this is still its prime role in modern medicine. It appears to be most effective where there is dry cough or asthmatic complication (there is a viscid mucus in some cases of the latter), when it is necessary to provoke and loosen obstructive secretions. On the other hand it is less advisable to use thyme in cases where there is already a surfeit of fluid mucus in the lung, e.g. in chronic bronchitis. In this sense thyme can be considered as a relaxing expectorant alongside the mucilage remedies. It has a particular application to the irritable coughs of children.

Thyme is used in France for liver disease and it has the appropriate bitter taste; this effect also points to a general stimulation of the upper digestive activities, and reinforces the suggestion that thyme is a good corrector of the environment of the gut, useful particularly in cases of enteric infections, where increased digestive secretions combine with the antiseptic effect.

Similar remedies: wild thyme (*Thymus serpyllum*); hyssop (*Hyssopus officinalis*).

Antitussives

These most often are members of the *Prunus*, or plum, genus, containing quantities of cyanogenic glycosides which act to suppress the cough reflex.

They are more symptomatic than others in this group, and care has to be taken not to use them to disguise underlying causes of coughs or as a substitute for more positive treatment.

WILD CHERRY BARK

Prunus serotina Ehrh.
Family: Rosaceae

Description: the bark occurring up to 4 mm thick, in flat or curved pieces; externally smooth, glossy, red-brown cork with white lenticels, sometimes exfoliated revealing greenish-brown cortex; the inner surface is brownish, striated longitudinally, sometimes with adherent patches of yellowish wood; rougher, darker bark pieces may be from older trees and are considered inferior. Odour of benzaldehyde when damp; taste is astringent and bitter.

Habitat: throughout North America.

Preparation: decoction.

Dosage: 3–10 g daily.

Constituents: cyanogenic glycoside (prunasin); benzaldehyde; tannins.

Pharmacology: the effect of the cyanogenic glycosides is to suppress the coughing reflex and they are respiratory depressants.

Toxicology: cyanogenic glycosides are moderately toxic, producing cyanic acid on hydrolysis: they clearly should not be taken to excess.

Temperament: warm.

Taste: bitter, sweet.

Action: reduces coughing.

Contra-indications: coughing of chronic illness and debility; diarrhoea.

Applications: a broad-acting remedy for coughing, especially when dry and non-productive. It is particularly effective in treating violent conditions where there is coughing to exhaustion.

Alteratives

This is a large and complex group of remedies widely used through-out history for their generally eliminative, detoxifying or cleansing roles. They have at various times been called 'depuratives', 'blood-cleansers', 'antiphlogistics' (meaning approximately 'anti-inflammatory'), dermatological agents (when applied specifically to skin disease), 'lymphatics' (when applied to lymphadenopathy – swollen lymph glands – or other lymphatic involvement) and 'detox' remedies.

As they are such a diverse group, there are few general statements to make: each remedy is a law to itself. However, they fit into this group mainly because they do not obviously make use of one of the eliminatory channels: they are not primarily laxatives, cholagogues, diuretics, expectorants or diaphoretics. They also tend to be rela-tively gentle in effect, although the clinical effects of 'dislodging' a congestive condition can sometimes be alarming if not approached carefully.

The main clinical indication for the use of alteratives is the chronic inflammatory disease, especially as it affects the skin (eczema, etc.), joints (arthritis), and other connective tissues.

The remedies classed as 'alterative' also include those used against infections and in the treatment of autoimmune diseases and tumours. Although independent pharmacological activities in these areas have been observed, most of the herbal remedies used for such problems almost certainly work to change the environment so as to depress such pathological disturbances as much as to directly attack pathogen or malignancy:

> **Anti-inflammatory** compounds have been widely found in the plant world. The sesquiterpene lactones and volatile oils are

two notable groups of plant constituents, and there is at least one recent screening showing that many plants themselves have anti-inflammatory effects as measured by conventional laboratory tests.[2] From a clinical point of view, however, such activities are likely to be secondary to broader alterative effects except in a minority of remedies.

Plants have, of necessity, had to be used for *antimicrobial* duties, and some seem to exhibit appropriate qualities, including those with antiseptic,[3] antifungal,[4] anti-amoebic and anthelmintic (antiworm) effects. All would have been classified in the past as cleansing, and even today those that are used in clinical herbal medicine, at doses perhaps too low for genuine antimicrobial activity, would be classed primarily as alterative. **Antitumour:** although several common plant constituents have been shown *in vitro* to have cytotoxic effects[5] it has only been in very rare cases, such as the extraction of vincristine and vinblastine from the Madagascar periwinkle (*Catharanthus rosea*), that new anticancer strategies have been established out of the plant world.

ECHINACEA

1: *Echinacea angustifolia* DC.
2: *E. purpurea* (L.) Moench.
3: *E. pallida* (Nutt.) Britt.
Family: Compositae
Synonyms: purple coneflower, rudbeckia, black sampson.

Description: 1: a perennial growing 15–50 cm high with simple rough stems, hollow near the base and thickening slightly close to the flower-head. The leaves are elongated, slightly elliptical with entire margins, covered in coarse hairs and protuberances, stalked at ground level and almost sessile up the stem. The flower is in the form of a high purple cone surrounded by roughly hairy bracts and then short spreading purple, crimson, pink or white ray florets.
2: similar to the above except that the leaves are broader, ovate to ovate-lanceolate and often toothed, the plant up to 2 m high.
3: narrow, linear leaves with long drooping rays, the plant up to 1 m high.
The taproot in all three species, when dried, is grey-brown or red-brown,

wrinkled and twisted longitudinally, often in a spiral; the fracture is fibrous and section reveals yellow medullary rays. It has an aromatic fragrance, with a sweetish taste leaving behind a slightly numb sensation.

Habitat: native of the prairies and open spaces in the USA; 1: Minnesota to Saskatchewan, Nebraska and Texas; 2: Pennsylvania to Alabama, Georgia, Michigan, Kentucky, Louisiana and Arkansas; 3: Illinois to Michigan, Alabama and Texas; preferring sandy soil; excessive demand in recent years has put a serious strain on natural populations and it is hoped a widescale programme of cultivation will be commenced; 2 is cultivated in Europe and elsewhere as an ornamental.

Parts used: the root and rhizome.

Cultivation: the roots are planted out in October to March; the seeds after cold-stratification for a month, sifted out and sown on the surface of a well-watered sowing bed in spring; the divided crown after harvesting in the autumn; plant in a sunny position in any fertile soil, preferably sandy and well drained.

Harvesting: in October or November when flowering has ceased.

Preparation: use the root in the form of a decoction, or a tincture at 1:5 in 45 per cent alcohol, rejecting samples that have lost their aroma or fragrant numbing taste.

Dosage: 0.5–1 g dried root three times a day.

Constituents: essential oil (incl. humulene in 1 and 3, caryophylene in 3); glycoside (echinacoside – only in 1); polysaccharide ('echinacin'); polyacetylenes (incl. echinalone in 1); isobutylalkylamines (incl. echinacein in 1); resin; betain; inulin; a sesquiterpene.

Pharmacology: evidence of immune and defence enhancement and antipathogenic action has accrued over many years from modern research. In 1950, a glycosidal fraction was shown to possess mild antibiotic activity; further work concentrated on the polysaccharide fraction indicating that this inhibited hyaluronidase activity, so reducing the ability of pathogens to penetrate tissues, and stimulated both fibroblast and macrophage activity: the mechanism is thought to involve polysaccharide-hyaluronic acid complex formation with a resultant increase in hyaluronic acid levels stimulating fibroblast activity; the polysaccharide was later found to have interferon-like antiviral activity *in vitro*, and immuno-stimulant activity, both effects suggested as following binding to cell receptors of T-lymphocytes by the polysaccharide, this stimulating interferon and other lymphokine production (all these polysaccharide effects will unfortunately be largely nullified when echinacea is taken by mouth, as polysaccharides are quickly broken down in digestion: at most a local effect on the throat and upper gut wall might be expected; in German medicine echinacin is most often administered as a purified intravenous injection); a compound isolated from the essential oil, pentadecadiene, was shown to have *in vitro* antitumour activity; polyacetylenes in general possess antibacterial and antifungal activity; echinacein provides the sharp taste and has local anaesthetic activity; it has also demonstrated insecticidal properties linked at least in part to its possessing hormonal growth regulators in juvenile insects; whole plant preparations were shown to be effective in the treatment of allergies.

References:

*Foster, S. (1984) *Echinacea Exalted*, New Life Farm Inc., Drury, Maryland

*Moring, S. E. (1984) '*Echinacea*', in *Botanica Analyticum*, Sunnyvale, California

Becker, V. H. (1982) *Deutsche Apotheker Zeitung*, Stuttgart, 122, p. 2323

Benigni, R., Capra, C. and Cattorini, P. E. (1962) *Piante medicinali: chimica farmacologia e terapia*, Inverni & Della Beffa, Milan, pp. 492–502

Bonadeo, I. *et al.* (1971) *Rivista Italiana Essenze, Profumi, Piante Officinali*, 53(5), pp. 281–95

Busing, K. H. (1952) *Arzneimittel-Forschung*, Aulendorf, Germany, 2, p. 467

Chone, B. (1976) *Arzneimittel-Forschung*, 11, p. 611

Farnsworth, N. *et al.* (1983) *Prog. Med. Econ. Pl. Res.*, vol. 1, Academic Press

Gilmore, M. R. (1911–12) *33rd Ann. Rep. Bur. Amer. Ethn.*, 63–4, p. 131

Haase, H. and Koch, E. (1952) *Arzneimittel-Forschung*, Aulendorf, Germany, 2, p. 464

Jacobsen, M. *et al.* (1975) *Lloydia*, Cincinnati, 38(6), pp. 473–6

Koch, E. and Uebel, H. (1954) *Arzneimittel-Forschung*, 4, p. 551

Orinda, D. *et al.* (1973) *Arzneimittel-Forschung*, 23(3)

Stoll, A. *et al.* (1950) *Helvetica Chimica Acta*, Basel, Switzerland, vol. 33(6)

Voaden, D. J. and Jacobsen, M. (1972) 'Tumor inhibitors. 3. Identification and synthesis of an oncolytic hydrocarbon from American coneflower roots', in *J. Med. Chem.*, 15, p. 6

Wacker, A. and Hilbig, W. (1978) *Planta Medica*, Stuttgart, 33, pp. 89–102

Wagner, H. and Proksch, A. (1981) *Zeitschrift für Agenwandte Phytotherapie*, 2(5), pp. 166–8

Temperament: warm to hot.

Taste: acrid; sweet.

Action: increases the body's resistance to bacterial, viral and fungal infections; stimulating and warming alterative; diaphoretic; reduces hypersensitivity reactions (e.g. allergies) and other immunological disturbances.

Applications: this plant comes with a formidable reputation from the annals of the settler tradition in North America, with many observing the native population using it as a 'remedy for more ailments than any other plant' (Gilmore), and reporting in often rapturous tones their own experiences with the remedy. In particular, it was recommended for the bites of snakes and other venomous creatures (to the extent that one researcher publicly volunteered to allow himself to be bitten by rattlesnakes to prove the point to his colleagues!), and for infected and poisonous conditions generally, to treat burns and wounds, and for toothache and sore throats. Septic problems were widely treated with nothing more than echinacea, and most herbalists of the day would go far to ensure a good supply.

The herbal practitioner today considers echinacea the finest blood-cleansing remedy for any infectious condition, and for a number of inflammatory conditions like skin disease, hypersensitivity reactions (e.g. allergies), inflammation and other immunological disturbances. There is reason to consider it as a useful agent in viral illnesses, and in cases of diminished or inappropriate immune responses as well, possibly because of its ability to enhance general defensive responses, host resistance and tissue repair. It is a specific remedy for boils, carbuncles and abscesses, for septicaemia, pyorrhoea and tonsilitis.

It has local antiseptic action in other areas, being the basis of successful douches for vaginal infections, suppositories, and external applications to skin ulcers, infected wounds and burns.

Its other influences are worth noting: it is a circulatory stimulant leading to increased blood flow through the tissues and a pronounced diaphoresis in febrile conditions. It has a digestive action that in certain cases acts to soothe dyspeptic conditions (particularly when there are digestive infections) but in other cases can lead to a feeling of nausea that might need additional carminative remedies.

Similar remedy: wild indigo (*Baptisia tinctoria*).

BURDOCK

Arctium lappa L.
Family: Compositae
Synonyms: great burdock, bardane, beggar's buttons, thorny burr.

NOTE: other species of burdock are used interchangeably with *A. lappa*.

Description: a stout biennial plant extending up to 2 m, marked out by its very large ovate-cordate leaves up to 45 cm across, though getting smaller up the stem; they are generally smooth above and with white cottony down underneath the borders. The other distinguishing marks are the flowers, borne in clusters at the top of the stems, globular in shape and covered with a dense array of stiff hooked bracts that cling to anything coming in contact with them; enclosed inside are purple florets, and, after fruiting, large achenes with a short pappus of stiff hairs on each. The long root, up to 1 m long, runs straight down into the subsoil; when chopped and dried it is covered externally with brown cork and longitudinally wrinkled, the inner surface mealy and buff-white; the taste of the root is mucilaginous and slightly bitter; the seeds are oblong, slightly incurvate, 7 mm long, 3 mm wide, grey with black spots, with a pungent taste.

Habitat: on roadsides and waste places and around field borders throughout northern China, Asian Russia, Europe, Britain and North America.

Parts used: the fruit (seeds) and root, the former mostly in Oriental medicine, the latter mostly in the West.

Preparation: decoction.

Dosage: the root is recommended at 1–6 g three times daily; in China, 3–10 g seed daily.

Constituents: *seed*: flavonoids (incl. arctiin, arctigenin); gobosterin; essential oil; fatty oil; *root*: bitter glycosides (incl. arctiopicrin); flavonoids (incl. arctiin); alkaloid; condensed tannins; volatile oil (trace); antibiotic substances (polyacetylenes – especially in the fresh specimen); inulin; resin; mucilage.

Pharmacology: arctiin is a CNS stimulant and smooth muscle relaxant; antibacterial and antifungal, oestrogenic, diuretic, hypoglycaemic and antitumour properties have been established for the plant.

References:

Benigni, R., Capra, C. and Cattorini, P. E. (1962) *Piante medicinali: chimica farmacologia e terapia*, Inverni & Della Beffa, Milan, pp. 129–32

Cavallito *et al.* (1945) *J. Amer. Chem. Soc.*, 67, p. 948

Fletcher Hyde, F. (1978) 'Burdock', in *Pharm. J.*, 9 Sept., p. 204

Leung, A. Y. (1980) *Encyclopedia of Common Natural Ingredients Used in Food, Drugs, and Cosmetics*, John Wiley, New York

Martindale The Extra Pharmacopoeia (1982), 28th edition

Morelli, I. *et al.* (1983) 'Selected medicinal plants', in *FAO Plant Production and Protection, 53/1*, FAO, Rome, pp. 10–13

Obata, S. *et al.* (1970) *Agr. Biol. Chem.*, 34(11), p. 31

Suchy, M. *et al.* (1957) *Collection of Czechoslovak Chemical Communications*, Prague, 22, pp. 1902–8

Temperament: cool.

Taste: acrid (seeds); bitter (root).

Action: *seed:* cooling diaphoretic; improves throat function; disperses congestions; detoxifier; *root:* detoxifier and cleanser; diuretic; mild laxative.

Applications: the seeds are used in traditional Chinese medicine for septic conditions, boils, abscesses, and especially for throat inflammations, tonsilitis, etc. It is also a diaphoretic with pronounced 'cooling' action used in fever management (for exanthematous, septic and other aggressive fevers) and a diuretic formerly applied to dropsy and other cases of oedema.

The concept of cleansing is certainly the dominant feature in the Western use of the root, traditionally applied for scrofulous skin conditions, septic disorders, boils and any chronic inflammatory state. Among modern practitioners burdock has the reputation of being one of the most active alteratives, having an often precipitous action on a condition (this leads to a certain caution in dosage: it does appear that the more congested and toxic the state of the tissues, the more likely it is that a transient toxaemia will ensue as the material is dislodged, this in turn producing a worsening of the symptoms). The root clearly has a more bitter effect than the seed, helping to improve digestion and also confirming it as a colder remedy. It has similar diuretic properties.

CLEAVERS

Galium aparine L.
Family: Rubiaceae
Synonyms: clivers, goosegrass, hedge-burs, sticky-willie, cleaverwort.

Description: a straggling annual plant closely related to bedstraws and to woodruff commonly seen scrabbling through bushes and hedges, clinging to them and to anyone brushing past them, by tiny curved prickles on the angles of the stems and the veins and edges of the leaves. The latter occur in whorls of 6–8, are linear-lanceolate and about 2–3 cm long. The flowers are borne in peduncles somewhat longer than the leaves, arising from the axils of each whorl; each peduncle bears a small loose cyme of 2–5 greenish-white flowers. The fruits are round, forming small burs of 4–6 mm covered with hooked bristles, clinging especially tightly to clothes and animals.

Habitat: throughout Britain and Europe as a very common hedgerow plant, and through the eastern half of the USA, all Canada and the Pacific Coast.

Parts used: the herb gathered just before flowering.

Cultivation: not necessary or feasible.

Harvesting: in spring and early summer before the plant gets too fibrous.

Preparation: infusion of the plant chopped before drying; a very effective juice may be obtained from the fresh plant with a juicing machine and preserved in glycerol up to 40 per cent; a tincture may be prepared at 1:5 in 25 per cent alcohol.

Dosage: 2–8 g dried herb three times per day.

Constituents: coumarin glycosides (incl. asperuloside); red dye containing an anthraquinone (galiosin); citric and other acids; tannins.

Pharmacology: galiosin is similar to the dye ingredient in cleavers' close relative, madder: this is known to have specific anti-inflammatory and spasmolytic effects on the urinary tract and may contribute to madder's litholytic (stone-breaking) action in the urinary system (it also stains the urine red); it has laxative effects.

Action: diuretic; lymphatic alterative.

Applications: cleavers is held in high repute in Europe as a blood cleanser with efficacy against such conditions as eczema and psoriasis and other chronic inflammatory conditions.

Its clinical reputation is that it has a dual effect on the urinary system and the lymphatic system, so that the plant is used in cases of lymphadenopathy (enlarged lymph nodes), oedema and urinary affections.

The name 'lymphatic' was given to those remedies used for inflammation of the lymphatic nodes: they were thought in naturopathic terms to improve the rate of flow through the lymphatic system and help tissue cleansing that way. There is some real doubt about the physiological reality behind such a concept but there is a clear effect on those forms of chronic inflammatory conditions marked by swollen lymph nodes.

The 'drying' effect claimed for cleavers in Galenic tradition reflected its apparent ability to reduce fluid congestive conditions. An image emerges of cleavers being primarily indicated for any toxic problem marked by lymphatic or oedematous symptoms. It is likely that the kidneys handle most extra wastes passed under the influence of cleavers, though a laxative effect is also likely.

There are other traditional uses: it was applied to jaundice, and was considered a good local wound-healing remedy.

SILVER BIRCH

Betula alba L.
Family: Betulaceae
Synonyms: *B. pendula* Roth., *B. verrucosa* Ehrh., white birch, paper birch.

Description: a well-known member of the catkin family of trees, recognized particularly for its silvery-white bark, peeling off in layers, along with its slender drooping branches. The leaves are broadly ovate, tapering to a fine point, toothed, but with a wide range of shapes around this pattern; they are smooth and shiny, but with minute glandular dots when young. The male catkins are drooping, 2–5 cm long, the female on short stalks but up to 15 cm long. The North American *Betula lenta* is medicinally close to *B. alba*.

Habitat: in woodlands throughout the whole northern hemisphere.

Parts used: the young leaves, the bark, the sap and the leaf buds.

Cultivation: the tree may be grown in larger gardens, but because of its shallow roots it should be at least 6 m away from any building; it is also susceptible to severe droughts for the same reason.

Harvesting: the buds in March, the leaves in April–May, the bark and the sap also in spring. The sap is obtained by boring holes into the trunk and tapping the flow through a pipe into a vessel for up to 2 days, preserving the fluid with alcohol.

Preparation: the leaves, buds and bark are dried in the usual way, though they take to being dried outside and this may be more efficient than using artificial heat. The leaves may be infused (adding a pinch of sodium bicarbonate aids extraction considerably), but the buds and bark will need varying degrees of decoction.

Dosage 1–4 g dried leaves, bark or buds three times a day; 10–20 ml sap preserved with 20 per cent alcohol three times per day.

Constituents: volatile oil and resin (together constituting 'empyreumatic oil of birch' – incl. betulin); saponins; flavonoids (mainly hyperoside); tannins; bitter glycoside.

Pharmacology: the mixture of volatile oils and resins has been found to be related in many ways to the oil of wintergreen (*Gaultheria procumbens*) used as an anti-inflammatory, both typically and systematically for arthritic and neuralgic conditions (however, although most commercial wintergreen oil is now, in fact, almost entirely obtained from distillation of the bark of the North American birch (*B. lenta*), this product does not actually exist in the original plant but is formed by interaction between constituents in the distilling process: thus there is no evidence of the presence of salicylates, so prominent in the oil, in the fresh sample). The effect of the oil is augmented by the saponins and flavonoids in a pronounced diuretic and urinary antiseptic action, and with bitter and other digestive stimulation.

References:

Ellianowska, A. and Kaczmarek, F. (1966) *Herba Polonica*, Poznan, Poland, 11, p. 47

Leclerc, H. (1938) *Revue de Phytothérapie*, Neuilly-sur-Seine, France, 2, p. 65

Ravanel, P. and Tissut, M. (1980) *Phytochemistry*, 19, p. 2077

Action: anti-inflammatory; diuretic; cholagogue; diaphoretic.

Applications: the many usable parts of the birch have a similar action: much of their influence is concentrated on the kidneys and urinary system, and they are applicable to kidney stones in particular and other disorders of the urinary tract. However, there are other actions: for example there is a stimulation of bile flow and birch is also slightly sedative and notably anti-inflammatory. Overall, therefore, it is found useful in the treatment of many complex inflammatory conditions such as rheumatic, arthritic and dermatological problems.

It may be used in arthritic conditions both internally and topically (when distilled to produce the liniment-like oil of wintergreen preparation). One sign of an internal effect is the diaphoretic property of birch, which is such that sweating is induced when it is taken in large doses: this points to a particular application in those cases of acute rheumatic symptoms associated with fever or serum sickness. Along with the better flushing through of the tissues that this suggests, there is an action in reducing oedematous states, and one of its specific indications is for oedema of renal and cardiac origins.

STINGING NETTLE

1: *Urtica dioica* L.
2: *U. urens* L.
Family: Urticaceae
Synonyms: 1: common nettle; 2: small nettle.

Description: two very similar-looking plants: 1: a perennial coarse plant with creeping invasive rootstock up to 1 m high, the toothed leaves covered with fine down, with stalked green hermaphrodite flowers; 2: a delicate annual rarely more than 30 cm high with smooth shiny leaves, no invasive rootstock, and sessile male and female flowers. Both plants have painful stinging hairs when living; when dried these are still visible on the wrinkled and rolled dark-green leaf fragments and may still cause slight irritation when handled.

Habitat: classic weeds of cultivation, occurring wherever humans have tilled the land and briefly turned their backs on it; both are extremely common in Europe; in the USA they are found in the states northwards from Colorado, Missouri and South Carolina.

Parts used: the young leaves with or without flowers.

Cultivation: undesirable.

Harvesting: spring or early summer; use gloves or grasp the nettle firmly from below to avoid stinging.

Preparation: infusion; the leaves may also be juiced or simply eaten in quantity as a cooked vegetable or soup; a tincture may be prepared at 1:5 in 25 per cent alcohol.

Dosage: 2–4 g dried leaves three times per day.

Constituents: acrid components in stinging hairs (incl. formic acid, histamine, volatile and resinous acids); glucoquinone; tannins; large quantities of minerals (especially iron and silica) and vitamins.

Pharmacology: the high nutrient value of this plant is notable and leads to its application to anaemic and other deficiency conditions. Research has indicated that nettles increase the excretion of uric acid from the body (a property likely to affect other acidic constituents as well). The tannins account for the astringent effect, and the glucoquinone helps to account for the perceived hypoglycaemic action. Extract of nettle has been found to slow the heart in experimental animals and dilate and constrict the blood vessels alternately under different conditions.

References:
Aliev, R. K. and Damirov, I. A. (1961) *Chemisches Zentralblatt*, Berlin, p. 4437.
Benigni, R., Capra, C. and Cattorini, P. E. (1964) *Piante medicinali: chimica farmacologia e terapia*, Inverni & Della Beffa, Milan, pp. 1056–63
Kirchhoff, H. W. (1983) 'Brennesselschaft als Diuretikum', in *Zeitschrift für Phytotherapie*, Stuttgart, 4, pp. 621–6
Lutomski, J. and Speichert, H. (1983) 'Die Brennesel in Heilkunde und Ernährung', in *Pharmazie in Unserer Zeit*, Weinhein, Germany, 6, pp. 181–6
Weiss, R. F. (1980) *Lehrbuch der Phytotherapie*, Hippokrates-Verlag, Stuttgart, p. 296

Action: nutritive; haemostatic and astringent; circulatory stimulant; diuretic; galactogogue; hypoglycaemic; eliminates uric acid.

Applications: like other invasive and piratical plants nettle is very efficient at extracting minerals from the soil and it contains high quantities of useful nutrients, including iron and vitamin C. Apart from thus being a good nourishing vegetable for convalescence and recuperation this quality adds to the others discussed below to give the plant a central restorative core.

Nettles have a reputation for the treatment of arthritic conditions. Like many other anti-arthritic remedies, it is a diuretic and in addition helps to remove uric acid and probably other acid metabolites from the body via the kidneys. There is certainly an application to gout, but these properties could also go a long way towards explaining the general alterative reputation of nettles, accounting for their effect in treating many joint and skin conditions.

The circulatory effects, supported by the findings noted in the pharmacology section above, are reflected in the traditional description of nettles as 'hot and dry in the second degree', and the more modern view that they help to improve circulation to the tissues. This obviously provides extra benefit in any detoxifying programme and adds to the indications for nettles' use.

Two hormonal effects are noted: nettles have an established ability to stimulate milk production in a nursing mother (and it makes an excellent fodder plant, when dried, for increasing production in milking farm animals and chickens); they are also one of several plants or foods that show an experimental lowering of blood-sugar levels in hyperglycaemics – a property which adds it to the list of desirable foods for late-onset diabetics.

Locally the action of nettles is appreciably astringent: they have been used for checking bleeding from external wounds, and from areas such as the nose and womb; they are also applied to haemorrhoids and even internally as a systemic agent for haemoptysis (coughing blood – the silica content might be useful here). The local action probably accounts for its use in the treatment of stomach and digestive problems as well, but the systemic action returns in the traditional use of the remedy for excessive menstruation (though again a hormonal action may be implicated).

There is one undoubted, if drastic, local action as a counter-irritant. The stings of the fresh plant produce weals and blisters (the term urticaria is directly translated as 'nettle rash'): in earlier times arthritic and other inflamed tissues were flayed with fresh nettles. The justification for such an approach to inflammation was discussed in the section. 'The Temperaments of Plant Remedies', on pp. 174–82.

Similar remedy: figwort (*Scrophularia nodosa*).

SWEET VIOLET

Viola odorata L.
Family: Violaceae
Synonyms: English violet, garden violet, blue violet.

Description: a perennial herb with a thick, short rhizome knotted and branched with the remains of old leafstalks and stipules, producing a rosette of stalked, broadly cordate leaves with crenate margins, covered in a light down. The long-stemmed violet-coloured or white flowers are 5-petalled and nodding, with a short spur on the lower petal, and obtuse-shaped. The whole plant is very small and delicately scented. Commercial samples contain curled or rolled light-green leaf fragments, occasional flowers with curled petals and pieces of pod containing yellow seeds.

Habitat: on banks and hedges, field borders and woods, patchily distributed around Britain, Europe, Asia and in the region of cultivated gardens elsewhere in the world. It is very unobtrusive and easy to miss among other plants.

Parts used: the whole herb when in flower.

Cultivation: propagated by cuttings from runners put out by the plants, struck in a damp rich compost until rooted; they are planted out in a semi-shaded position if possible; they prefer lime-rich soil.

Harvesting: flowering is from February to April.

Preparation: infusion; a tincture may be made at 1:5 in 25 per cent alcohol.

Dosage: 1–6 g herb three times per day.

Constituents: saponins; methyl salicylate; alkaloid (odoratine or violine); essential oil; flavonoids (incl. rutin).

499   Alteratives

Pharmacology: the salicylate provides the plant with a clear basis for its anti-inflammatory action, and this is possibly augmented by the saponin component; the latter also accounts for its expectorant properties and with the flavonoids for its diuretic actions. The alkaloid has been implicated as having hypotensive properties, a feature which may support the view that the plant is vasodilatory.

Action: anti-inflammatory; stimulating expectorant; diuretic; anti-neoplastic.

Applications: this remedy is primarily a stimulating expectorant, used for bronchial and congestive pulmonary complaints, helping to make coughing more productive.

The anti-inflammatory action is seen in its application for treating certain migraines, rheumatic and skin problems, and as a mouthwash for inflammations of the mouth and throat.

However, it is as a standard adjunct remedy for the treatment of cancer that sweet violet has become most well known, especially in treating tumours of the lung, breast, throat and intestine. This reputation goes back to the early years of this century and has remained today, though without independent assessment of the claims.

Similar remedy: red clover flowers (*Trifolium pratense*).

MYRRH

Commiphora mol-mol Engl. spp.
Family: Burseraceae

Description: the oleo-gum-resin obtained from the stem of shrubs, or small trees; obtained as either rounded or irregular tears, 1.5–2.5 cm in diameter or in agglutinated masses of such tears; reddish-brown to yellow, dry and often dusty; it has a brittle fracture exhibiting a granular translucent surface, rich brown in colour and often with whitish spots or veins. The odour is aromatic.

Habitat: north-eastern Africa and southern Arabia.

Parts used: the resinous sap.

Preparation: the resin is not soluble in water so must be prepared in alcohol, and used as a tincture, 1:5 in 90 per cent alcohol.

Dosage: 0.1–1 g resin three times per day.

Constituents: 25–40 per cent resin (containing triterpenes, alcohols and esters); around 60 per cent gum; up to 14 per cent volatile oil (containing primarily sesquiterpenes and some monoterpenes); steroidal constituents have been isolated from another species of *Commiphora*.

Pharmacology: *in vitro* antimicrobial activity has been reported for the resin, and there are suggestions that it stimulates phagocytosis *in vivo* as well; it also appears to reduce cholesterol and fat levels in the bloodstream.

References:
British Pharmaceutical Codex (1973)
Delaveau, P. *et al.* (1980) *Planta Medica*, Stuttgart, 40, p. 49
Govindachari, T. R. (1977) 'Steroidal constituents of *Commiphora
    mukul*', in *New Natural Products and Plant Drugs with
    Pharmacological, Biological or Therapeutical Activity*, Wagner, H.
    and Wolff, P. (eds.), Springer-Verlag, Berlin, p. 222
Leung, A. Y. (1980) *Encyclopedia of Common Natural Ingredients Used
    in Food, Drugs, and Cosmetics*, John Wiley, New York, pp. 214–42
Martindale The Extra Pharmacopoeia (1989), 29th edition
Pernet, R. (1972) 'Phytochimie des Burseracées', in *Lloydia*, Cincinnati,
    35, pp. 280–87
Rombi, M. (1987) *Phytotherapy: A Practical Handbook of Herbal Medicine
    for the Practitioner*, Herbal Health Publishers, Hindhead, UK, p. 52
Srivastava, M. *et al.* (1984) *J. Bio. Sci.*, 6 (3), p. 277
Steinegger, E. and Hänsel, R. (1988) *Lehrbuch der Pharmakognosie und
    Phytopharmazie*, Springer-Verlag, Berlin, p. 348

Temperament: warm.

Taste: acrid, bitter.

Action: astringent and antiseptic topically and on mucosal membranes; carminative; hypocholesterolaemic.

Applications: tincture of myrrh is a powerful ingredient in many herbal mixtures for the treatment of infections and inflammations in the mouth and throat. It is dramatically effective in reducing gum inflammations and sore throats and tonsillar infections. As well as a direct antiseptic action the resin seems to provoke increased activity by phagocytes in the locality. This may account for

501 Alteratives

its long-term benefit in many cases: it is as though it works to enhance the body's own defences as well as attacking troublemakers, and so promotes beneficial activity after treatment has finished.

The resin in the tincture sediments as soon as it is mixed with water solution, so it is best taken in a suspending agent. Fluid extract of liquorice is recommended for this purpose, and it is also recommended to reduce the acrid astringency of the myrrh.

Neat tincture of myrrh, perhaps mixed with that of calendula (also an anti-inflammatory resin), is an excellent topical lotion for application to fungal infections of the nails and skin. Over exposed surfaces and mucous membranes, it is usually too irritating for comfort.

There is a tradition, especially in France, for using myrrh to reduce blood-cholesterol levels. This would presumably involve other principles than that of mucosal provocation.

RIBWORT

Plantago lanceolata L.
Family: Plantaginaceae
Synonyms: English plantain, jackstraw, ribgrass, snake plantain.

Description: a short, thick, often branched rootstock gives rise to a rosette of erect spreading lanceolate leaves, 5–25 cm long, each with 3–5 prominent longitudinal ribs, the basal-leaf stems covered with woolly hairs. The flowerstalks are longer than the leaves, erect, furrowed and leafless: they support an elongated or almost spherical flowerspike up to 2.5 cm long, greenish at first but turning brown-black on ripening; the flowers are very small and indistinct with ovate bracts and sepals and very prominent pale-yellow or purple anthers. The seeds are about 1 mm long, blackish-brown and oval. There is no odour, and a mucilaginous taste. It is to be distinguished in particular from its near-relative, *Plantago major*, the rat's-tail, or common broad-leaved plantain, marked by ovate instead of strap-like leaves.

Habitat: very common in pastures, roadsides, banks, waste places, preferring dry sandy soil, throughout Britain, Europe and temperate zones in Asia; it is also introduced to North America and Australasia.

Parts used: the leaves.

Cultivation: rarely necessary, but best done from seed in a dry, sunny spot on lightish soils.

Harvesting: during early to mid-summer: it flowers from spring to autumn.

Preparation: drying should be done quickly at temperatures of 40–50°C (or 104–122°F), otherwise the remedy will discolour and lose its effectiveness; in making an infusion the fact that the plant is mucilaginous will be obvious. The tincture is made at 1:5 in 25 per cent alcohol.

Dosage: 2–4 g three times per day.

Constituents: mucilage; glycosides (incl. aucubin); tannins; minerals such as silica, zinc and potassium.

Pharmacology: the aucubin appears to be anticatarrhal and antibiotic, and increases the excretion of uric acid by the kidneys; silica promotes lung tissue repair, zinc aids healing and defences, the mucilages provide a relaxing expectorant action and they and the tannins provide a good local soothing and healing effect on the gut lining and skin.

Temperament: neutral.

Taste: bland.

Action: restorative to respiratory mucous membranes; astringent and demulcent; soothing diuretic.

Applications: this plant is one of a number (see below) that are used in dealing with a range of catarrhal conditions and have sometimes been called 'anticatarrhal'. This, however, seems to be rather a misnomer: rather than suppressing catarrh production the action of this and of the other plants seems to be more restorative and gradualist in effect. In Europe, for example, ribwort is applied as much to hay fever and other allergies, where the mucous membranes are dry and hypersensitive, as to respiratory catarrh. Furthermore its action seems to be long-term, leading to an improvement in respiratory health after treatment.

It may thus be recommended for all forms of respiratory congestion, such as nasal catarrh, bronchitis, sinusitis and middle-ear infections. It is particularly useful in treating such conditions in children.

As a mucilaginous remedy it also acts as a relaxing expectorant and will soothe irritating coughs and tightness in the airways. It was used, as Parkinson noted, to 'stay the spitting of blood', a symptom usually referring to tuberculosis, but also an extreme sign of mucosal irritation.

The mucilaginous effect, combined with the tannins and other constituents, gives ribwort appreciable healing effect and it has been both used as a wound herb and taken internally for 'staying all manner of fluxes in man and woman . . . bleedings at the mouth . . . by having a veine broken in the stomacke' (Parkinson). This action is also transferred to the urinary system so that ribwort can be used for painful urination from a range of causes, from stones to infection (or, in the words of Parkinson, for 'bloody or foul water by any ulcer in the kidney or bladder').

Similar remedies: ground ivy (*Nepeta hederacea*); eyebright (*Euphrasia officinalis*); golden rod (*Solidago virgaurea*); wood betony (*Stachys betonica*).

Tonics and Hormonal Remedies

This is a diverse group of remedies having in common a restorative and adaptogenic effect on body functions and structures. Their broad remit of action is summed up in the chapter 'Physiology', namely in the sections 'Integration', on pp. 126–9, and 'Reproduction', on pp. 130–31, and the latter part of the chapter 'Therapeutics'.

The word 'tonic' is not a precise one. In the European tradition the word tends to mean an influence close to that of food or a food supplement, i.e. that it simply nurtures the part of the body concerned. In the sense used in Chinese medicine and briefly illustrated in the following pages, it is a more dynamic quality, with thus a series of contra-indications for various types of debility.

LIQUORICE

Glycyrrhiza glabra L.
Family: Leguminosae
Synonym: *Liquiritia officinalis.*

Description: a tall erect perennial with light, gracefully spreading foliage presenting an almost feathery appearance from a distance. The leaflets hang down at night, are dark green and lanceolate. From the leaf axils grow long-stemmed spikes of numerous bluish-purple-to-white butterfly-shaped flowers, followed by small leguminous seedpods, smooth-skinned in this species rather than the more normal hairy (hence *glabra* = smooth) kind. The roots are a mixture of taproots, long branch roots and stolons. In commerce these are cylindrical pieces, up to 1 cm thick and 15 cm long, externally brown. The cork is coarsely fibrous and longitudinally striated, the inner surface white or yellow and fibrous. The odour and taste are characteristic.

Habitat: a native of south-east Europe and of south-west Asia including Iran, growing in open fields and moorland, generally near running water.

Parts used: the roots and stolons (runners).

Cultivation: plant out runners in early spring in light or sandy but well-manured soil in an open sunny situation in districts free from heavy frosts (cold weather reduces the production of good sap).

Harvesting: in the autumn of the fourth season after planting, the plant is surrounded by a trench up to 1 m deep and the whole enclosed area dug up and exhaustively sifted for roots, etc.

Preparation: the chopped root may be prepared by decoction; it is often advantageous to use a more concentrated form, available from wholesalers as either a hard stick of dried solid extract, the same as a desiccated (and hygroscopic) powder, or as a thick black fluid (liquid) extract.

Dosage: 1–4 g three times per day.

Constituents: glycyrrhizin (the calcium and potassium salts of glycyrrhizic acid); triterpenoid saponins; flavonoids (incl. liquiritegol); bitter principle (glycymarin); oestrogenic substances (probably incl. α-sitosterol); asparagin; volatile oil; coumarins; tannins (trace).

Pharmacology: central to the activity of this remedy is the presence of glycyrrhizin, which on hydrolysis in the gut yields glycyrrhetinic acid and two molecules of glucuronic acid. The glycyrrhetinic acid has a triterpenoid structure and this may account for its close interaction with the hormones of the adrenal cortex. Thus it has been shown to have anti-inflammatory and anti-arthritic effects similar to hydrocortisone, to resemble the activity of ACTH in causing aldosterone-like retention of water and sodium at the kidney, and consequently hypokalaemia (lowered potassium levels), raised blood pressure and decreased haemoglobin levels. It enhances the immunosuppressive action of cortisone, but on the other hand inhibits its antigranulomatous action and its effects in increasing liver glycogen storage. The action of glycyrrhetinic acid is dependent on there being a functioning adrenal cortex and there appears to be a direct ACTH-like effect increasing adrenal production of all steroids produced there; but there is in addition an effect reducing breakdown of steroids in the liver and kidney. The results can be dramatic: there is recorded the case of a physician maintaining a woman with Addison's disease on liquorice extract only, and moreover reducing the initially high dose to a low maintenance regime – suggesting a degree of recuperation on the part of the adrenal cortex under the influence of liquorice.

Other actions noted are the ability of the remedy as a whole to produce a highly viscous adherent mucus over the stomach wall, to reduce gastric secretion, to have an antipyretic effect (due to glycyrrhetinic acid) comparable to that of sodium salicylate, an increase in the secretion of bilirubin in the bile (possibly due to increased haemoglobin turnover) and a reduction in the spasm of visceral smooth muscle. Glycyrrhizin is weight for weight 50 times sweeter than sucrose (without stressing pancreatic responses) and this accounts for the widespread use of the plant as a disguise for unpleasant-tasting prescriptions. Asparagin is a potent diuretic, and this has led to speculation that its presence may reduce the chance of the whole plant increasing blood pressure compared with isolated glycyrrhetinic acid.

References:
*Gibson, M. R. (1978) 'Glycyrrhiza in old and new perspectives', in *Lloydia*, Cincinnati, 41, 4, pp. 348–54
Anon. (1980) *Gastric and Duodenal Ulcers, Reflux Oesophagitis and Aphthous Ulcers: Biogastrone, Duogastrone, Pyrogastrone, Bioral Gel*, Winthrop Laboratories, Surbiton, Surrey, UK
British Pharmacopoeia (1988)
Chandler, R. F. (1985) 'Liquorice, more than just a flavour', in *Canad. Pharm. J.*, pp. 421–4
Epstein, M. T. *et al.* (1978) 'Liquorice raises urinary cortisol in man', in *J. Clin. Endocrinol. Metab.*, 47, pp. 397–400
   (1977) 'Effect of eating liquorice on the renin-angiotensin aldosterone axis in normal subjects', in *BMJ*, 1, pp. 488–90
Evans, W. C. and Trease, G. E. (1989) *Pharmacognosy*, 13th edition, pp. 495–8
Glick, L. (1982) 'Deglycyrrhizinated liquorice for peptic ulcer', in *Lancet*, ii, p. 817
Hänsel, R. and Steinegger, E. (1988) *Lehrbuch der Pharmakognosie und Phytopharmazie*, Springer-Verlag, Berlin, pp. 188–91
Hatano, T. *et al.* (1988) 'Anti-human immunodeficiency virus phenolics from liquorice', in *Chem. Pharm. Bull.*, 36, pp. 2286–8 (coumarin derivative licopyranocoumarin)
Hattori, M. *et al.* (1983) 'Metabolism of glycyrrhizin by human intestinal flora', in *Planta Medica*, Stuttgart, 48, pp. 38–42
Hikino, H. (1985) 'Recent research on Oriental medicinal plants', in *Economic and Medicinal Plant Research*, H. Wagner, H. Hikino and N. R. Farnsworth (eds.), Academic Press, 1, pp. 55–61
Kiso, Y. *et al.* (1984) 'Mechanism of antihepatotoxic activity of

glycyrrhizin. I: Effect of free radical generation and lipid
    peroxidation', in *Planta Medica*, Stuttgart, 50, pp. 298–302
Leung, A. Y. (1980) *Encyclopedia of Common Natural Ingredients Used
    in Food, Drugs, and Cosmetics*, John Wiley, New York, pp. 200–23
Martindale The Extra Pharmacopoeia (1989), 29th edition

Temperament: neutral.

Taste: sweet.

Action: soothing and healing on the gastric and duodenal mucosa;
balanced expectorant; anti-inflammatory (applied especially to
chronic inflammation of the joints, liver and vasculature); diuretic;
supporting stress response.

Applications: liquorice is one of the most widely used plants among
traditional practitioners throughout the world, and it comes with a
long list of indications. Many of these have received backing from
modern investigation.

The remedy has received much attention as a treatment for
peptic ulcers and a fragmented form of the plant is used in conventional medicine in the UK for this effect (Biogastrone). It appears
to work initially by producing a thick protective adherent mucus
over the gut wall, by tempering acid production, and finally almost
certainly by exerting a local anti-inflammatory and healing effect.
This action is applicable to other gut problems, and its effects on
the tract can be summarized as soothing and healing. Liquorice is
also a significant but very gentle laxative, and is often applied
primarily for this effect.

On the respiratory system liquorice acts like a mucilaginous
remedy: it is thus a relaxing expectorant, helping to soothe tickling,
irritable and harsh coughs, and bronchospastic conditions (such as
asthmatic breathlessness). There is more to this, however: the saponins are likely to exert something of a stimulating expectorant
effect to counterbalance the relaxing action; the steroid-enhancing
action of the remedy is likely to underpin its strong reputation as a
remedy for asthma and allergic conditions of the respiratory tract,
and as a potent healing agent after tuberculosis (where its effects
have been compared to hydrocortisone). A central action on respiratory mucosa can be postulated in its widespread use in limiting
catarrhal conditions.

Most modern interest in the plant derives from its demonstrated actions in support of the adrenal cortex, as outlined in the pharmacology notes above. Clinical experience strongly suggests that it may help those coming off steroid drugs. If steroids have been taken for a long time, a degree of adrenal suppression is certain and this proves to be a major inhibition to withdrawal (the body cannot produce comparable levels itself). Liquorice not only stands in for cortisone at its peripheral sites of operation and reduces the breakdown of existing hormone, but it seems to encourage a degree of endogenous production by the adrenal cortex itself. This ACTH-like activity represents a therapeutic goal long sought after in conventional medicine. It does however lead to the major criticism of liquorice: that it encourages also the activity of aldosterone, with a resulting increase in water retention, sodium retention and potassium loss. However, these findings were initially made with isolated glycyrrhetinic acid and with liquorice candy. Without minimizing the risks involved, and whilst still warning about the use of the plant in hypertension and cardiovascular disease, it may be pointed out that in the whole plant there is appreciable diuretic action that is likely to offset the aldosteronal effect, apart from the fact that, as in all plants, there are appreciable levels of replacement potassium in liquorice as a whole.

The anti-inflammatory effect that is observed in liquorice probably accounts for its traditional place in the treatment of chronic inflammations, such as arthritic and rheumatic diseases, chronic skin diseases and autoimmune diseases in general. It may also be used with profit as an eyebath in conjunctivitis and other inflammatory conditions of the eye surface.

Underlying the benefits of liquorice in treating inflammatory conditions is a general improvement in the ability to withstand stresses of other sorts. It is a classic saponin-containing remedy, in the same group as ginseng and the 'Harmony' remedies. Like these it can genuinely be said to restore equilibrium in the functions it affects. It is however more cooling than ginseng, more likely to moisten and nourish, for example. The European tradition clearly emphasizes its gentle disposition ('the nearest unto our temper', according to Culpeper) and its facility for soothing and moistening. This would make it a valuable component of any regime geared to recuperation after a particularly exhausting phase or disease. Its balancing virtues have been compared unfavourably with those of Chinese liquorice, Gan Cao (*Glycyrryhiza uralensis*), but this is not borne out by its traditional European reputation nor by personal experience of its benefits.

A key point is in its effect on fluids. On the one hand it is a notable moistening remedy, soothing dryness in the respiratory tract, relieving irritations in the urinary tract, and actually being used to relieve thirst in earlier times. However, its Chinese relative is contra-indicated in conditions of 'damp', and today we are concerned about its aldosteronal action. Nevertheless, it is also indicated for catarrhal conditions and its Chinese counterpart is indicated for clearing *Phlegm* conditions. The key may be in the latter point: *Phlegm* arises from deficiency in *Spleen*, allowing conditions of 'damp-heat' to develop, and resulting in the production of a thick phlegm as part of what in the Western tradition would be seen as a wider toxic condition. The central point may, after all, be the tonification of *Spleen* as understood in Chinese physiology.

The final point follows: liquorice is universally seen as the prime balancing remedy in a herbal prescription. It was seen in China as a harmonizing influence among many other remedies; in Western practice it might find favour for no more than making a prescription palatable, and it is perhaps the only herb that will allow the herbal treatment of children.

OATS

Avena sativa L.
Family: Graminaceae
Synonym: groats.

Description: a major plant food derived from the wild oat (*A. fatua*); the flowers are arranged in loose panicles of spikelets, each bearing 3–5 flowers with lanceolate glumes, the outer tapering to a fine point, the inner one smaller and cleft in two.

Habitat: in fields and farmland the world over; particularly happy in temperate to cool climates.

Parts used: the whole flowering plant (oatstraw) and seed in the form of oatmeal.

Cultivation: the seed from wild oats can be collected after weeding cultivated fields, to be sown in early spring by dense broadcasting.

Harvesting: the straw is collected in midsummer, the seed somewhat later (agricultural sprays are a major hazard).

Preparation: the straw will need relatively little drying and is quite robust; a decoction may be made or a tincture at 1:5 in 25 per cent alcohol (both preparations, if allowed to sediment and the liquid decanted off the top, should be free of gluten). The oatmeal may be prepared and consumed in the usual culinary way.

Dosage: 1–4 g three times a day of oatmeal or straw.

Constituents: saponins (incl. avenacosides A and B); alkaloids (incl. indole alkaloid, gramine, trigonelline and avenine); sterol (avenasterol); flavonoids; silica; starch and protein (incl. gluten); minerals (esp. calcium), and other nutrients.

Pharmacology: the presence of saponins and alkaloids probably accounts for some of the clinical benefits observed, but little pharmacological work is to hand; the presence of silica will aid its local healing effects.

References:

Becker, H. and Förster, W. (1984) 'Biologie, Chemie und Pharmakologie pflanzlicher Sedativa', in *Zeitschrift für Phytotherapie*, Stuttgart, 5, pp. 817–23

Temperament: neutral.

Taste: sweet.

Action: a sure and effective restorative to the nervous system.

Applications: this plant represents the classic bridge between foods and medicine, and is a notable representative of the simple restorative tonic in the Chinese 'sweet' sense. Oats can be considered as a superb nourishing food for any state of debility and exhaustion and during convalescence, or as a simply sustaining ingredient through the day.

It has a particular application to the nervous system, seeming to provide raw materials of specific benefit to that tissue and also seeming to 'direct' them there in an active sense. It is extremely useful as long-term measure in any nervous debility, making for real sustained, though slow, progress in fighting off such 'neurasthenias' as shingles and other forms of herpes (including the genital kind), neuralgias, neuritis, and even chronic depression. As a relaxing influence it will also steady the system in chronic anxiety states as well. It is generally the remedy of choice in any restoration or convalescent programme where the nervous system is involved.

Gluten may be a problem in some otherwise appropriate indications (one example is that many cases of multiple sclerosis have been linked with a gluten sensitivity). This should present no problem to the use of a tincture or decanted decoction.

Oats has been used as a local healing remedy, as a poultice for burns, wounds and neuralgias.

Similar remedy: vervain (*Verbena officinalis*).

ST JOHN'S WORT

Hypericum perforatum L.
Family: Hypericaceae

Description: an erect perennial about 30–60 cm high with cylindrical or oval smooth stems, branching in their upper parts, bearing opposite sessile oblong leaves with entire margins: on inspection against a light source they are seen to be marked with tiny translucent pinpricks (hence *'perforatum'*), and also with a few black spots on the underside; the veins are opaque. The bright-yellow 5-petalled flowers are borne in a terminal corymb, the long lanceolate petals and shorter sepals both marked with black dots; the numerous stamens are bunched into three bundles, and there are three styles.

Habitat: throughout Britain and the whole of Europe well into Asia, and introduced into many other parts of the world, for example North America; on roadsides, banks, woods and hedgerows, preferring open situations and relatively dry and ideally calcareous soils.

Parts used: the flowers and herb; for the 'oil', fresh flowers.

Cultivation: easily grown by sowing the capsulated seeds in any open situation in the garden; alternatively root cuttings may be taken. It will seed itself and spread once established.

Harvesting: the herbs and flowers are picked in summer and early autumn.

Preparation: drying can be achieved at medium temperatures without too much risk of damage to the active principles. One of the characteristic features of the flowers is that when handling them the fingers are marked by red pigment; this has been shown to be medicinally useful, and may be extracted in the following way: the fresh flowers are pressed in a little sunflower oil, and then a total of 500 ml of sunflower oil is poured over 100 g flowers. These are placed in a glass container and fermented in the warmth for a few days, then put out in direct sunlight for two weeks until a bright-red liquid has formed in the bottom. The herb is pressed through muslin, and any watery layer decanted off. The oil is then used externally for pains and slight burns as outlined below.

Dosage: 1–4 g three times per day.

Constituents: flavonoid glycosides (incl. in the red pigment: hypericin); dianthron; volatile oil (with sesquiterpenes); tannins; resin; carotene; pectin.

Pharmacology: an explanation for the use of this remedy on the nervous system is not so far forthcoming; there is, however, an effect in stimulating the rate of formation of granulation tissue (the intermediate tissue produced at the first stages of wound healing). German and Russian work has demonstrated antibacterial properties, and it has *in vitro* antispasmodic activity.

Action: anti-inflammatory and tissue healer; relaxing restorative.

Applications: St John's wort has been used throughout Europe for a number of symptoms of nervous tension: insomnia, cramps, intestinal colic and irritable bowel, dysmenorrhoea (menstrual cramps), bed-wetting and anxiety. As noted above the plant has been shown to have direct antispasmodic action. It also has a reputation for relieving pain, and is taken internally, as well as applied topically, for neuralgic pain and for the pain of mild burns and contusions.

The plant also has a traditional use as a restorative treatment for melancholic conditions, depression and the convalescence following concussion and other trauma. This combination of restorative and relaxant effect is not contradictory, and underlies the plant's recommendation for the treatment of a number of such conditions where tension and exhaustion combine.

One particular example is menopause, and St John's wort has a specific application for the various symptoms of that change. Most of the symptoms of menopausal syndrome, the hot flushes, night sweats, depression, fatigue, irritability, lack of concentration, fluid retention and so on, were recognized as symptoms of debility long before a hormonal factor was implicated. The modern practitioner still finds advantage in treating menopausal problems primarily as symptoms of depletion, requiring restorative and convalescent measures. St John's wort seems to have an ideal balance of qualities for this task: it is even felt by many of those who use it that it has a hormonal influence as well.

The red oil of St John's wort brings appreciable relief in the topical treatment of wounds and burns. The whole plant extract has also been used as a wound healer, and has been taken internally for inflammation of the upper digestive system, including oesophagitis, gastritis and peptic ulceration.

KELP

Fucus vesiculosus L.
Family: Fucaceae
Synonyms: bladderwrack, kelp-ware, black-tang, rockweed.

Description: this is a seaweed, actually an alga, in the form of long ribbons or thalli, about 1 m long and up to 5 cm across. When fresh, it is a leathery shiny olive-green to yellow-brown, with an entire margin. Down the centre of each thallus is a midrib on either side of which are air-containing bladders which keep the alga floating up from its anchorages on stones in the tidal region (and incidentally ensure that it is one of the most common species washed up on beaches and coasts after storms). There are other species called 'kelp', including *Macrosytic purifera* and *Alaria esculenta*; although seaweeds are generally rich in nutrients and probably represent an underdeveloped medicinal strategy, all that is said here applies only to *Fucus vesiculosus*.

Habitat: the coasts of the Atlantic Ocean and the Baltic, Irish and North Seas.

Parts used: the whole thallus.

Harvesting: from unpolluted coastlines at low tide, especially after gales which tear it from its moorings and wash it up to the tideline; at any time of the year.

Preparation: the kelp is dried in the open after washing off excess sand and mud; it forms brittle brownish-black strips which can then be chopped and preferably ground up for storage. The taste is rather salty but it makes an acceptable infusion; however, the best way of taking it is to eat it whole as a tablet or capsule. A tincture (actually fluid extract) may be prepared at 1:1 in 25 per cent alcohol.

Dosage: 5–10 g dried thallus three times per day.

Constituents: mucilage; iodine and many other minerals in large amounts; pigments: fucosterin, fucoxanthin, zeaxanthin.

Toxicology: kelp is extremely non-toxic under normal circumstances; however, as a collector of minerals it is likely to accumulate levels of toxic metals in polluted waters – there is a particular concern about arsenic and many commercial stocks are now automatically screened for traces of this metal.

References:
Benigni, R., Capra, C. and Cattorini, P. E. (1964) *Piante medicinali: chimica farmacologia e terapia*, Inverni & Della Beffa, Milan, pp. 1179–83
Bezanger-Beauquesne, L. (1982) *Plantes médicinales et phytothérapie*, Angers, France, 1, p. 73
British Pharmaceutical Codex (1949)
Hänsel, R. and Steinegger, E. (1988) *Lehrbuch der Pharmakognosie und Phytopharmazie*, Springer-Verlag, Berlin, pp. 569–70
Larson, B. and Medcalf, D. G. *Carbohyd. Res.*, 59, 2, p. 531
Martindale The Extra Pharmacopoeia (1982), 28th edition

Taste: salty.

Action: general metabolic stimulant; nutritive; thyroid restorative; detoxifier.

Applications: as a seaweed, this remedy contains a rich store of minerals, particularly iodine. This is certainly nourishing for the thyroid, and it is thought to supply in total an ideal diet for this gland. This would account for some of its reputation in treating thyroid diseases, but there appears to be more to it. In some thyroid-deficiency diseases, for example, the problem is not in the supply of iodine, but in the inability of the thyroid tissues to use it. From traditional usage, moreover, we may draw the conclusion that kelp has an action for states of both hyper- and hypothyroid difficulties, in other words, it is a restorative to thyroid function generally, an adaptogen. Having said this it should be emphasized that the action is very gentle rather than dramatic, and the best way to see the remedy is as a back-up, a long-term course of slow restoration, particularly when thyroid trouble is associated with nutritional deficiencies (as is particularly likely with hypo-thyroidism, but possible also when the thyroid is too active).

Like other seaweeds, kelp is an excellent bulk laxative, and powder may be taken for this effect at 3 teaspoonfuls daily – it swells many times in the gut and is very gentle on the bowel lining by comparison with cereal roughage. Whether for this reason or for others, the remedy has a reputation as a detoxifying agent.

DAMIANA

Turnera diffusa Willd. var. *aphrodisiaca* Urb.
Family: Turneraceae
Synonym: *Damiana aphrodisiaca.*

Description: a shrub up to 2 m high, the much-branched stems are smooth, straight and yellow or reddish-brown. The small leaves are alternate or in bunches; their upper surface is pale green, the underside lightly covered with pale hairs, and they have toothed margins. Small yellow flowers grow in the leaf axils. The fruits are small capsules, tripartite and slightly curved; the leaves have a strong pleasant aroma, reminiscent of chamomile.

Habitat: a native of Texas, Mexico and Central America, preferring hot humid climates.

Parts used: the stem and leaves.

Preparation: an infusion may be made from the herb or a tincture made at 1:5 in 60 per cent alcohol.

Dosage: 1–4 g dried herb or equivalent three times per day.

Constituents: volatile oil (incl. tricyclic sesquiterpene α-copaene, Δ-cadi-nene, thymol, calamenene, α- and β-pinene, cineol, arbutin, cymene); alkaloids; bitter (damianin); flavonoids; cyanogenic glycosides; tannins; gum; resins.

Pharmacology: the alkaloids are thought to have a testosteronal effect (they are similar to those of sarsaparilla, which has the same reputation) and to contain constituents similar to caffeine. The cyanogenic glycosides on the other hand are likely to provide a relaxing influence to the whole plant to compensate for the stimulating action otherwise expected.

References:

Benigni, R., Capra, C. and Cattorini, P. E. (1962) *Piante medicinali: chimica farmacologia e terapia*, Inverni & Della Beffa, Milan, pp. 428–9

British Pharmaceutical Codex (1934)

Hänsel, R. and Steinegger, E. (1988) *Lehrbuch der Pharmakognosie und Phytopharmazie*, Springer-Verlag, Berlin, p. 630

Leung, A. Y. (1980) *Encyclopedia of Common Natural Ingredients Used in Food, Drugs, and Cosmetics*, John Wiley, New York

Lowry, T. P. (1984) 'Damiana', in *J. Psych. Dr.*, 16 (3), pp. 267–8

Merck Index (1976) 9, pp. 249 and 1599

Temperament: warm.

Taste: bitter aromatic, acrid.

Action: testosteromimetic, providing a generally stimulating and enhancing influence on those functions related to the reproductive system, especially in the male; euphoric and nervous restorative; laxative.

Applications: although there is no scientific evidence for an appreciable effect, this plant has been tested in other arenas. It has a reputation that passes the purely medicinal into the world of recreational drug use: as a tea inducing a mild euphoria and particularly as an aphrodisiac. In traditional medicine, in 'sub-euphoric' doses(!), it has been highly regarded as a prophylactic against disease and to improve stamina, and it was used as a tonic for the central nervous system, and specifically for sexual inadequacies with a strong psychological or emotional element, especially in the male. It is also a mild laxative and is applicable to cases of atonic constipation.

Damiana may be recommended in any debilitated condition of the central nervous system (from depression to neuralgias and problems such as herpes – it has a particular use in containing genital herpes). Although male-orientated it is not contra-indicated for women with debilitated conditions: its main contra-indications are in the very excitable and those with irritable bowel syndrome. Otherwise, it often fills a desirable place in a prescription for those simply too *sad*.

SAW PALMETTO

Serenoa serrulata Hook.
Family: Palmae
Synonyms: sabal, *Serenoa repens* Bartr., *Sabal serrulatum* Roem and Schult.

Description: a low scrubby palm with a largely subterranean trunk; above the ground this is covered with the bases of withered leaves: these will often remain stunted or form twiggy branches growing along the ground. The stiff leaves are around 60 cm long, spreading out in fans. The ivory-coloured flowers grow in fragrant clusters; the stone fruits are about 25 mm long when fresh, dark purple to black, with light-brown flesh, growing in bunches; when dried the flesh contracts to give the surface large angular depressions and the hard stone occupies most of the bulk. The odour is aromatic and very pungent.

Habitat: sand dunes and coastal regions of Florida, Texas and Georgia.

Parts used: the berries.

Preparation: an infusion may be prepared from the berries: for this purpose the stones are taken out, the better to extract the fleshy material left; a tincture may be prepared at 1:5 in 45 per cent alcohol.

Dosage: 1–2 g dried berry pulp three times per day.

Constituents: volatile oil; steroidal saponins (incl. α-sitosterol); possible alkaloid; resin; tannins; fixed oil.

Pharmacology: although unconfirmed, the presence of the saponins lends weight to claims that the remedy may be used for prostatic and hormonal disorders. The volatile oil is likely to have the main urinary antiseptic action.

References:
Boshamer, K. (1951–2) *Therapiewoche*, Karlsruhe, Germany, 2, p. 236
British Herbal Pharmacopoeia (1983)

Feriz, H. (1960) *Ars Medici*, Leistal, Switzerland, 50, p. 407
Scultéty, S. (1961) *Zeitschrift für Urologie*, Leipzig, 54, p. 219
US Pharmacopoeia (1906)

Action: tones the male reproductive system and particularly the prostate gland; urinary antiseptic; acts to reduce congestive catarrhal conditions of the respiratory system; relaxant.

Applications: this plant is passed on from North American history with a number of recommendations. It was used for catarrhal conditions of the respiratory system, especially where this was chronic and congestive.

It is also used for urinary infections, especially when these involve the prostate. It is for the prostate in general indeed that the remedy is most used today. It is specific for benign prostatic hypertrophy, a common accompaniment of ageing, and it extends beyond that to have a supportive effect on the male reproductive system as a whole, especially when combined with damiana. The two remedies are recommended for debility and senility in men, and to improve reproductive performance when this is flagging.

Although apparently paradoxical there is no contradiction in the relaxing influence of the remedy reported in the *US Pharmacopoeia* of 1906. This and its widespread consumption by both humans and animals in its habitat simply support the contention that the remedy is essentially supportive rather than aggressively dynamic.

SEVEN BARKS

Hydrangea arborescens L.
Family: Saxifragaceae
Synonyms: hydrangea, wild hydrangea.

Description: a shrub up to 3 m high, the stems of which are covered with thin layers of multicoloured bark; there are opposite, serrate, ovate leaves and clusters of small creamy flowers; the rhizome is obtained in pale-yellow woody chumps with fragments of thin brown cork, along with short pieces of thin, fibrous roots.

Habitat: woodland and stream banks of south-eastern and central North America.

Parts used: the rhizome and roots.

Preparation: decoction or a tincture prepared at 1:5 in 25 per cent alcohol.

Dosage: 1–4 g three times per day.

Constituents: glycoside (hydrangin); saponins; resin.

Action: diuretic.

Applications: this remedy is reputed to be effective in a large range of urinary problems such as urinary stones and infections; however, it is for prostatitis that it has been most recommended. It may be seen as a useful complement to saw palmetto and/or damiana in supportive prescriptions for senescence and infirmity in men.

HELONIAS ROOT

Chamaelirium luteum (L.) A. Gray
Family: Liliaceae
Synonyms: false unicorn root, blazing star, devil's bit, *Helonias dioica* Pursh., *H. lutea* Ker-Gawl., *Veratrum luteum* L., *C. carolianum* Willd.

Description: a herbaceous perennial about 30–100 cm high, the stem smooth and angular, leaves alternate, spatulate below, lanceolate above, radical, about 2 cm by 20 cm, narrow at the base and formed into a whorl; numerous flowers small, greenish white, in a dense terminal raceme. The rhizome is bulbous and terminates abruptly: it gives off fine wiry pale roots; the commercial sample of rhizome is up to 1.5 cm in diameter with grey-brown closely annulated exterior and a grey-white interior with scattered fibro-vascular bundles; the taste is astringent at first, bitter later.

Habitat: a native of the Mississippi area growing on low moist ground.

Parts used: the rhizome and roots.

Harvesting: flowers in May–June, the rhizomes are best collected in September.

Preparation: a decoction of the rhizome and roots is probably the most effective preparation; a tincture may be prepared at 1:5 in 25 per cent alcohol.

Dosage: 1–2 g dried rhizome and roots three times a day.

Constituents: steroidal saponins (incl. chamaelirin).

Pharmacology: although there is almost no experimental evidence reported, it is possible to conjecture that the presence of the steroidal saponins is the key to the effects of the plant: they appear to justify comparisons with the effect of ginseng, also containing such molecules, although in this case the observed action is on the steroidal hormone production by the ovary, rather than the production by the adrenal cortex. There is certainly a similar amphoteric action.

References:

Benigni, R., Capra, C. and Cattorini, P. E. (1962) *Piante medicinali: chimica farmacologia e terapia*, Inverni & Della Beffa, Milan, p. 548

Horhammer, L. and List, P. H. (1972) *Hagers Handbuch der Pharmazeutischen Praxis*, Springer-Verlag, Berlin, p. 831

Action: improves the secretory responses and cyclical functions of the ovary, appears to have an adaptogenic action on that organ.

Applications: this remedy is one of a number of promising gynaeco-logical remedies reaching us from the native American tradition. The recorded medicine of the Indian is notable for the emphasis placed on treating gynaecological and obstetric conditions: else-where, and particularly in Europe, these matters seem to have been less well recorded (perhaps because most archivists and scholars were men, and most treatment of women was conducted on an informal intimate basis by women).

It has been claimed as a remedy in a broad range of female symptoms, including amenorrhoea, dysmenorrhoea, irregular men-struation, vaginal discharge, pelvic congestion and structural laxity of the pelvic organs. It is used traditionally to prevent miscarriages in pregnancy, and has a striking reputation for improving fertility generally (to the extent that early practitioners discouraged its use if the patient did not wish to get pregnant!); the physiomedicalists emphasized the tonifying effects on the uterus – 'for all depressed conditions of the uterus and ovaries' (Lyle).

For modern conditions, helonias root commends itself as an 'ovarian tonic', applicable as in tradition to a full range of gynaeco-logical and even obstetric problems. It finds particular application to chronic pelvic inflammation (e.g. chronic salpingitis) where it combines favourably with echinacea (*Echinacea angustifolia*), for amenorrhoea from any cause, for infertility as a remedy of first choice, for dysmenorrhoea, especially of the type that accompanies menstruation rather than precedes it, for irregular menstrual cycles, and for the hormonal adjustment problems sometimes marking menopause. One may also recommend it, with discretion, in morning sickness of pregnancy or in case of threatened miscarriage – there seems practically no stimulating influence on the gravid uterus. From the subjective point of view the remedy is particularly indicated in conditions accompanied by a low dragging feeling in the lower abdomen.

The impression received is that the effect of helonias root is to encourage the ovary to perform and respond in its hormonal choreography more appropriately. In menstrual or sex hormone disturbances, there is most often a predictable prognosis: treatment is recommended continuously for three months; in the first month or two the menstrual cycles are likely to be considerably transformed in ways that are always unpredictable and not always pleasant or convenient. By the third cycle, however, it appears that a new order is emerging from the chaos, this order being close to the normal subtle but robust cycle that most women have, and which can be left to run itself without further treatment once established. It seems, in other words, as though the remedy has enabled the ovary to shake itself out of its old irregularities and to find itself its usual pattern.

AGNUS CASTUS

Vitex agnus-castus L.
Family: Verbenaceae
Synonyms: chaste tree, monk's pepper.

Description: the fruit (drupe) of a shrubby plant: a lignified ovary of 2 carpels each containing one seed, roughly ovoid about 3 mm across, 4 mm long, dark-grey in colour, yielding when crushed a dark powder of characteristic aroma and fragrant slightly acrid bitter taste.

Habitat: countries bordering the Mediterranean and western Asia.

Parts used: the fruit.

Preparation: decoction or tincture at 1 : 5 in 25 per cent alcohol.

Dosage: 0.2–2 g fruit three times a day.

Constituents: volatile oil; bitter principle (castine); alkaloids.

Pharmacology: considerable research work in Germany during the 1940s and 1950s pointed to an effect on pituitary hormone activity, with an apparent effect in mimicking the activity of the corpus luteum, the transitional endocrine gland left in the ovary for about 10 days after ovulation; changes in women's endometrium, basal temperature and vaginal secretions were confirmed. There was also support for the lactation-promoting reputation of the plant.

Temperament: warm.

Action: regulates female hormonal activity: relieves premenstrual tension; stimulates lactation.

Application: this remedy has achieved considerable popularity among both herbal practitioners and women generally in Britain in recent years, and has been at least as well known in West Germany. Its major reputation now is in relieving symptoms of tension occurring either before a menstrual period or during the menopause, but it has been used with acclaim for a whole range of gynaecological conditions, particularly menstrual disturbances.

An association with such matters is well established. Parkinson noted: 'it also procureth milke in womens breasts, it procureth their courses, and the urine stopped' ('courses' referred to menstrual flow), and: 'the decoction of the herbe and seede is very good for women troubled with the paines of the mother, or inflammations of the parts'.

Its traditional reputation was always intriguingly paradoxical, a fact that herbalists often take to point to an amphoteric effect. Thus Parkinson takes Galen to task: 'although so famous a writer and Physician contraryeth himselfe in this one place . . ., for having affirmed before that the seede hereof is hot and dry . . ., he saith that the seede of Vitex doth refraine Venerous desires, and giveth little nourishment to the body, and that because it is cooling and drying'. He himself concludes that of the two positions the temperament of *Vitex* is 'a meane between them both'. Another contradiction is found in the two common names for the plant: 'chaste tree' is a title recalling Parkinson's statement that it 'refraineth also the instigations of Venery in any manner used and taken'; yet its other name 'monk's pepper' may refer to an aphrodisiac reputation.

A balancing action on the activity of the female sex hormones has in fact been a widely accepted interpretation of the effect of agnus castus among herbal practitioners in Britain, a tradition deriving from the literature provided by the leading supplier of the retail remedy in West Germany (Dr Madaus and Co.) quoting several medical papers published in the 1940s and 1950s in that country. The idea is that the herb in some way affects the balance of follicle-stimulating hormone (FSH) and luteinizing hormone (LH) production by the anterior pituitary so as to effectively support the corpus luteum in its own endocrine production in the second half of the menstrual cycle. There is, in fact, very little evidence for this conclusion but clinical experience is that the remedy does seem more progesteronal than oestrogenic, and that it is more effective for troubles building up to menstruation rather than starting with or following it, both pointing to an effect in support of or mimicking the corpus luteum.

Agnus castus has a relaxing and calming quality. It is popular among women suffering menopausal and premenstrual tensions, and can be relied on to soothe in any context.

BLUE COHOSH

Caulophyllum thalictroides (L.) Mich.
Family: Berberidaceae
Synonyms: papoose root, squaw root, blue ginseng.

Description: a perennial plant up to 1 m high with large 3-lobed leaves and racemes of small yellow-green flowers; the rhizome is hard and knotted with masses of fibrous roots below and large cup-shaped scars above; taste bitter-sweet becoming acrid.

Habitat: in moist rich ground in eastern North America.

Parts used: the rhizome and roots.

Preparation: decoction or a tincture made at 1:5 in 60 per cent alcohol.

Dosage: 0.2–1 g of rhizome and roots three times per day.

Constituents: steroidal saponins (incl. caulosapogenin); lupin-type alkaloids (incl. methylcystisine, anagyrene and baptisine) and quaternary apophine alkaloids (incl. magnoflorine).

References:

Anderson, L. A. and Phillipson, J. D. (1984) 'Herbal remedies used in sedative and antirheumatic preparations: part 2', in *Pharm. J.*, July 28, pp. 111–15

British Pharmaceutical Codex (1934)

Leung, A. Y. (1980) *Encyclopedia of Common Natural Ingredients Used in Food, Drugs, and Cosmetics*, John Wiley, New York

Action: antispasmodic, particularly on the female reproductive system; tonic effect on the womb and Fallopian tubes.

Contra-indications: it is probably unsafe to take in pregnancy until labour has commenced.

Applications: this remedy was traditionally used to facilitate childbirth, and given during labour itself. It is most beneficial both to ease pain in the latter stages of labour and for the hours immediately afterwards, including the passing of the placenta.

It is however also well suited to functional menstrual disturbances, particularly those involving spasm or disturbance of the womb and Fallopian tubes. Thus it is applied to help with dysmenorrhoea and other pains of the menstrual cycle and menopause, with especial benefit on the spasmodic dysmenorrhoea marked by pain starting with menstruation (and usually occurring in girls and women before childbirth). It will help in some cases of functional amenorrhoea.

BETH ROOT

Trillium erectum L.
Family: Liliaceae
Synonyms: birth root, wake robin, *T. pendulum* Willd.

Description: a stout erect perennial herb with a simple stem bearing a whorl of 3 broad rhombic pointed leaves and terminating in a large terminal flower with 3 petals, purple, pale green or pale brown; the rhizome is obtained as hard fragments, transversely ringed and with numerous fibrous rootlets. Taste is bitter and acrid.

Habitat: rich woodland in central and western states of the USA.

Parts used: the rhizome and roots.

Preparation: decoction or a tincture made at 1:5 in 45 per cent alcohol.

Dosage: 0.5–2 g three times per day.

Constituents: steroidal saponins (incl. trillarin); steroidal glycoside; tannins; fixed oil.

Action: antihaemorrhagic, with particular action on the female reproductive system; *partus praeparator*; astringent.

Applications: another traditional birth-facilitating remedy applied also, in modern times at least, to heavy menstrual or menopausal bleeding (but always ensure in the latter case that organic disease has been eliminated). It has always been applied to blood loss, including that from the lungs and urinary system, and it may be used as a palliative for these cases as well, at least until the real problem has been sorted out. There is certainly a local astringent effect, recognized in the use of the remedy as a vaginal douche for infections and discharges, but this does not explain the systemic action on internal bleeding, nor the use of the remedy internally for discharges from the reproductive system.

SQUAW VINE

Mitchella repens L.
Family: Rubiaceae
Synonyms: checkerberry, partridge berry.

Description: a small prostrate perennial evergreen herb with opposite ovate-orbicular entire leaves and 2 sessile white flowers at the tip, these giving way to red and occasionally white berries. The commercial samples occur as loosely matted masses of branched light-yellow-to-brown filiform rhizomes and fine roots together with aerial quadrangular or flattened green stems and leaves. The taste is slightly bitter.

Habitat: on woodland floors in eastern North America.

Parts used: the whole plant.

Preparation: infusion of the plant or a tincture made at 1 : 5 in 25 per cent alcohol.

Dosage: 1–4 g three times per day.

Constituents: saponins; bitter principle; mucilage; tannins.

Action: nervous tonic and restorative; *partus praeparator*, uterine relaxant.

Applications: this remedy is traditionally applied in later pregnancy to facilitate labour and delivery, having much the same reputation in former North American times as raspberry leaves have today.

It is also recommended for dysmenorrhoea and other painful and irritant conditions of the female reproductive tract.

A separate tradition had the remedy applied to nervous debility (or neurasthenia) and exhausted conditions in both sexes, as an aid to convalescence.

Chinese Tonic Remedies

These remedies are essentially restorative. They are indicated for depletion of energies, where illness, prolonged stress or constitutional weakness has so drained resources that the person's ability to cope with a situation is significantly impaired.

Unlike most other traditional remedies, the tonics are designed for long-term prescription and chronic disease. In times when most indications were acute they had the useful role of supporting a traumatized constitution, aiding convalescence or maintaining health into old age.

In modern times, when most vigorous manifestations of vital resistance have been successfully suppressed, low-grade, chronic reactions are increasingly the norm, and the tonic remedies are becoming ever more central to prescription making.

In Chinese medicine, the tonics are generally divided into four groups, depending on whether they are seen to particularly support *qi, yang, xue* or *yin*. The first two groups tend to be warming, the last two cooling.

Although generally supportive in influence, it is appropriate to insert a word of caution about tonics. They support energy, but are not always beneficial. It is important that they should support only the vital sphere and not the disturbance. It is quite possible for tonics to actually support a disease if mis-prescribed: note should therefore be taken of their temperament, contra-indications and other qualities.

Finally, it is worth emphasizing that the tonics are all individual remedies: their differences are greater than any similarities between them.

Qi tonics support active energies; they are used for depletion of *qi*, particularly in the *Spleen* and *Lungs*.

In the first case, possibly as a result of prolonged illness or constitutional weakness, disturbance is likely to affect the functions of assimilation and distribution, to be associated with such symptoms as fatigue and depression, with depressed digestion, diarrhoea, abdominal pain or tension, visceral prolapse, pale-yellow complexion with a tinge of red or purple, pale tongue with white coating, and/or languid, frail or indistinct pulses. This may lead in turn to a 'damp' condition developing.

In the second case, extreme or prolonged stress or disease, or chronic pulmonary disease, leads to depletion or cold in the *Lungs*, with easy fatigue and prostration associated with disturbances of regulation, shortness of breath or shallow breathing, rapid, slow or little speech, spontaneous perspiration, pallid complexion, dry skin, pale tongue with thin white coating, weak and depleted pulses.

Ginseng is a well-known *qi* tonic.

Yang tonics support the active energies, particularly those of the *Kidneys* (but also of the *Heart* and *Spleen*).

Deficient *Kidney yang* leads to listlessness with a feeling of cold, and cold extremities, back and loins; there may be weak legs, poor reproductive function, frequency of micturition, nocturia, diarrhoea (especially early in the morning), pale complexion and submerged, weak pulses.

Deficiency affecting the *Heart* involves poor performance and co-ordination associated with profuse cold sweating, asthmatic states, thoracic or anginal pain on exertion, palpitations and fear attacks, cyanosis, white tongue coating and/or diminished, hesitant or intermittent pulses.

Fenugreek is one of the best-known *yang* tonics.

Xue tonics support more substantial energies, those manifesting in substantial disturbances or pathologies. By definition such disturbances are serious and profound, and treatment will need to be prolonged. Symptoms of depletion of *xue* may include cyanosis, pallor, vertigo or tinnitus, palpitations, loss of memory, insomnia or menstrual problems.

Dang Gui and rhemannia are both known as *xue* tonics.

Yin tonics replenish the body fluids and essence, supplying condensed energies and nourishment, for the most depleted conditions. Areas in most need of support are the *Kidneys, Liver, Lungs* and *Stomach*.

Deficient *Kidney yin* often follows very serious debilitating disease, or alternatively extended sexual or alcoholic abuse or overwhelming nervous stress. It may manifest as a deficient Fire condition, marked by a pale complexion with red cheeks, red lips, dry mouth, dry but deeply red tongue, dry throat, hot palms and soles, palpitations, vertigo or tinnitus, pains in the loins, night sweats, nocturnal emissions, nightmares, urinary retention, constipation, accelerated though weak pulses.

Deficient *Liver yin*, usually following the above, is often associated with dry eyes, poor vision and vertigo or tinnitus, deafness, muscle twitching, sleeplessness, hot flushed face with red cheeks, red dry tongue with little coating, diminished, stringy and accelerated pulses.

Deficient *Stomach yin* is marked by anorexia, regurgitation, thirst, abdominal rumbling, red lips and red tongue with no coating.

Deficient *Lung yin*, often following prolonged exposure to dryness or chronic pulmonary disease, is marked by dry cough, haemoptysis, hoarseness and loss of voice, strong thirst and/or restlessness and insomnia.

Asparagus root and lycium are both considered to be *yin* tonics.

GINSENG

Panax ginseng C. A. Meyer
Family: Araliaceae
Synonyms: Asiatic ginseng, Ren Shen

NOTE: there are many species of ginseng recorded, notably the American ginseng *P. quinquefolium* L., *P. pseudo-ginseng* var. *notoginseng* Burk., found wild in the Yunnan and Kwangsi provinces of China, and *P. pseudo-ginseng* var. *japonicus* C. A. Meyer, or Japanese ginseng; not to mention so-called 'Siberian ginseng', actually *Eleutherococcus senticosus*. All these plants have different constituents and activities and only *P. ginseng* is discussed here.

Description: a perennial herb up to 1 m tall with simple erect red stem bearing at the top compound leaves with 5 leaflets, the 3 terminal ones larger than the lateral ones, and a single small terminal umbel of pink flowers giving way to a small red berry; the bifurcate fusiform roots grow down from a short rhizome giving rise to a number of fine rootlets. When dried they are found as fusiform or cylindrical pieces 6–10 cm long and 0.5–2 cm across; externally they are light yellow-brown, annular in the upper (rhizome) portion, terminated at the crown by one or more stem scars; the lower portion is longitudinally wrinkled and marked by a number of root scars; the fracture is short, internal surface light yellow-brown, marked by a distinct brown cambium line, radiate wood, oil secretion canals in the cortex. The odour is slightly aromatic, taste initially sweet and slightly bitter. The root is sometimes cured soon after harvesting, a process involving steaming, sun-drying and smoking, this producing so-called 'red ginseng', a deep-red root with a glassy fracture.

Habitat: north-eastern China and North Korea in mountainous forests; extremely rare in the wild form and now cultivated.

Parts used: the root with rhizome.

Preparation: decoction, or the root chewed whole or made up into pills or tablets. It is wise to presume that any sample bought in the West is of inferior quality unless having authoritative evidence to the contrary.

Dosage: 1–9 g daily; a single dose of 30 g for emergency use. Practical use in the West suggests a daily dose of 1–3 g for short-term use (for up to 14 days), with a longer-term regime taking 0.5–0.8 g daily.

Constituents: triterpenoid saponins (incl. ginsenosides R_b, R_g and R_c); panax acid; glycosides (panaxin, panaquilin, ginsenin); α-sitosterol;

stigmasterol; campesterol; a sesquiterpene (pancene); polyacetylenes (α-elemene; panaxynol); kaempferol; choline; an anti-oxidant ('maltol'); essential oil. There are in fact many ginsenosides discovered, but they are generally divided into two groups, based on two dammarine-type core triterpenes called protopanaxadiol and protopanaxatriol, called for this reason 'diols' and 'triols' (ginsenosides R_b and R_c are diols, ginsenoside R_g is a triol).

Pharmacology: a substantial body of research has supported many of the traditional claims for ginseng and moreover found such activity closely linked to the presence of the triterpenoid saponins. Most interest has focused on those of the 'triol' group which have been found to be the most arousing, the 'diols' being more sedative. (Incidentally diols predominate in the American ginseng – *Panax quinquefolium*.) Trials have shown that both ginseng and other mixtures of triol saponins effectively help the body to withstand stresses better, whatever these stresses might be (extremes of temperature, excessive exertion, hunger, battle conditions, mental strain, emotional excess, and so on). For a review of the body's ability to adapt to stress see 'How Strong are the Body's Reserves?', on pp. 209–12. The structural similarity of the triterpenoid saponins to the steroid hormones and the observed link experimentally between their activities have led to the thesis that some at least of the saponins interact with steroid receptors, perhaps including those in the key switching mechanisms controlling steroid production in the hypothalamus: in the case of ginseng at least (and possibly other members of the Araliaceae) the result is an improvement in both positive reinforcement, leading to increased secretion of hormones when needed, and negative reinforcement curtailing their secretion when not. This adaptogenic behaviour accords with the clinical findings that ginseng has neither an excessively stimulating nor a sedating effect, but switches between the two depending on individual circumstances. In addition to these actions of the ginsenosides, ginsenoside R_b especially increases RNA, protein and cholesterol production in the liver, with the plant as a whole increasing hepatic rough endoplasmic reticulum (these effects on liver function have great significance in postulating a widespread metabolic action for the plant, and may also help to explain experimental evidence suggesting ginseng helps the liver resist hepatotoxins and radiation); there is an inhibitory effect on glycogen utilization in white skeletal muscle during exercise (suggesting a carbohydrate-sparing and stamina-increasing action locally at the muscle site); an increase in enzymes mobilizing and utilizing fatty acids; an increase in adrenal cholesterol by about 20 per cent. Increased sperm production has been reported in men, and increased vaginal moisture and libido in post-menopausal women; reduction in bone-marrow depression in an anticancer drug regime has been reported, and in another trial a wide range of health criteria improved in a population of geriatric patients. Non-saponin constituents have been found to have activity in isolation: panax acid stimulates the heart and metabolic rate, panaxin stimulates the heart and brain stem centres, ginsenin is hypoglycaemic.

References:

* Fulder, S. (1980) *The Root of Being*, Hutchinson, London

Brekhman, I. I. and Dardymov, I. V. (1969) 'New substances of plant origin which increase nonspecific resistance', in *Ann. Rev. Pharmacol.*, 9, pp. 419–30

'Pharmacological investigation of glycosides from Ginseng and Eleutherococcus', in *Lloydia*, Cincinnati, 32, pp. 46–51

D'Angelo, L. *et al.* (1986) 'A double-blind placebo-controlled clinical study on the effect of a standardized ginseng extract on psychomotor performance in healthy volunteers', in *J. Ethnopharmacol.*, 16, pp. 15–22

Hallstrom, C. *et al.* (1982) 'Effects of Ginseng on the performance of nurses on night duty', in *Comparative Medicine East and West*, VI, 4, pp. 277–82

Lee, F. C. *et al.* (1987) 'Effects of Panax ginseng on blood alcohol clearance in man', in *Clin. and Exp. Pharmacol. and Physiol.*, 14, pp. 543–6

Leung, A. Y. (1980) *Encyclopedia of Common Natural Ingredients Used in Food, Drugs, and Cosmetics*, John Wiley, New York, pp. 186–8

Martindale The Extra Pharmacopoeia (1989), 29th edition

Owen, R. T. (1981) 'Ginseng: a pharmacological profile', in *Drugs of Today, Medicamentos de Actualidad*, XVII, 8, pp. 343–51

Petkov, V. D. *et al.* (1987) 'Effects of standardised Ginseng extract on learning, memory and physical capabilities', in *Amer. J. Chin. Med.*, XV, 1–2, pp. 19–29

Shibata, S. *et al.* (1985) 'Chemistry and pharmacology of Panax', in *Economic and Medicinal Plant Research*, Academic Press, London, 1, pp. 217–84

Singh, V. K. *et al.* (1984) 'Immunomodulatory activity of Panax ginseng extract', in *Planta Medica*, Stuttgart, 50, pp. 462–5

Temperament: warm to neutral.

Taste: sweet, slightly bitter.

Action: adaptogenic: improves the body's ability to adapt to a wide range of stresses; improves stamina; reduces some of the symptoms of senescence. (In Chinese medicine: replenish *qi*, tonify *Spleen* and *Lungs*.)

Contra-indications: anxiety and nervous tension; cardiovascular disease; disturbed menstruation.

Applications: in traditional Chinese medicine, ginseng was applied to deficient *qi*, marked by the restlessness of debility, irritability, insomnia and/or palpitations, leading on to severe sweating with cold extremities, breathlessness, very weak pulses. These were the sort of symptoms that might arise after debilitating illness or severe injury.

It was also applied to deficiency in the *Lung*, with difficulty in breathing especially on exertion, little stamina, coughing, reluctance to speak, cold perspiration; and also to deficiency of the *Spleen* and *Stomach* with severe weakness, anorexia, chronic diarrhoea, prolapse and tension in the lower abdomen. As with the previous paragraph, both these patterns of disharmony would tend to arise after severe debilitating illness: both would be particularly likely to follow such illness when it had persisted for a long time.

These applications have become channelled into new patterns in the modern Western context. We now see ginseng as having roughly two main types of application. The first to short-term treatment of the effects or anticipated effects of stress, whether so far as treating shock or collapse, or simply to reduce generally the damage sustained during a stressful period. Under this heading would be placed the use of ginseng by soldiers in a battle situation and by cosmonauts, and its use in convalescence from surgery or serious illness, in anticipation of a stressful work period, to sit examinations, to treat jet-lag, or other short-term needs. (One insight: ginseng seems to help raise the threshold over which a stress stops becoming life-enhancing and becomes life-threatening.)

The second type of application is in generally, and over a long period, reducing the impact of the ageing process. The plant has been called a longevity herb, and it does seem to have the ability to maintain the adrenal cortex in maximal responsive condition. It has certainly been highly favoured by the bureaucratic classes in China for many centuries as a component of a graceful passage through the twilight years. There is also no doubt that ginseng becomes increasingly impressive the more depleted the person taking it, and that it is by contrast increasingly likely to be stimulating when consumed by those younger and more vigorous in spirit.

These last considerations contribute to the cautions that should attend the use of ginseng. It should not be taken for too long by those of young, active or robust constitution; it should not be mixed with caffeine or other stimulant consumption. In addition, there are question marks over its use by women during their reproductive years, and in general it should be avoided unless the menstrual and associated hormonal cycles are fully stable. Last, but not least, ginseng should not be taken in the case of cardiovascular disease.

Other *qi* tonics: Dang Shen (*Codonopsis pilulosa*); Huang Qi (*Astragalus membranaceus*); Bai Zhu (*Atractylodes macrocephela*); Jujube – Da Zao (*Zizyphus jujuba*); Chinese liquorice – Gan Cao (*Glycyrrhiza uralensis*).

FENUGREEK

Trigonella foenum-graecum L.
Family: Leguminosae
Synonym: Hu Lu Ba.

Description: an annual herb up to 45 cm high with petiolate trifoliate leaves and solitary sessile whitish flowers in the leaf axils; the seeds are light to dark yellow-brown, rhomboidal, nearly smooth, 5–7 mm long and about 2 mm thick; on one side runs a diagonal depression, dividing the radicle and 2 yellow cotyledons; the odour is characteristic, the taste mucilaginous and slightly bitter.

Habitat: indigenous to the Mediterranean area; cultivated in India, China and other places.

Parts used: the dried ripe seeds.

Preparation: decoction.

Dosage: 3–10 g daily.

Constituents: alkaloids (trigonelline); steroidal saponins (incl. diosgenin, yamogenin); mucilage; aromatic hydrocarbons; fixed oil; proteins.

Pharmacology: the presence of a steroidal saponin diosgenin, the same as that used as a raw material for the synthesis of synthetic oestrogens, is of immediate significance, although there is no pharmacological investigation into its contribution to the actions of the remedy; the plant is however oxytocic *in vitro* and is also hypoglycaemic.

References:
Abdo, M. S. and Al-Kafawi, A. A. (1969) *Planta Medica*, Stuttgart, 17, p. 14
British Herbal Pharmacopoeia (1983)

Temperament: hot.

Taste: bitter.

Action: warming tonic; resolves 'cold' and 'damp' illnesses; relieves pain.

Contra-indications: depleted reserves, pregnancy.

Applications: in traditional European medicine fenugreek is a convalescent remedy for the stimulation of appetite and the improvement of assimilation in the recovery from debilitated conditions; it also is prominent for its gentle bulk laxative effects.

In traditional Chinese medicine fenugreek was applied to deficient cold conditions of the *Kidney* with such symptoms as hernia and stabbing pains in the lower abdomen, and others as might arise in congestive period pains in women, low-grade pelvic inflammation and congestion.

A persistent tradition has fenugreek being used to stimulate milk production in lactating women, and incidentally in domestic animals as well. (Its oil and protein content make it a favourite highly nourishing cattle food in many countries.)

Fenugreek also had considerable local healing benefits, acting as the basis of a poultice for boils, wounds, myalgia, ulcers, and so on.

Other *yang* tonics: Ba Ji (*Morinda officinalis*); Walnut – Hu Tao Ren (*Juglans regia*); Du Zhong (*Eucommia ulmoides*).

DANG GUI

Angelica sinensis (Oliv.) Diels.
Family: Umbelliferae
Synonym: *A. polymorpha* var. *sinensis* Oliv.

NOTE: *Angelica acutiloba* (S. and Z.) Kitag. and *A. gigas* Nak. have often been used as substitutes for this plant under the title of Dang Gui; the properties appear the same, but they are likely to be inferior.

Description: a perennial herb with smooth erect stem; lower leaves tripinnate, superior leaves simply pinnate – segments oval or oval-lanceolate, sharply toothed – on long sheathed petioles; the flowers are in umbels with 9–13 irregular rays. The root is much divided into numerous rootlets; when dried these are obtained peeled, in thin slices: the outer surface pale yellow-brown, a deep bark layer with pronounced cambium line; the interior is pale-whitish and of amorphous consistency; the fracture is short and granular. Odour is aromatic, taste sweet.

Habitat: China, Japan, Korea; cultivated at high altitudes in west and north China.

Parts used: the root.

Preparation: decoction.

Dosage: 3–10 g daily.

Constituents: essential oil (incl. carvacrol, safrol, isosafrol, cadinene, n-dodecanol, ligustilide); furanocoumarins (incl. bergapten).

Pharmacology: experimentally shown to be stimulating to the uterus, and to the smooth muscle of bladder and small intestine; action on the uterus is compounded by a complementary relaxing influence possibly associated with an increase in local circulation; certainly, there is evidence of a dilating action on the coronary vasculature and a peripheral vasodilatory action potentially useful in the treatment of arteriosclerosis throughout the body; it lowers blood-cholesterol levels and, in addition, has a cardiac stabilizing effect comparable to quinidine (experimentally applied to the treatment of auricular fibrillation); it is said to potentiate vitamin E activity; the whole remedy has been shown to possess immunoregulating properties, reducing experimentally induced hypersensitivity reactions; there are reported antibacterial and sedative properties. No oestrogenic substances have been found in the remedy. *A. gigas* has been shown to antagonize caffeine-induced stimulation, and antispasmodic action has been observed in *A. acutiloba* as well.

References:

Mosig, A. and Schramm, G. (1955) 'Der Arzneipflanzen und Drogenschatz Chinas . . .', in *Beitrage zur Pharmazie Heft*, Berlin, 4, pp. 1–71

Read, B. E. and Schmidt, C. F. (1923) *Proc. Soc. Exp. Biol. Med.*, 20, pp. 395–6

Sung, C.-P. *et al.* (1982) *Lloydia*, Cincinnati, 45 (4), pp. 398–406

Tanaka, S. *et al.* (1977) *Arzneimittel-Forschung*, Aulendorf, Germany, 27/11, pp. 2039–45

Temperament: warm.

Taste: sweet, acrid and bitter.

Action: supplements and stimulates *xue*; regulates menstrual cycle; relieves pain; aperient.

Contra-indications: damp *Spleen* conditions with abdominal fullness and diarrhoea.

Applications: this remedy is highly regarded in traditional Chinese medicine as an excellent tonic for substantial debilities, for those severely weakened by trauma or stresses.

Dang Gui is revered as a superb gynaecological remedy applicable to all types of dysmenorrhoea, amenorrhoea, irregular menstruation and infections (as, for example, marked by vaginal discharge).

It is applied also to excess *xue* symptoms marked by such conditions as congestion, swellings, contusions, bruising, traumatic injury, and also in complications of labour and birth.

It was additionally used to treat 'damp-wind' conditions with joint and muscle pain and inflammation.

Modern usage has emphasized the potential of Dang Gui for such circulatory problems as angina, coronary heart problems and thromboangiitis obliterans.

Its aperient properties were noted in the recommendation that it be applied to conditions of 'dryness' as manifested by constipation.

REHMANNIA

Rehmannia glutinosa (Gaertn.) Libosch.

Family: Scrophulariaceae

Synonyms: *R. chinensis* Fisch. et Mey., *Digitalis glutinosa* Gaertn., Chinese foxglove; 1: **Sheng Di Huang,** *Rhizoma (radix) rehmanniae viride,* fresh rehmannia; 2: **Shu Di Huang,** *Rhizoma (radix) rehmanniae praeparata,* prepared rehmannia.

Description: an erect perennial herb up to 60 cm high with a basal rosette of dentate petiolate leaves and alternate oval or spatulate dentate leaves up the stem; the axillary solitary or cymose flowers are purple-orange in colour; the rhizome or root is large, fleshy and brownish-yellow in colour; when prepared it is tarry-black and soft and malleable, obtained in slices or smaller root pieces; the taste is slightly sweet.

Habitat: north-western China and Inner Mongolia.

Parts used: the rhizome or root.

Preparation: decoction.

Dosage: 9–30 g daily.

Constituents: iridoid glycosides (incl. catalpol); rehmannin; mannitol; sterols.

Pharmacology: experimental and clinical evidence points to an anti-hepatotoxic action and a potential effect in some cases of hepatitis; clinical work also suggests an antirheumatic and anti-eczema action; cardiotonic and hypoglycaemic effects have also been detected; the prepared form lowers blood pressure and cholesterol levels in clinical work.

Temperament: cold.

Taste: sweet, bitter.

Actions: 1: cooling, especially for *xue*; moistening; producing body fluids; 2: tonifying *xue* and *yin*.

Contra-indications: deficient 'damp' conditions of the *Spleen*, with abdominal tension, diarrhoea; all signs of deficient *yang*.

Applications: the raw or dried remedy is primarily used for 'heat' problems with impairment of the *yin* energies such as *xue* or *jing*, with symptoms like fever, blood in the sputum or nasal discharge, symptoms of internal deficiency, scarlet tongue; exanthemata, infections, throat infections. Diabetes was a traditional indication, but one probably with only partial justification.

There are tonifying actions as well with a wider application for 'heat'-induced damage to the *yin* with such signs as dry mouth, persistent pyrexia (high temperature) and constipation. A particular cooling application is to 'heat' in the *Heart* with malar flush, irritability and insomnia, and mouth ulcers.

The most popular form of the remedy (and it was always very popular), however, was the prepared root, which was cooked in wine. This was seen as a major tonifying remedy, valuable for any deficiency state of *xue* or *yin*: thus for deficient *Kidney yin* problems such as night sweats and nocturnal emissions, and for deficiency of *xue* such as vertigo, palpitations, insomnia and pallor, and, for women, menorrhagia, irregular menstruation and post-partum haemorrhage.

Other *xue* tonics: paeony root – Bai Shao (*Paeonia lactiflora*); mulberry fruit – Sang Shen (*Mori alba*).

ASPARAGUS ROOT

Asparagus cochinchinensis (Lour.) Merr.
Family: Liliaceae
Synonyms: Tian Men Dong, *A. lucidus* Lindl., shiny asparagus.

Description: a low shrub with extensive fine cylindrical branches, reflected spines and numerous very fine midribs; polygamous solitary or paired white flowers occur in the axils of the leaf-like cladophylls; the dried roots occur as yellowish pieces 7–8 cm long with gelatinous consistency and appearance; its taste is sweetish, with bitter aftertaste.

Habitat: southern China, Korea, Japan, Indochina.

Parts used: the roots.

Preparation: decoction.

Dosage: 6–20 g daily.

Constituents: asparagin; mucilage; α-sitosterol.

Pharmacology: asparagin is a notable diuretic; the whole plant has demonstrated experimental antitumour activity.

Temperament: cool.

Taste: bitter, sweet.

Action: moistens the *Lungs*, and loosens a dry cough; regulates *yin*, tonifying the *Kidneys*, the source of the body fluids.

Contra-indications: *Spleen* and *Stomach* deficiencies with dia-rrhoea.

Applications: the traditional view of asparagus was as a moistening tonic remedy with particular reference to the respiratory system.

It was seen principally to moisten the *Lungs*, to counteract those conditions of 'heat' or deficient *Lung yin* manifested as dry cough, haemoptysis, fever, thirst and dry throat.

Supplementary applications were to constipation (again a moistening action), and other conditions where body fluids were unduly depleted, such as long-term night sweats and nocturnal emissions. These latter point to a wider tonic action on the *Kidneys*.

LYCIUM

Lycium chinensis Mill.
Family: Solanaceae
Synonyms: Gou Qi Zi, Chinese wolfberry.

Description: a small shrub with pendulous, often spine-covered branches; petiolate oval-lanceolate entire leaves with small purple flowers, single or in clusters, in the leaf axils; the fruit is an ovoid orange-red berry 1.25–2.5 cm long with a sweet taste.

Habitat: China, Japan and eastern Asia.

Parts used: the fruit and root bark.

Preparation: decoction.

Dosage: 3–12 g daily.

Constituents: solanaceous alkaloids; betaine; physaline; carotene.

Pharmacology: a close relative (*L. barbarum*) has shown experimental hypoglycaemic effects; this species is a CNS stimulant and has the usual atropine-like parasympathetic-blocking action of the Solanaceae; it influences fat transport mechanisms so as to reduce fat deposition in the liver and atheroma formation, and promotes regeneration of liver tissue.

Temperament: neutral.

Taste: sweet.

Action: tonifies the *Kidneys* and *yin*; maintains the *Liver* and improves the vision.

Contra-indications: superficial excess 'heat' conditions; deficient 'damp' *Spleen* conditions; diarrhoea.

Applications: this is a tonifying remedy applied specifically to deficient conditions of the *Kidneys* and *Liver* with such symptoms as impotence, pains in the loins or legs, general muscle weakness and aching, and vertigo. This tonification effect is augmented by indications for generalized deficient *yin* conditions such as sterility or frigidity, and poor eyesight or hearing.

Diabetes used to be seen as an example of such a deficiency, and an indication for lycium, and there is some pharmacological evidence of the remedy having some effect on the levels of blood sugar under experimental conditions. It would be wise to proceed with caution in actually using such a remedy with confirmed diabetes, especially if conventional hypoglycaemics are being prescribed.

Other *yin* tonics: American ginseng (*Panax quinquefolium*); Mai Men Dong (*Ophiopogon japonicus*); Nu Zhen Zi (*Ligustrum lucidum*); sesame seeds – Hei Zhi Ma (*Sesamum indicum*).

Healing Remedies

The following remedies are all used principally to promote tissue healing and reduce inflammatory damage, usually at the point of application. They often exhibit mucilaginous or tannin properties (see the chapter 'Traditional Pharmacology'), but in one or two cases there is a systemic effect as well.

CALENDULA

Calendula officinalis L.
Family: Compositae
Synonyms: marigold flowers, pot marigold, mary bud.

Description: this plant is recognized most easily for its bright orange single flowerheads, on which many complex garden varieties are based. It is, however, to be firmly distinguished from all such cultivars. It is an annual plant with an angular branched stem, with a pithy hollow core 30–60 cm high; the leaves are spatulate or oblanceolate, sessile, with widely spaced tiny teeth on the borders, and the whole covered with very short fine hairs. The flowers are borne on elegant crown-shaped receptacles, and as the petals drop off, a circular corona of seeds remains in view.

Habitat: a native of Egypt and the Mediterranean area, it has escaped from garden cultivation throughout the temperate regions of the world, and is easily naturalized. It prefers previously cultivated positions.

Parts used: the flowerheads or flower petals alone.

Cultivation: easily grown from seed in any sunny position; sow in spring; it will spread rapidly in subsequent years.

Harvesting: the flowers are collected throughout the long flowering season on dry sunny days.

Preparation: the flowers should be carefully dried so as to avoid both overheating and the retention of dampness. Bleaching of colour is a sign of poor drying technique. An infusion can be made of the dried flowers, but a tincture made at 1:5 in 90 per cent alcohol will be the only way to dissolve the important resinous fraction. Alternatively, a good calendula lotion may be made by simmering anhydrous wool fat (lanolin) with as much dried flower material as it will carry for 20–30 minutes, then sieving off the flowers and agitating until the ointment is cool and set.

Dosage: 1–4 g three times per day.

Constituents: triterpenoid saponins (sapogenin: oleonolic acid); resin; carotenoids; bitter glycosides; essential oil; sterols; flavonoids; mucilage.

Pharmacology: although not containing any tannins, this remedy is locally astringent, due mainly to the resin component but probably to other water-soluble constituents as well. One substance has been found to promote blood clotting and the whole plant acts to reduce capillary effusion; the plant clearly acts against fungal, amoebic, bacterial and even viral infections and also has potent local anti-inflammatory action as well. There are some hormonal influences stemming probably from the sterol fraction.

Action: non-tannin astringent; anti-inflammatory; local tissue healer; antipathogenic; antispasmodic.

Applications: the essential action of this remedy is in its antiseptic and anti-inflammatory healing astringency: sufficient astringency to make it an effective stauncher of bleeding. It thus finds use on its own, or with comfrey, where there are infected or slow-healing wounds or lesions, or ones discharging or bleeding too extensively. Its effectiveness (as a compress) in healing bullet wounds was reported enthusiastically by a Dr R. G. Reynolds in the American West in 1886.

For the digestive system calendula is indicated wherever there is unresolved infection or erosion in the upper tracts, particularly if there is evidence of bleeding into the gut (classically the dark stools of melaena). Obviously, in all such cases, energetic measures to establish the underlying problem will be made, but calendula tincture will help contain it in the meantime. Benefits here are augmented by the bitter quality of the plant, as evidenced by its use for jaundice and liver disease in some traditions.

There is also apparent a systemic anti-inflammatory action and it is particularly called for wherever there are swollen lymph nodes.

Calendula tincture (especially combined with another high resin tincture, myrrh) makes an effective addition to local applications to combat fungal and other infections of the vagina, or to treat broken skin surfaces in inflammatory or fungal skin conditions. It makes a powerful mouthwash to check infections of the gums, mucous membranes and throat, and in infusion form only, as an eyewash. In ointment form it is an excellent cosmetic remedy for repairing minor damage to the skin such as subdermal broken capillaries or sunburn.

COMFREY

Symphytum officinale L.
Family: Boraginaceae
Synonyms: knitbone, boneset, blackwort, bruisewort.

Description: a herbaceous plant notable for its large broadly lanceolate leaves up to 30 cm long, arising as a rosette from ground level: each has a very rough texture and is covered with short stiff hairs. From the base of the rosette arise the flowering stems reaching up to 130 cm, bearing sessile opposite leaves, each decurrent down the stem to the next leaf below. The flowers are borne in cymes on forked stalks above the top leaf, each stalk supporting short one-sided racemes of pedicillate bell-shaped mauve or white flowers curving downwards. The root is thick, quite short and very much branched from the crown, black outside with a white interior. The whole plant, and especially the root, is extremely mucilaginous on cutting and tasting. The Russian comfrey, *S. peregrinum*, is one widely grown in gardens in Britain and elsewhere, and it hybridizes freely with the common variety: it has similar clinical properties.

Habitat: on moist banks, field borders, ditches and pondsides throughout Britain, Europe and western Asia and the USA.

Parts used: the leaves and roots.

Cultivation: from the rootstock struck into almost any position, though it prefers damp and well-fertilized soil; it takes very readily, and then spreads freely to take over its corner of the garden. It is sufficient to leave only very small fragments of the root after harvesting for it to remain and grow the following year.

Harvesting: the root is best taken in the autumn, the leaves throughout the summer.

Preparation: the root should be cut into small pieces before drying, then both it and the leaves can be dried quite briskly. The root can then be decocted, the leaves infused, or a tincture may be made with either at 1:10 in 25 per cent alcohol. The plant is notable for its external applications and for this purpose the root can be incorporated into an ointment, or the leaves or root made into a poultice. An excellent form is to make a tincture or a strong decoction of the root into a 'jelly' (see 'Pharmacy', on pp. 365–87).

Dosage: 1–4 g dried root or leaves three times per day.

Constituents: allantoin; tannins; mucilage; gum; resins; pyrrolizidine alkaloids (incl. symphytine, cynoglossine, echinidine, consolidine); inulin.

Pharmacology: much of the healing effect of comfrey is known to be due to the effect of the allantoin: this promotes the constructive activity of the fibroblasts in producing connective tissue, and their near-relatives chondroblasts (cartilage) and osteoblasts (bone) and even neural cells; it promotes keratin dispersal and has been used topically with some success for the treatment of psoriasis. It thus aids the regeneration of all tissues in the body, including bone, but with the possible exception of skeletal muscle. In addition allantoin is very highly diffusable through the body and can be relied on to reach deep tissues from external application. On the surface its action is aided by the phenomenal contracting 'plaster' effect of comfrey's mucilage, tannins and resins as they dry. The aqueous extract of the plant increases the release of prostaglandins of the F series from the stomach wall, pointing to a direct action in protecting the gastric mucosa from damage.

Toxicology: the presence of hepatotoxic pyrrolizidine alkaloids in comfrey has provoked concern about the toxicity of the remedy; there is no doubt that these alkaloids are toxic, and there are even claims of toxicity of the whole plant in laboratory rats; similar experiments have also shown a protective antitumour effect in mice. Much depends on the species of comfrey used – the one discussed here is low in alkaloids; and there is the suggestion that drying and metabolizing the plant reduces the availability further. In any case the dosages used in such experiments (10–40 per cent of total diet) are vastly greater than any likely to be consumed by humans for therapeutic purposes. The leaf has been shown to have negligible quantities of the alkaloids. There are many who advocate that therapeutic use of comfrey is usually safe (see 'Are Herbs Safe?', on pp. 249–58).

References:

*Awang, D. V. C. (1987) 'Comfrey', in *Canad. Pharm. J.*, pp. 101–4

*Bone, K. M. (1984) *Studies in Materia Medica. Part 1:* Symphytum *species*, The School of Herbal Medicine, Bodle Street Green, Hailsham, Sussex, UK

Editorial in *BMJ*, 30 March 1979, p. 598

Goldman, R. S. *et al.* (1985) 'Wound healing and analgesic effect of crude extracts of *Symphytum officinale* in rats', in *Fitoterapia*, LVI, 6, pp. 323–9

Hironon, I. *et al.* (1978) 'Carcinogenic activity of *Symphytum officinale*', in *J. Nat. Cancer Inst.*, 61, 3, pp. 865–9

Kaplan, T. (1937) *JAMA*, 108, p. 968

Leung, A. Y. (1980) *Encyclopedia of Common Natural Ingredients Used in Food, Drugs, and Cosmetics*, John Wiley, New York, pp. 142–4

Loots, J. M. *et al.* (1979) *S. Afr. Med. J.*, 55, p. 53

Martindale The Extra Pharmacopoeia (1982), 28th edition

Pembury, J. A. (1982) *The Safety of Comfrey*, Henry Doubleday Research Association, Bocking, Braintree, Essex, UK

Spychalska, M. (1966) *Czasopismo Stomatologiczne*, Warsaw, 19, pp. 1297–1300

Stamford, I. F. and Tavares, I. A. (1983) 'The effect of an aqueous extract of comfrey on prostaglandin synthesis by rat isolated stomach', in *J. Pharm. Pharmacol.*, 35, pp. 816–17

Taylor, A. *et al.* (1963) *Proc. Soc. Exp. Biol. Med.*, 114, p. 772

Welsh, A. L. and Ede, M. (1959) *Ohio St. Med. J.*, 60, p. 124

Young, E. (1973) *Dermatologica*, 147, pp. 338–41

Action: stimulates tissue repair; soothing and astringent; relaxing expectorant.

Applications: comfrey is possibly the most effective healing mucilaginous remedy in the materia medica. It is very widely used to treat all manner of lesions and injuries, from small cuts and abrasions, to large wounds, bone fractures, torn cartilage, tendons or ligaments (although these last three have notoriously slow regeneration rates under any circumstances). The constant reference to bone healing in the local names of the plant bears witness to centuries of use as a poultice over broken bones in humans and domestic animals, to produce a verifiable improvement in bone healing rates.

The astringent and contracting effects of the tannins, mucilage and resins draws wounds together on the surface, and reduces the need for stitching; moreover, the allantoin stimulation of regeneration makes scar tissue formation much less likely.

Such local action is also referred to the wall of the gut. It is not surprising to find comfrey being used in the healing of ulcers and other erosive damage of the tract (oesophageal damage, inflammatory diseases of the bowel and diverticulitis are examples) where the action of the mucilage and tannins combines with other healing effects (one notes the healing prostaglandin release mentioned in the pharmacology above).

Traditional claims extended to using the plant to help 'those that spit blood, or that bleede at the mouth, or that make bloody urine: as also for all inward hurts, bruises and wounds ... the fluxes of blood, or humours by the belly, womens immoderate courses, as well the reds as whites' (Parkinson): such distal healing effects are not excluded when the high diffusibility of allantoin is taken into account. Certainly a healing effect on the lungs, as put again by Parkinson, 'helpeth the ulcers of the lungs, causing the fleagme that oppresseth them, to be easily spit forth', and can easily be explained by the mucilaginous relaxing expectorant effect we would expect.

Comfrey is also widely regarded in folklore as a treatment for arthritic conditions, taken internally as an infusion of the leaves.

WITCH HAZEL

Hamamelis virginiana L.
Family: Hamamelidaceae

Description: a small deciduous tree growing to a height of up to 5 m, with alternate elliptical, coarsely toothed leaves with prominent veins, often finely hairy underneath; drooping axillary clusters of yellow flowers appear in the autumn when the leaves are falling and give way to a woody capsule ejecting two shiny black seeds the following year. The bark is obtained as thin channelled pieces, pink-brown in colour and up to 15 cm long and 2 cm wide; occasionally covered with ash-grey fissured and scaly cork, darker in older pieces; the inner surface is pale pink and longitudinally striated, sometimes with adherent small pieces of white xylem; fracture is short in the cortex and fibrous in the phloem. The leaves are dark greenish-brown, darker on the upper surface, 5–12 cm long, brittle and fibrous, broadly oval to rhomboid-ovate; petiole 1–2 cm long, margin coarsely crenate to sinuate, with straight lateral veins. The taste of both leaves and bark is astringent and bitter.

Habitat: in damp woodland throughout eastern and central North America.

Parts used: the bark and leaves.

Cultivation: the tree may be propagated from hardwood cuttings struck in the autumn or the seeds may be planted in the autumn.

Preparation: a decoction or a tincture made at 1:5 in 25 per cent alcohol. The distilled witch hazel commonly available by definition contains no tannins.

Dosage: 1–4 g bark or leaf three times per day.

Constituents: hydrolysable and condensed tannins; flavonoids; bitter principle; volatile oil.

Pharmacology: this is a classic tannin-containing remedy exhibiting most of the properties of these constituents; there is also a toning action on the peripheral vasculature probably due to a combination of leuco-anthocyanin-like condensed tannins and the flavonoid fraction. The fact that the distilled preparation maintains some astringency suggests that there are other astringent principles not so far detected.

References:
Bernard, P. (1977) *Plantes médicinales et phytothérapie*, Angers, France, 11, p. 184
Friedrich, H. and Kruger, N. (1974) *Planta Medica*, Stuttgart, 26, p. 327

Taste: sour.

Action: astringent; toning vascular walls.

Applications: witch hazel can be applied whenever an astringent remedy is required. It thus makes an ideal application for wounds, ulcers and abrasions in any accessible location, as a wash, ointment, douche or other preparation. It makes an excellent base in eyebaths, gargles for mouth ulcers, gum problems and sore throats, and a nose-drop or snuff for hay fever and nasal catarrh and even nasal polyps.

It can also be considered a prime remedy for toxic conditions of the gut. It checks gut-wall irritation, infection and inflammation (and thus incidentally reduces the major effect of these conditions: diarrhoea) and significantly checks the virulence of pathogenic and other gut toxins. It thus finds application in enteritis, gastritis and diseases of the bowel, and even in some cases of food poisoning. (Tannins in quantity are also a standard treatment for poisoning incidents, especially those involving alkaloids.) In acute cases it may be sufficient in itself (or with the help of other remedies) to treat the problem: in chronic conditions it is obviously only a management therapy, but nevertheless very valuable in this role.

Its overall effect on the bowels is thus a relaxing one, acting to reduce activity and remove irritation. It can therefore be used as a troubleshooter for bowel upsets, helping with mucilages to control nervous bowel, helping modify the stimulating effect of an-thraquinone laxatives, and teaming very well with the aromatic carminatives in reducing colic and flatulence (for more information see 'Tannins' on pp. 282–6).

Similar remedy: tormentil root (*Potentilla erecta*).

ICELAND MOSS

Cetraria islandica (L.) Ach.
Family: Parmeliaceae
Synonym: Iceland lichen.

Description: a dried lichen with loose branching, fringed segments, 5–10 cm long and about 0.5 cm wide, with pale olive-coloured upper surface and greyish-white undersurface, the pieces curled and springy; the taste is slightly bitter and mucilaginous with little odour.

Habitat: throughout northern regions of the northern hemisphere.

Parts used: the whole lichen.

Preparation: decoction or by tincture at 1:5 in 40 per cent alcohol.

Dosage: 1–2 g three times per day.

Constituents: polysaccharides (lichenin 40 per cent, isolichenin 10 per cent); bitter lichen acids (incl. fumaroprotocetraric, protocetraric, cetraric and usnic acids).

Pharmacology: some antibiotic effects have been adduced to this remedy, the lichen acids generally considered as the main active principles; the principle action is as a straight mucilage, with the polysaccharides exerting their predictable physical properties.

References:
Huoven, K. *et al.* (1985) *Acta Pharmaceutica Fennica*, Helsinki, 99, p. 94

Temperament: neutral.

Taste: bland; slightly bitter.

Action: mucilaginous; anti-inflammatory on the gastric membrane; relaxing expectorant.

Applications: this is a prime remedy for inflammation of the stomach wall, as seen in such cases as gastritis, gastric ulceration, hiatus hernia and reflux oesophagitis. It is notably indicated in cases of low-grade stomach infections seen when there is low stomach acid production, but it is also useful in ameliorating the effects of excess stomach acid secretion.

It seems very well tolerated by even the most sensitive stomach and may also have minor nutritive benefits as well. It is difficult to find cases where it cannot be safely used.

Similar remedies: slippery elm (*Ulmus fulva*); meadowsweet (*Filipendula ulmaria*).

APPENDIXES

Clinical Index

The following clinical index summarizes a herbal approach to the treatment of many common diseases. The comments are brief and are intended to complement the more detailed descriptions in the text. *Referral to the main index is thus also recommended*, although cross-referencing within this list can also be productive. The herbs referred to are largely those described at length in the book: where other herbs are mentioned their botanical names are added.

The assumption is always made that other forms of treatment, dietary, manipulative and conventional medical as well as exercise will be applied concurrently where necessary, and none of the recommendations should be seen as substituting for a thorough appraisal of each individual patient.*

To help grade conditions for their severity and the appropriateness of herbal treatment a code of symbols is applied. *These are for general guidance only and must not be taken as a recommendation for treatment or otherwise in any individual case.*

Symbols

* **generally not serious and often self-correcting; quite suitable for home treatment but care is necessary if the symptoms persist longer than usual or if they develop into others that are more severe – they should then be referred to a doctor or well-trained medical**

---

*For a comparison of the different approaches to particular problems, covering the major complementary therapies as well as conventional medicine, with comments on a range of common medical problems by a herbalist, homoeopath, acupuncturist, osteopath/naturopath, chiropractor and a doctor, see: Mills, S.Y. (ed.) (1988) *Alternatives in Healing*, Macmillan, London.

herbalist; some in this category are not considered medical problems at all and would not usually get treatment from a doctor;

** often not serious but possibly difficult to treat; it sometimes disguises a problem that is dangerous: any reluctance to clear up should lead to referral to a doctor or well-trained medical herbalist;

*** potentially dangerous: any home treatment should only proceed after an expert diagnosis and prognosis has been established, and then if possible only after consultation with the doctor and an expert medical herbalist;

**** serious condition that needs immediate medical treatment or close attention by doctors: not for home treatment at all.

abscess **/****

All but the most simple should be referred to medical treatment, as in some parts of the body (especially the head area) they can be critically dangerous. Chronic abscesses are often tubercular or may follow malignancy or other serious conditions. Expert herbal treatment might include the use of myrrh, echinacea, wild indigo, marigold and arbor-vitae.

acne *

Herbal treatment usually concentrates on providing eliminative remedies, checking bile and bowel function in particular; if the condition persists after adolescence, then hormonal adaptogens might be used.

acne rosacea **

May be linked with disturbed digestive and liver and hormonal functions, and herbal treatment will tend to concentrate on these areas; alcohol and tea are often exacerbatory.

Addison's disease ***

Atrophy of the cells of the adrenal cortex which produce steroidal hormones, including the stress hormones such as cortisone. The symptoms are severe anaemia and debility, wasting and pigmentation. Originally described in 1855, it has become much more common in modern times as a result of over-prescription of steroid drugs. A case has been reported of the condition being reversed with the administration of large amounts of liquorice.

adenoid trouble *
Will tend to obstruct breathing through the nose but removal should be considered the measure of last resort and there are usually effective herbal approaches. See also **throat problems** and **catarrh**.

alcoholism ***
Bitter and other hepatic remedies are often prescribed with some success for both the immediate effects of alcohol consumption and as part of the often rigorous drying-out and recuperative regime; they may also optimize damaged liver functions in those seriously affected.

allergy */**
Allergic syndromes include allergic eczema, hay fever, nettle rash, asthma or classic food allergies. Even when not immediately implicated, isolation of an early food allergy can often help reduce other allergic symptoms; the herbalist will look at other digestive functions as well, and bitters are often indicated.

alopecia areata **
Patches of sudden hair loss, mainly in adolescents and young adults; the cause is unknown. Spontaneous recovery is usual although regrown hair may be lighter. Herbal treatment concentrates on improving any debilitated conditions, and notably diseases of the teeth, gums or throat; signs of hormonal turbulence might also point to appropriate treatment, and relaxants and nerve restoratives might be indicated.

anaemia **
There are many possible causes: the most notable is excessive loss of blood, as in excessive menstrual bleeding, childbirth and gastro-intestinal disease. Replacement of even normal blood turnover may also be inadequate if dietary iron intake is low or there are factors interfering with its assimilation. In all such cases an improved iron

intake is essential, either through foods or supplements. Green turnip tops and parsley are notable sources from the plant world. Anaemia may also be caused through some other disease, such as haemolytic disease, poisoning or disease of the bone marrow. An inability to metabolize vitamin B12 leads to the formerly fatal pernicious anaemia.

angina pectoris ***
Although primarily a functional disorder, there is always the risk of permanent damage to the coronary muscle, so-called coronary infarction, or heart attack. A qualified herbal practitioner might use hawthorn or motherwort (*Leonurus cardiaca*) as part of a wider regime of treatment which takes account of all other medical priorities.

ankylosing spondylitis ***
A form of autoimmune disease rather like rheumatoid arthritis which affects particularly the spine and ribcage, sometimes with progressively debilitating results; young men make up the majority of sufferers. An inherited white-blood-cell type is a known factor but other unknown factors are also involved. Cross-reactivity with sub-clinical infections involving the bacteria *Klebsiella* has been established as a cause; elimination of starch products from the diet is worth trying for several weeks. The medical herbalist will in any case look for evidence of any prior infection anywhere in the body, especially in the urinary system, lungs and gut and for any sign of disturbance in the functions of the latter. Remedies and strategies aimed at cleansing such trouble spots can have benefit for the course of the disease. See also **autoimmune disease**.

anorexia **
Loss of appetite, an accompaniment of many diseases. It is a positive sign in acute conditions like fever, a worrying complication in chronic debilitating illness. Use of bitters is often indicated to improve both the appetite and the underlying digestion.

anorexia nervosa ***
A loss of appetite resulting from a complex disturbance of self-image and emotional relationships. It most often affects adolescent girls and young women; it can be serious, even fatal. Treatment

should be very broad-based, emphasizing support and care for the sufferer; herbs like condurango (*Marsdenia condurango*) or other bitters, or the relaxants may be used profitably if the patient will accept them.

anxiety */**
A range of symptoms that can result from unduly high levels of adrenaline in the blood. If excessive or long-standing, they may be relieved by the use of relaxants combined with such restorative remedies as oatstraw, vervain and damiana.

appendicitis ***
Typically of sudden onset with severe pains in the umbilical region moving to the right lower abdomen; it may however be less dramatic and may occur intermittently, with sensitivity midway between the umbilicus and hip bone on the right side (McBurney's point) as a classic indication. 'Grumbling appendix' is probably diagnosed more often than is justified. Where the condition is not acute it may be appropriate to provide herbal treatment: agrimony (*Agrimonia officinalis*) is a classic remedy for the intermittent condition, especially in children; other astringents and carminatives are also indicated.

appetite, lack of see anorexia

arrhythmia ***
Variation in the regular rhythm of the heartbeat, including fibrillation, extrasystole and tachycardia. May vary from the fatal condition to just reducing maximum heart capacity in exertion and stress. Conventional heart drugs will most often be prescribed and any herbal treatment will have to be most cautiously administered, and only by an expert medical herbalist: in practice hawthorn and lily-of-the-valley will be among the most widely used.

arteriosclerosis ***
Apart from attending to dietary factors the herbalist might use peripheral vasodilatory remedies, particularly hawthorn, lime-flowers and ginkgo, for their ability to improve circulation and oxygenation. Garlic has a combined vasodilatory and fat- and cholesterol-reducing action that makes it an obvious candidate: the

odourless capsules may be used for this purpose.

arthritis **/***

As it is a feature of many types of inflammatory disease the herbal approach will not be standard. It can range from symptomatic anti-inflammatories to the concerted and subtle assessment and treatment of underlying causative factors. A frequent approach is to use eliminative remedies, particularly those with diuretic properties, and circulatory stimulants (sometimes powerful examples applied locally as counter-irritants). See also **autoimmune disease**.

asthma ***

Symptomatic relief of asthma used to rely on the smoking of members of the deadly nightshade family such as datura and henbane, but conventional inhalants have made these potentially dangerous remedies unnecessary. Medical herbalists may still apply them with extreme discretion but will usually use lobelia or Ma Huang as tinctures for a symptomatic relief of tension; grindelia (*Grindelia* spp.), skunk cabbage (*Symplocarpus foetidus*), euphorbia (*Euphorbia hirta*), bloodroot and sundew (*Drosera rotundifolia*) are other professional tools. General application of relaxing expectorants and antispasmodics is also likely and a wide review of background factors will be useful. See also **allergy**.

atherosclerosis see **arteriosclerosis**

athlete's foot *

Usually responds to external treatment with tincture of myrrh, calendula or arbor-vitae. If it does not, then a more deep-seated difficulty will have to be assumed.

autoimmune disease ***

The herbal approach is to start with the obvious pathology and then work backwards and outwards, looking for prior or parallel disturbances that might provide exacerbation to the inflammation. Signs of clinical or sub-clinical infections or other alterations of tissue microclimate are especially promising and echinacea, wild indigo, calendula and specific antimicrobials are then likely to be applied. Other eliminative remedies usually figure large; digestive, hepatic and circulatory remedies may also find a useful place.

babies' problems */****
For babies still feeding from the breast the herbalist has always preferred to treat the mother, relying on the high extraction rate from blood to milk for the remedy to reach the baby that way. Aromatic remedies with high volatile oil content are most favoured and mother-to-baby transmission is assured. If direct prescription is necessary, only the most gentle remedies are applied, with relaxants like chamomile and limeflowers finding especial favour. Dosage should be a quarter of the adult dose or less.

backache **
The herbalist complements manipulative treatment by administering remedies to reduce muscle tension and/or any inflammation. This might be either through topical application with embrocations or liniments or by treating it as a systemic problem (as for arthritis, for example).

baldness *
Most often an unavoidable ageing symptom in men. It is occasionally possible to defer loss by vigorous steps to increase scalp circulation and a number of irritative plant extracts have sometimes been used for this purpose: general prospects must however be poor. Scalp hygiene and care is always advantageous and sage and rosemary infusions are useful rinses; quillaia, or soap bark (*Quillaia saponaria*), has an especial reputation as a cleanser. Treatment of any concurrent eczema is particularly useful, and baldness may of course be the result of disease or hormonal disturbance. See also **alopecia areata** and **dandruff**.

bed-wetting **
The use of herbal relaxants may usefully reduce the effect of ambient anxiety, antispasmodics like cramp bark may reduce bladder irritability; providing gentle diuretics early in the day, like couch grass, corn silk, marshmallow or horsetail can be an effective component of a wider regime aimed at co-ordinating bladder diurnal rhythms.

bilious attacks see **gastritis** and **migraine**

bladder problems see **urinary infections** and **urinary stones**

boils **

Treated in the first instance with such eliminatives as burdock and echinacea, as part of a broader regime that encourages resolution from within. If boils are persistent, the possibility of kidney disease or diabetes must be eliminated and other causes of debility should be tackled: disturbances of digestion and liver function are particularly frequent.

breast disease ***

This complex glandular tissue is prone to many types of inflammatory problems ranging from simple fibrous changes, chronic cystic mastitis, fat necrosis, cysts, papilloma, to carcinoma in its many forms. Expert diagnosis is always essential. If there is scope for conservative treatment, a range of alteratives and eliminatives with long popular traditions may be selected, including sweet violet leaves, red clover flowers, marigold flowers, wild thyme and arbor-vitae. The professional practitioner should pay close attention to the wider landscape, with particular regard for other toxic and hormonal conditions. Acute mastitis, found commonly in lactating mothers, may be treated with soothing poultices of linseed, and internally with echinacea, marigold or fresh garlic. See also **cancer**.

bronchiectasis ***

Usual postural drainage and other lung-clearing techniques can be augmented by the use of warming or stimulating expectorants. See also **bronchitis**.

bronchitis ***

The aim of herbal treatment is to promote the clearing of congested mucus and, if possible, reduce its production. To this end warming and stimulating expectorants are used, often in considerable quantities: remedies such as fresh garlic, fresh ginger, cinnamon, horseradish, angelica root, elecampane and, by practitioners only, lobelia; these are often combined for good effect with liquorice. Relaxing expectorants are not generally encouraged, although there are some, such as mullein flowers, coltsfoot flowers and thyme with other redeeming properties that might be applied. There are usually other predisposing weaknesses and especial care is needed with the cardiovascular system. Dietary measures would include a tight restriction on consumption of alcohol, caffeine, milk products and refined carbohydrates. Smoking should of course be banned.

Buerger's disease ***

A potentially serious disease of the circulation, most often affecting the legs. Herbal remedies might include hawthorn, limeflowers, angelica and wild yam for the immediate symptoms. See also **Raynaud's disease.**

bulimia nervosa see anorexia nervosa

burns */****

For first-degree burns relief may be had (after immediate immersion in cold water) by applying the red oil obtained from steeping St John's wort flowers in sunflower seed oil in sunlight for two weeks. For more serious burns medical treatment should be sought immediately; as a first-aid measure when no such facilities exist, washing the wound with a strong lukewarm solution of tannins will form a seal, or eschar, to protect against infections and fluid loss. A decoction of oak bark, oak galls or the bark of many other broad-leaved trees will be effective.

calculi see urinary stones and gall-bladder disease

cancer ***

As part of a broad strategy to promote body defences against malignant cells, the herbalist may call on the full range of treatments according to the needs of the individual patient. Most often such treatment will be given alongside conventional chemo- or radio-therapy; in some cases the patient will have made a decision not to pursue conventional treatment. This is a serious decision and should be supported by the most fair advice: the professional medical herbalist will not claim too much for the herbal option. Prominent in herbal prescriptions will be eliminative and alterative remedies, particularly violet leaves, red clover, cleavers, marigold, echinacea and (particularly where radiotherapy is being employed) arbor-vitae and buckwheat leaves. Tonics for the digestion, circulation and nervous system are also often employed. Care should be taken to choose only such remedies as the constitution can take: cancer is often debilitating, some conventional treatments for it even more so; many of the more vigorous remedies may upset a weakened constitution and be counter-productive. The choice should thus be left to the experts.

Candidiasis see **thrush**

carbuncles see **boils**

catarrh */**
When accompanying an acute condition like a common cold or flu, excessive mucus secretion is most often the mark of a vigorous defence in the airways and need not always be considered a problem as such. It is often very uncomfortable and there is a big market in conventional antihistamines to relieve such symptoms: herbal relief can be had either by treating the cold as a whole, or by inhalations, in steam or directly, of volatile oils like aniseed and pine (menthol and eucalyptus are also effective but should not be used for too long). When catarrh is persistent other factors clearly operate and treatment should be fundamental. There are two distinct approaches, each appropriate to a different type of catarrh. The first, and more common, was traditionally termed 'cold': it is found in those of sluggish metabolism who like stodgy and sweet food and dairy products; the catarrh tends to be watery and non-coloured, the mucous membranes pale and puffy; it is often associated with bronchitis. Treatment will emphasize circulatory stimulants, often of a vigorous nature. The second type of catarrh, the 'hot' type, is linked with an active constitution and high metabolic rate, possibly a nervous or anxious personality; the catarrh is thicker and more scanty and often coloured; the mucous membranes more inflamed. A concurrent hay fever, asthma or other allergic condition is frequent. Background treatment may concentrate on giving bitters, relaxants or even sedatives. In all cases of catarrh, bowel elimination is critical and should be checked for; any prior source of infection or inflammation in the body must also be positively vetted. General remedies for catarrh, to accompany any of the above strategies, might include ground ivy, wood betony (*Stachys betonica*), hyssop, eyebright (*Euphrasia officinalis*), elderflower, ribwort, and golden rod (*Solidago virgaurea*). Attention to diet is rarely wasted effort.

cervical problems **/***
Apart from excluding and perhaps attending to possibly serious

underlying disease the herbalist will often employ astringent and healing herbs as douches. See also **vaginal problems**.

chicken pox **
Usually self-limiting, although the virus can give rise to shingles in adults; treatment is on the whole conservative, with fever management and convalescent strategies predominating; relaxants and topically soothing remedies may help reduce itching.

chilblains *
The treatment of this minor form of frostbite aims to reduce spasm of the small blood vessels: measures to reduce dramatic changes in temperature can be reinforced by the use of peripheral vasodilators and moderate circulatory stimulants.

children's illnesses */****
Herbs are often very appropriate for the treatment of everyday children's problems, combining supportive gentleness with firm effect; the main difficulty can be in getting children to accept their taste. It is particularly important to monitor children's diseases closely: their constitution predisposes to sharp changes in fortune; their diseases are more likely to be acute and rapidly shifting. On the other hand there is no greater need to counter tendency for a condition to become chronic: the widespread use of antibiotics and other conventional drugs in the treatment of acute children's conditions has led to a new and depressing wave of persistent problems for which drugs are almost counter-productive. The goal in herbal treatment is to combine restorative and appropriately relaxing remedies to both nurture and calm, using those herbs with sufficient gentleness in appreciable doses; for many the adult dose is quite possible, though a general guide would be to start with a quarter of the adult dose up to the age of two years, going up to a third to half the adult dose around the ages of eight to ten, then quickly rising to the adult regime soon after puberty. For most complaints relaxing remedies like chamomile, limeflowers, lemon balm and peppermint are almost central to treatment; liquorice is recommended as a valuable flavouring agent with particular benefits for chest and stomach conditions; for coughs hyssop and elderflowers are also recommended; for stomach upsets also chamomile, lemon

balm, peppermint, cinnamon, fennel and dill; catarrhal conditions will often respond to ground ivy, ribwort and elderflower; urinary problems to couch grass or corn silk; nervous exhaustion to oats and oatstraw, vervain, angelica and chamomile; cold and 'cold illnesses' to angelica, cinnamon, cardamom and fresh ginger; constipation must never be treated with stimulating laxatives: chamomile, fennel, peppermint and other relaxants are indicated instead.

cold, common *

Although viruses are the usual precipitating agents the herbal approach to the cold is as a weakness in mucosal defences, with the symptoms themselves as evidence of a vigorous counter-attack by the body. Constitutional evidence is thus more important than focusing on infective organisms. Initial treatment is as for catarrh, with the emphasis most likely to be on the 'cold' type: in practice such a cold may be held at bay or even eliminated by frequent sipping of a cup of hot water with cinnamon and fresh ginger with fresh lemon juice.

cold sores see herpes

colic **

This may be of simple origin, treated as a symptom of flatulence or nervous bowel, or may indicate a more serious condition such as gut infection, adhesions, appendicitis, strangulated hernia, lead poisoning, gall-bladder disease, urinary stones, painful menstruation or the complications of pregnancy.

colitis, mucous see nervous bowel

colitis, ulcerative ***

As an autoimmune disorder this should be treated as of much wider origin than a bowel pathology, and herbal treatment can thus be complex: for the pathology itself astringent and mucilaginous remedies may be combined with visceral relaxants. Conventional drug treatment is generally used to contain more violent symptoms and will only be withdrawn if the condition subsides. Close examination of the possibility of food intolerances and a strict exclusion of abrasive foods are usually essential.

constipation *
Lack of bowel movement through poor tone is best treated with a combination of high, though not necessarily rough, fibre intake and short-term use of stimulating laxatives like cascara, senna and alder buckthorn; constipation arising as a result of visceral tension responds much better to relaxants like wild yam, hops, peppermint and chamomile, given with soft mucilaginous fibre such as psyllium seed and linseed.

cough */**
The herbalist does not view coughing as essentially a problem: rather it is seen as a vigorous effort by the body to expel congestion or irritation in the airways of the lungs. If a cough is persistent, this suggests that it is not being successful: rather than stopping the cough the herbalist seeks to make it more efficient. Expectorants are remedies that make the cough more productive and thus less necessary. Stimulating and warming expectorants like ginger, garlic, angelica, elecampane, squills, cowslip, white horehound and ipeca-cuanha are applied to congested bronchial and catarrhal, 'cold' chestiness; relaxing expectorants like thyme, hyssop, and the mucila-ginous remedies such as ribwort, marshmallow, comfrey and colts-foot are better applied to tight, dry, irritable coughs; liquorice, mullein flowers and, in expert hands, lobelia have a broad range of expectorant properties. If a cough is clearly counter-productive (as in solely nervous coughing or when there is an immovable irritant such as an injury or tumour), then antitussive remedies like wild cherry bark may be justified.

Crohn's disease ***
The approaches outlined for ulcerative colitis are appropriate here.

croup see laryngitis

cystitis see urinary infections

dandruff *
Scalp hygiene can be improved by using quillaia or soap bark (*Quillaia saponaria*) infusion after washing, but the herbalist will concentrate on internal treatment to reduce the excessive secretions from the hair root that sustain the bacterial infection: appropriate alteratives are used.

dental problems **

In support of conventional tooth hygiene and dentistry the herbalist is able to offer a number of antiseptic and astringent mouthwashes with remedies such as thyme, blackberry leaf (*Rubus fructicosus*), witch hazel, tormentil root and strong alcoholic tinctures of myrrh and marigold blended with fluid extract of liquorice. These are likely to be especially effective for gum disease and accessible infections.

depression **

The traditional view of clinical depression was as a whole-body disorder (the Greeks chose the word '*melancholia*' from their words for black and bile). The herbalist will be keen to help digestive and metabolic functions as well as to attend to the neurological symptoms. In this latter case the emphasis is on restorative remedies rather than on conventional ideas of antidepressants (actually having a sedative effect): herbs such as oatstraw, vervain, St John's wort and damiana are used consistently for weeks or months; Asiatic ginseng and other Oriental adaptogens may be used productively with more discretion.

diabetes mellitus ***/****

When contracted earlier in life diabetes is usually relatively dramatic and dependence on insulin injections more likely: the nature of the balance in blood-sugar control means that intervention in the condition without close monitoring by the patient's physician is inadvisable. Late-onset diabetes is often more gradual in its course: dietary control is often sufficient to avoid insulin administration; at this stage herbal treatment may be valuable. Supplementing a high-fibre intake with selective use of bitters and aromatic digestive remedies, and such hypoglycaemic foods as leafy greens, nuts and root vegetables can be particularly productive; the fibre from the guar bean has been established as particularly able to retain sugar in the gut.

diarrhoea **/***

The single most common cause of death in the world, particularly among children in developing countries; the main dangers of dehydration and electrolyte loss are less likely risks in affluent countries. In fact, a transient bowel looseness is often seen as a healthy sign of elimination in herbal treatment. Nevertheless, care should be exercised that the symptom does not become prolonged or excessive, and if this is the case the possibility of such diseases as ulcerative colitis, Crohn's disease, diverticulitis or bowel cancer (the existence of food poisoning, gastro-enteritis or dysentery is usually obvious from other signs) should be considered. If the diarrhoea is benign, it may be managed with the use of astringents such as tormentil root, witch hazel, oak bark or galls, rhatany (*Krameria triandra*) and the many others containing appreciable quantities of tannins.

diverticulitis **
Apart from avoiding rough fibre like bran, rough grains and nuts, the most effective treatment for the bowel with this condition is mucilaginous and astringent herbs applied whole in capsules or tablets: comfrey, ground linseed and marigold are especially recommended.

drug addiction **
The use of herbal 'detox' regimes is well established in some clinics, especially in the USA. Hepatic remedies, cholagogues and laxatives feature strongly, although any eliminative remedy may be used. Valuable support in the period of withdrawal and afterwards may be had in the use of Chinese tonic remedies, nervous restoratives and with discretion such stimulants as kola; the Indian remedy gotu kola (*Centella asiatica*) has been particularly favoured.

dysentery ***
Although ulcerative colitis is sometimes referred to as non-infective dysentery, this condition usually involves bacillary or amoebic infection. It is a potentially very serious condition and blood tests are necessary afterwards to rule out the possibility of long-term amoebic infection. Aftercare with garlic, bitters and mucilaginous and astringent healing remedies is often helpful. See also **diarrhoea**.

dyspepsia */**
If following a non-serious condition of the digestive system, it should be readily relieved with one or more of the following strategies: bitter digestive remedies; carminatives and aromatic digestive remedies; mucilaginous healing herbs such as marshmallow, Iceland

moss, liquorice, meadowsweet, comfrey or marigold; relaxants such as chamomile, lemon balm or peppermint. The last two categories are generally the most predictably effective: the first two are the most effective in the long term if the right combination can be found. Gastritis, peptic ulceration, hiatus hernia, liver or gall-bladder disease or cancer are among the serious and intractable causes of dyspepsia.

ear problems **
There are three chambers of the ear: practical treatment is only possible for the outer, open to the exterior, and the middle ear on the further side of the eardrum, connected to the throat by the Eustachian tube. The inner ear, containing the sensory apparatus and connected directly to the balance organs and the brain, is generally inaccessible to direct herbal treatment. Infections, inflammations and irritation in the outer ear, as well as catarrhal problems of the middle ear, may be treated with ear-drops. Olive oil, or similar, is used as a vehicle: to this may be added such agents as mullein flowers, garlic, marigold, comfrey or chickweed (*Stellaria media*), according to the problem. Care is necessary in all such applications to ensure that the eardrum is undamaged. Congested conditions of the middle ear and Eustachian tube, often giving earache, should be treated as variations of upper respiratory catarrh: inhalations may be particularly effective here. See also **catarrh**.

eczema **
The herbalist looks principally for internal factors in skin inflammations, even those which have an obvious allergic component: this means that medicines are more likely to be prescribed than just external lotions. Traditional remedies were often eliminatives and alteratives, and 'blood cleansing' was most often considered to be indicated for skin disease: such remedies still dominate in treatment today; relaxant remedies are appropriate where nervous and emotional tension are exacerbatory. External applications emphasize the use of soothing and anti-inflammatory herbs: a great many have been traditionally applied. Dietary experiments, especially geared towards establishing the presence of masked food allergies, are often productive, notably in children.

571 Clinical Index

enuresis see **bed-wetting**

epilepsy ***/****
Herbs with relaxant and sedative effects have been used to contain both *petit mal* and *grand mal* attacks but their performance in controlling the condition is not always assured, and particular care in their prescription is necessary.

eye problems **/***
Treatment of the eye is best confined to problems of the surface, such as conjunctivitis, blepharitis and styes. Eyebaths are applicable, using such remedies as eyebright (*Euphrasia officinalis*), liquorice, fennel, agrimony (*Agrimonia officinalis*), chamomile, raspberry leaves and marigold, all prepared by decoction and applied fresh. Where such problems are due to allergic conditions, colds, debility or other illness, these should be treated as well. Iritis, or inflammation of the iris, is often an extension of a wider inflammatory disease, especially autoimmune disease, gonorrhoea, diabetes and tuberculosis, or even infection of the mouth, gums, throat or sinuses: it will only be affected by the successful treatment of such root causes. Problems of the internal eye, such as glaucoma, cataracts, retinal problems and other sources of blindness are not easily approached by herbal treatment.

fever **/***
The essential goal in the herbalist's treatment of feverish conditions is management rather than suppression: the treatment is geared to helping the body through its fever, shortening the process by improving its efficiency, reducing uncomfortable symptoms associated with it, and providing convalescent support in its aftermath. There are well-established nursing techniques that should be applied, and these are particularly well suited to combining with herbal strategies. Peripheral vasodilatory remedies are well suited to the early stages of temperature control (aiming to maintain a body temperature of 38–39°C (approx. 101–102°F) through the course of the fever); bitters may be used to cool more firmly; circulatory stimulants are used to stir up a sluggish febrile response (as often seen in modern affluent conditions); relaxants and antispasmodics are often indicated for the tensions, pain, spasms and even convulsions sometimes found;

expectorants and diuretics may be used to ease appropriate eliminations; bitters are often effective in reducing gut-centred toxicities; astringent remedies may reduce the virulence of any diarrhoea. After the fever has broken satisfactorily, a considerable period of convalescence is advisable, using restorative and tonic herbs accordingly.

fibroids **

Containment and, occasionally, reduction of fibroids can be achieved by the use of such remedies as helonias root, blue cohosh, agnus castus, damiana, motherwort (*Leonurus cardiaca*) and black cohosh. Surgical removal is sometimes unavoidable.

fibrositis see myalgia

fissure **

Treatment is the same as for an open wound or ulcer, though the position of the fissure may cause difficulties; if there is an anal fissure, mucilaginous bulk laxatives may help to soften the stool.

flatulence */**

If of short-term duration, as when it is the result of dietary indiscretion, the use of carminatives is indicated. Other causes may have to be deduced from other clues and treated at source. Unconscious air-swallowing is one of the most common causes and may be helped by relaxant remedies. Nervous dyspepsia, nervous bowel, poor digestion, excessive laxative use and food intolerances are other common causes. Gall-bladder disease, gastritis, ulcers or other serious diseases may be implicated, though usually with other symptoms.

food allergies **

To complement food elimination strategies, the herbal practitioner will often have recourse to bitter and aromatic digestives to help support digestive secretions and other functions; astringent herbs, such as those containing tannin, or marigold or golden seal may also be used where there is any suggestion of damage to the gut-wall lining.

food poisoning **/***

Bacterial or other pathogenic infection of the gut may be prevented in countries where there is a high risk by eating hot spices or bitters. Many of the incidents of such infection pass off spontaneously, if painfully; others are serious and require expert care. In all cases recovery can be aided by digestive tonics such as yarrow, agrimony (*Agrimonia officinalis*), bayberry, angelica, elecampane, garlic and slippery elm. Toxic or chemical food poisoning usually requires immediate medical help: taking emetics or large quantities of tannin-containing remedies may be options in certain cases.

fractures ***
External application of comfrey is specific, provided of course access is possible to the site.

gall-bladder disease **
Infection (cholecystitis) and the formation of gallstones are the two most common conditions affecting the gall-bladder. Both are linked to biliary constituents or contaminants and the herbal strategy has traditionally been to provoke an increased bile flow, thereby diluting and reducing their impact. Cholagogues, that are often also bitters, are used around the world for these problems: notable examples include dandelion root, yellow dock root, barberry bark, greater celandine, golden seal, artichoke and boldo (*Peumus boldo*). Several of these herbs are powerful and the treatment of these conditions often requires care, particularly if gallstones are liable to be flushed out.

gastritis **
Inflammation of the stomach wall may be transient or mild, or may herald more serious conditions like ulceration or cancer. Particular care should be given to dietary measures and the sharp restriction of smoking, alcohol and caffeine. Herbal soothing remedies with particular reputation for gastritis include Iceland moss, meadowsweet, liquorice, marigold, gum myrrh, comfrey, golden seal and cinnamon.

glandular fever **
Seriously underestimated by many modern doctors this viral infection can leave a long legacy of debility, compromised immunity and vulnerability to illness unless recuperation is ensured. This involves a programme of convalescence over weeks or even months, including substantial bedrest wherever possible, and other supportive measures. Herbal remedies with especial benefit in boosting

recovery include echinacea, marigold, angelica, cleavers, wild indigo and fenugreek.

goitre see **thyroid disease**

gout **
Apart from dietary measures, levels of uric acid in the bloodstream may be reduced by celery seed and nettles; other diuretic and anti-inflammatory herbs may also be used.

gravel see **urinary stones**

gum disease **
An improved general mouth hygiene is a high priority. There is also often a requirement for broad-based systemic treatment, especially if tooth roots or bone are involved. Effective mouth-washes that reduce inflammation and improve gum health include thyme, tormentil root, witch hazel, sage, blackberry leaf (*Rubus fructicosus*), and tinctures of gum myrrh and marigold mixed with liquid extract of liquorice.

haemorrhoids *
There are two main approaches to pursue. Topically, astringent herbs, such as tormentil, witch hazel, pilewort (*Ranunculus ficaria*), rhatany (*Krameria triandra*) and comfrey, applied especially in the form of gel, will help contain and possibly shrink the varicose swelling. The use of gentle aperients or bulking laxatives, along with dietary and other measures, will help the haemorrhoids in the long term by easing bowel movements.

hay fever *
The medical herbalist will supplement other prophylactic measures by the use of herbal remedies with a tradition for improving mucosal health such as ribwort, ground ivy, golden rod (*Solidago virgaurea*), cudweed or golden seal: this builds on the assumption that penetration of the mucosal barrier by the allergen is a necessary first step. Ma Huang may also be used to reduce sensitivity, but the priority will be to develop systemic constitutional treatment to reduce inherent susceptibility.

headache */***
Most cases are transient, even if frequent, but some headaches may
be a sign of more dangerous conditions and any frequent and
severe headaches should be checked. Strategies for the less severe
cases might include remedies that regulate peripheral blood vessels,
like limeflowers, yarrow, wood betony (*Stachys betonica*), self-heal,
rosemary and other peripheral vasodilators. Oil of lavender applied
externally will have comparable effects. Relaxants, antispasmodics
and sedatives may be used as appropriate. Feverfew may be used
symptomatically for migrainous headaches marked by vascular constriction, possibly augmented by other warming remedies; 'hot'
headaches may by contrast be better treated by bitter herbs and,
for short periods, stimulating laxatives. Other eliminative remedies
may be effective in other cases where a toxic factor can be implicated.

heartburn see **hyperacidity**

heart problems ***
Well-qualified herbalists may use a number of herbs with established effects on the heart: lily-of-the-valley is the herbalist's
favoured alternative to digoxin derived from foxglove. More gentle
and sustained remedies such as hawthorn, motherwort (*Leonurus
cardiaca*) and rosemary are indicated for arrhythmias and anginal
conditions. Non-qualified persons are well advised to leave such
conditions well alone.

hepatitis ***
The first approach to most cases, whether viral, bacterial or toxic
in origin, is to apply gentle hepatic remedies such as dandelion,
milk thistle seed, artichoke or yellow dock root. These will be
unlikely to provoke the condition and should be effective. More
definitely bitter cholagogues (see **gall-bladder disease**) should be
used only by expert practitioners. Sustained convalescent care after
the attack is often important.

herpes **
More specifically, herpes simplex, to distinguish it from herpes
zoster, or shingles. Most often seen as 'cold sores' around the

mouth, but in another variant as sexually transmitted genital herpes. Herbal treatment is directed mainly to restorative strategies, using such remedies as oatstraw, vervain, damiana, and the adaptogens like ginseng and other such Oriental herbs. Echinacea is useful in promoting the body's defences, and may be augmented by eliminative remedies where appropriate. The prognosis is that outbreaks may be contained quite successfully.

herpes zoster see **shingles**

hiatus hernia *
Reduction in the irritation and reflux resulting from acid spilling into the gullet may follow the taking of slippery elm after meals. See also **hyperacidity**.

high blood pressure ***
Herbal approaches to this mysterious condition include the use of relaxing vasodilators like hawthorn, limeflowers, yarrow and cramp bark, diuretic herbs, and calming remedies like passionflower, valerian and hops. The use of herbs that improve liver-bile and bowel function where appropriate can be surprisingly effective.

hives see **nettle rash**

hot flushes see **menopause**

hyperacidity *
Several herbs will directly help to reduce acid production in the stomach, such as slippery elm, meadowsweet, marshmallow, liquorice and Iceland moss. They may be usefully augmented by relaxants like chamomile, lemon balm and peppermint in tea form. Dietary and other intake should be carefully vetted, but often more broad-based systemic treatments are necessary to get to the root of the problem.

hypoglycaemia (reactive) *
Low blood-sugar levels especially soon after eating (as witnessed by cravings for sugar, sweets and chocolate), may be directly eliminated by taking strong bitters during an attack. These may usefully complement a dietary programme aimed at substituting complex, wholegrain carbohydrates for refined flour and sugar.

impetigo ∗∗
As this is notoriously infectious, isolation from other children is essential; it will generally correct itself anyway but attention to nourishment and the use of herbal eliminatives and alteratives will probably help recovery.

impotence ∗∗
In a number of cases restorative remedies like damiana, saw palmetto and ginseng can be perhaps surprisingly effective, best used in short-term regimes; they may also be combined with appropriate relaxants in cases where tension is a factor.

indigestion see **dyspepsia**

infectious parotitis see **mumps**

infertility ∗∗
In the woman, infertility due to ovarian dysfunction (as manifested perhaps in irregular or upset periods) can often be corrected with the use of helonias root, agnus castus and Dang Gui. Where pelvic inflammation is a factor, this may also be relieved (see **pelvic inflammation (chronic)**). In the man, damiana, saw palmetto, oatstraw and sarsaparilla have a reputation for increasing fertility.

inflammation ∗∗
The herbalist sees this as essentially a healthy defence and cleansing response. Problems arise if it is excessive, and particularly if it becomes a chronic, and thus ineffective, response. Even in such cases, the concern is not to suppress the inflammation but to help make it unnecessary. The herbal treatment of such examples as arthritis, skin disease, chronic 'infections', the autoimmune diseases and diverticulitis is marked by an emphasis on remedies that improve circulation to the area (circulatory stimulants or rubefacients), or have alterative or eliminative properties (such as digestive stimulants, laxatives, diuretics and expectorants) – these often directed to toxic conditions at places other than the immediate problem.

influenza ∗∗
Herbal treatment primarily involves normal fever management with special emphasis on herbs such as elderflowers, garlic, ginger, horseradish, echinacea and expectorant remedies.

insomnia *

Although the herbalist will have recourse to relaxant and sedative herbs to help sleeping, a more long-term strategy will be the preferred aim. This will often involve the use of restorative herbs (such as oatstraw, vervain and St John's wort), especially if the difficulty is worse in the early morning, attention will have to be paid to all other health matters.

intermittent claudication **

Treated as an aspect of arteriosclerosis with peripheral vasodilators prominent. Hawthorn and prickly ash (*Zanthoxylum americanum*) have particular reputations. Also see **arteriosclerosis**.

itching see **pruritus**

jaundice ***

A common symptom of hepatitis or other liver disease, it may follow blockage of the bile ducts from stones or, less frequently, cancer; it may also result from drug prescription or abuse or from poisoning and may occasionally accompany pneumonia or yellow fever. In babies it is very common and usually harmless. Treatment will obviously be tailored to the cause so must depend on an expert diagnosis.

kidney diseases ***

Damage to the kidney structures presents particular problems for the herbalist as many herbal products are excreted through this route and have diuretic effects. Several are positively contra-indicated in kidney disease, so this is a case where only expert herbal treatment is recommended.

labour ***

It is against the law in the UK to attend a woman in childbirth without medical supervision unless a certified midwife or registered nurse (one of the few such proscribed areas in British law). Having satisfied such criteria it is nevertheless the case that herbal tradition provides a number of effective remedies to ease labour. Raspberry leaves, beth root and squaw vine are notable *partus praeparaturae* but there are a host of others recovered from folk tradition. In general all such remedies are best, and most safely, taken in the last stages of pregnancy. It must be re-emphasized that this is not an area for the inexperienced: only raspberry leaves can be freely re-commended.

laryngitis **
Apart from other predisposing factors this may be treated in the same way as catarrh, throat problems and bronchial conditions. Steam inhalations may be particularly effective. A stubborn problem should be sent for specialist examination to exclude growth formation.

liver disease ***
Ranging from the life-threatening to the potentially serious this is an area to be handled very carefully. Nevertheless, herbalists have powerful strategies available and may, if informed of the issues, produce remarkable results. They will choose from either hepatic, cholagogue or aperient herbs, depending on the problem (the latter reflecting the close working relations between the liver and the bowel).

malaria ***
Herbs that have been used at various stages of the disease include cinchona bark (*Cinchona succirubra*) – the source of quinine – chiretta (*Swertia chirata*) from the Himalayas and barberry bark. Recent research points to a Chinese herb, *Artemisia argyi*, as also helpful but none can be assured of providing complete protection.

measles **
A major source of death in developing countries, it is a usually mild condition in affluent communities. As such it is treated as other fevers, with perhaps particular use of expectorants and eyebaths.

menopause *
Essentially not a problem, the change in hormonal landscape may nevertheless produce unpleasant symptoms. The traditional view of most of these symptoms is that they represent a generalized debility, and although we now know about the role of hormones in many of them this is still a productive viewpoint. The herbalist's strategy therefore is to provide restorative and supportive remedies,

tonics with a particular reputation for this type of debility. St John's wort, life root (*Senecio aureus*) and oatstraw are notable; vervain and damiana may also be useful, and many other herbs have a good reputation. Those with a relaxant effect, particularly chamomile and black haw bark, may also find application.

menstrual disorders */**

These range from the minor irregularity of menstruation on the one hand to heavy and painful periods on the other, and include premenstrual syndrome, intermittent bleeding, and pelvic pain at times of the cycle. Causes may be mild or serious ovarian hormonal malfunction, infection or inflammation of the reproductive tissues, fibroids, poor circulation or circulatory activity to the pelvic structures, pelvic congestion, or a number of other more remote factors. The success of treatment will often thus depend on a proper diagnosis being made. There are many herbs with a remarkable effect in many cases. Helonias root, agnus castus, blue cohosh, shepherd's purse, white deadnettle (*Lamium album*), parsley, rosemary, beth root, lady's mantle (*Alchemilla vulgaris*), black haw, mugwort, squaw vine, motherwort (*Leonurus cardiaca*) and chamomile: all have strong reputations among the herbalists (traditionally mostly women) of Europe and North America. Dang Gui is a remedy from China that is proving popular as well.

migraine *

Although sometimes unbearably painful this is rarely a serious condition and may respond well to gentle sustained treatment with herbal remedies. It is however a notoriously variable condition, often pointing to a generally unstable metabolism: apparent improvements can be followed by nasty relapses and a new range of sensitivities. Herbalists will thus treat gently and gradually, having due regard for background constitutional factors, particularly evidence of the type of vascular activity in the head. 'Hot' migraines are marked by being temporarily relieved by cold packs; 'cold' migraines, the majority, are relieved by heat. The former will most often respond to treatments that include bitter and other digestive, hepatic or bowel remedies; the latter will tend to improve with vasodilatory remedies and others with warming effects. Feverfew is one of the latter.

miscarriage, threatened ***

With due caution it is possible to use a number of herbal remedies to reduce the risks of miscarriage in pregnancy. Helonias root, cramp bark and black haw have such traditional use in North America; while all medicines must be treated with suspicion in pregnancy, these at least have a good safety record.

mononucleosis see **glandular fever**

morning sickness (in pregnancy) */**

Early-morning nausea and sickness in the first months of pregnancy is common. It is often exacerbated by low blood-sugar levels (and may thus be relieved by eating), but is usually mysterious. Chamomile and black horehound are very useful general remedies, but gentle bitters like dandelion root may also be valuable. If the sickness proceeds past the first three months, or becomes excessive, then expert treatment is essential.

mumps **

Remedies used in managing any fever are augmented by mouthwashes with tinctures of thyme, gum myrrh in liquorice, lymphatic herbs such as marigold flowers and cleavers and anti-infectives like echinacea and wild indigo. It is especially important to be careful if the infection strikes after adolescence, in which case the testes or ovaries may be threatened.

myalgia **

Muscular rheumatism, fibrositis or lumbago, is a generalized inflammation of the muscles or their coverings or tendons. It has similarities to rheumatism in being a generalized inflammatory condition and should be treated on a broad basis. Specific remedies sometimes included in such prescriptions include wild yam, buckbean (*Menyanthes trifoliata*), black cohosh and devil's claw (*Harpagophytum procumbens*). External liniments using warming herbs and oils are usually productive.

nausea *

Symptomatic relief with Iceland moss, cinnamon, black horehound and chamomile should be backed by attention to possible underlying causes, including migraine, liver disease, food poisoning, stomach disease and infections.

nervous bowel *
There are several effective herbal relaxants that can be used to reduce ambient tension in the large bowel and encourage a natural rhythm. Notable are peppermint, hops, wild yam, chamomile, and the carminatives like fennel, dill (*Anethum graveolens*), caraway (*Carum carvi*) and cardamom.

nervous breakdown **
Herbal treatment can be useful in helping recovery from such an event, using nervous restoratives like oatstraw, St John's wort and vervain, and other convalescent strategies.

nettle rash *
A condition most often so transient that it passes before treatment can be tried; if recurrent or persistent, then the search should begin beyond immediate reactions to foods for general digestive dysfunction.

neuralgia **
This form of inflammation of the nervous system is seen traditionally as a mark of debility and as an indication for nervous restoratives like oatstraw, St John's wort and circulatory stimulants like ginger and prickly ash bark (*Zanthoxylum americanum*). Topical applications of lavender oil and wintergreen oil may help to reduce the immediate pain.

neurosis **
The conventional use of herbal medicine is not ideally suited to the immediate treatment of nervous problems, although nervous restoratives and relaxants provide approaches not matched elsewhere for their long-term recuperative effects. In the past, however, plants figured largely in the hands of shamans and others charged with chaperoning the human spirit through its world. There are many psychoactive herbs, like cannabis, peyote, coca, opium poppy, datura, johimbe and several fungi, now quite inappropriate in modern therapeutic conditions, which used to be applied as agents in a form of guided psychodrama.

night sweats see **perspiration, excessive**

osteoarthritis **

As part of a wide-ranging programme herbal remedies are often chosen to remove metabolic accumulations in the tissues and because of their reputation in reducing inflammation in the joints. Parsley seed, celery seed, wild carrot, lignum-vitae, birch, dandelion root, devil's claw (*Harpagophytum procumbens*), juniper berries and wall germander (*Teucrium chamaedrys*), most of which are seen primarily as eliminatives, especially diuretics, have all been used in attempts to contain this condition. Chances are quite promising in the early stages, but as joint damage occurs the prospects for genuine repair reduce.

otitis see ear problems

palpitations *

Reassurance that this symptom is generally harmless is often the priority: it generally reflects thoracic tension and can be treated with herbal relaxants supplementing breathing and other relaxation exercises; limeflowers are almost specific.

pelvic inflammation (chronic) **

Usually following acute pelvic infection, or as a consequence of IUD insertion or abortion, this condition is becoming more widespread among younger women. Conventional treatments are not very successful in containing the condition and infertility is a very real risk. A qualified herbal practitioner may have better prospects, using especially North American remedies helonias root and echinacea, combined where appropriate with blue cohosh, wild indigo, beth root and agnus castus, as well as others individually indicated.

period problems see menstrual disorders

perspiration, excessive *

In traditional medicine this symptom was seen as a mark of debility, especially when occurring at night ('night sweats'). It was thus seen as an indication for restorative regimes, often with an emphasis on bitter herbs, as well as other tonics as appropriate. Sage, boneset, life root (*Senecio aureus*) and, in the hands of expert practitioners only, deadly nightshade (*Atropa belladonna*), all have their own specific effects in this area.

piles see **haemorrhoids**

pleurisy ***
Often requiring emergency treatment, and occasionally linked to tuberculosis, but herbal remedies can nevertheless be useful in this case. Expectorants like pleurisy root (*Asclepias tuberosa*), comfrey, mullein flowers, thyme and liquorice have been used successfully, associated perhaps with anti-infective agents like fresh garlic, echinacea and wild indigo, and fever management strategies as required. External poultices have also been effective: linseed and cabbage leaves are particularly popular.

PMT see **premenstrual tension**

pneumonia ***
The seriousness of this condition does not rule out the use of herbal remedies in many cases, provided of course that medical priorities have been addressed (pneumonia is still a major killer). Management of the fever may be an important contribution but the use of appropriate expectorants, like garlic, liquorice, lobelia, thyme, ginger and ipecacuanha with echinacea is always necessary. Attention to convalescence for a considerable time afterwards is especially important and herbs like angelica and elecampane will come into their own.

poliomyelitis ***
Although potentially devastating this viral infection is most often diagnosed as flu and has no more impact than that. Normal fever management techniques may thus be sufficient. Sore neck and back and muscle tenderness are warning signs, the more so if there is a relapse after apparent recovery from the initial fever. With a minimum of muscular activity even this advance need not be crippling but the need for care is obvious and in practice referral to acute medical supervision is necessary.

post-natal depression *
There is a likely hormonal basis for this distressing condition (usually linked to precipitate drops in progesterone levels), so that loving support and counselling can be supplemented by the use of agnus castus, with nervous restoratives and galactogogue herbs.

pregnancy, problems with **/***
Apart from morning sickness (see above), most problems within pregnancy need cautious handling; the herbalist has even more reason to be careful as many herbs have the potential to stimulate the womb in pregnancy.

premenstrual tension *
Like post-natal depression there are probable hormonal reasons for premenstrual tension, with premature slumps in progesterone levels most likely; such appropriate herbal remedies as agnus castus and evening primrose oil have particular benefits, and diuretic remedies such as parsley seed and nettle have been used effectively as well.

prostate disease **
The most common prostatic problem is simple benign enlargement, so common with age as to be almost universal; nevertheless, any enlargement must be positively vetted to eliminate the risk of it being malignant, and there is also the possibility at any age in a man's life of prostatitis. The following points assume an expert diagnosis has been made and are concerned only with benign enlargement and prostatitis. The first has traditionally been treated with male 'tonics': remedies with a strong association with improving conditions for elderly men. Examples include notably saw palmetto, damiana and seven barks from North America, ginseng from the Far East, and pumpkin seeds. Each has potential benefits although ginseng at least will need expert assessment. Prostatitis is treated in similar ways to other urinary infections, with urinary antiseptics, possibly augmented by horsetail and seven barks, eryngo (*Eryngium maritimum*), or gravel root (*Eupatorium purpureum*).

pruritus *
This may follow any one of a wide variety of conditions, such as eczema, liver disease, shingles, diabetes mellitus, kidney disease, worms, vaginal infections, haemorrhoids and allergies. Obviously, treatment of the underlying cause is the priority. Other things being equal, using bitters and/or relaxants in the prescription can be productive; externally chickweed (*Stellaria media*) ointment is almost specific and a soothing relief from the itching.

psoriasis **
Treated, as with other autoimmune conditions, as the manifestation of a very complex series of inflammatory disturbances, with no simple suggestions possible. However, once the wider predispositions are tackled, remedies such as Oregon grape (*Berberis aquifolium*), curled dock, red clover, burdock root and sarsaparilla often recur in successful prescriptions.

pyelonephritis ***
Infection of the kidney most often as a complication of urinary infection, but also possible after septic infections elsewhere in the body. It is potentially serious, with the possibility of complications in treatment, so should not be treated by the non-expert. Soothing urinary remedies like couch grass root, corn silk and horsetail may be combined with buchu and anti-infective remedies; there is almost certainly a need for a degree of fever management and other constitutional remedies.

quinsy see **throat problems**

Raynaud's disease **
As a manifestation of autoimmune or allergic disturbances, the treatment of this spasmodic constriction of the peripheral blood vessels will be broadly based. Circulatory stimulants and peripheral vasodilators such as ginger and hawthorn may be used to alleviate the symptoms and cramp bark may also help relax the vascular muscle walls.

rheumatic fever ***
A potentially dangerous over-reaction to streptococcal infections. As long as expert medical care is involved it may be possible to apply fever management strategies with especial use of garlic and/ or echinacea. Convalescence after the attack is important and eliminative and restorative herbs may play a useful part.

rheumatism, muscular see **myalgia**

rheumatoid arthritis **
Recent evidence, establishing the principle of immunological

cross-reactivity between tissues attacked in rheumatoid arthritis and such micro-organisms as *Proteus*, adds further support to the traditional approach to such autoimmune conditions. Herbalists have always looked to signs of prior infection and inflammation (or toxicity), paying particular attention to the lungs, urinary system and gut, applying such herbs as are appropriate in each case. Isolation and treatment of food allergies may be productive and there is sometimes a hormonal factor, i.e. disturbed menstruation or menopause, that may merit its own attention. There is a role for specific anti-inflammatory herbs and lignum-vitae, arbor-vitae, buckbean (*Menyanthes trifoliata*), black cohosh, wild yam, gotu kola (*Centella asiatica*), and sarsaparilla all have reputations for this task.

ringworm *
A combination of topical treatment with tincture of marigold or gum myrrh and systemic treatment with eliminative and anti-infective remedies is the usual approach to any fungal infections of the skin and nails.

rosacea see **acne rosacea**

salpingitis see **pelvic inflammation**

schizophrenia see **nervous breakdown**

sciatica **
Although manipulative treatment and bedrest are primarily indicated, the use of herbal relaxants and remedies that might treat inflammations of the affected tissues can be helpful. The condition may also be treated as a form of neuralgia (see above).

shingles **
Although the result of an infection (with the chicken-pox virus) of the nerve fibres, there is considerable value in the traditional approach which treats shingles as an example of a neuralgia or neurasthenia and applies nervous restoratives to correcting the problem. The use of remedies like oatstraw, damiana, vervain and St John's wort is particularly appropriate in those cases where the original infection passes into a clear 'post-herpetic neuralgia', with severe pain persisting sometimes for many months.

sinusitis**
This is treated as a form of catarrh (see above) with the particular use of remedies like wood betony (*Stachys betonica*), ground ivy and ribwort. Given the location of the problem it is often useful to use steam inhalations with chamomile flowers or oils of pine and aniseed to accentuate the action of the prescription. Circulatory stimulants are also often effective.

sprains *
External application of comfrey or arnica will help healing time and reduce pain.

stomach problems see **dyspepsia, gastritis, ulcer, peptic** and **hyperacidity**

stroke ***
The usual cause for treatment is the attempt to improve recovery rates from strokes (prevention is much more a dietary and lifestyle factor): yarrow, hawthorn, limeflowers, buckwheat and other peripheral vasodilators may be combined with nervous restoratives.

throat problems */**
Effective gargles for infections of the pharynx or tonsils may include sage, balm of Gilead (*Populus gileadensis*), thyme, blackberry leaves (*Rubus fructicosus*), catechu (*Acacia catechu*), bistort (*Polygonum bistorta*), cranesbill (*Geranium maculatum*) and tormentil; particularly effective is a mixture of fluid extract of liquorice and tinctures of marigold and gum myrrh. Soothing mucilaginous remedies like liquorice, marshmallow root or leaf, and ribwort may help with dry and irritable surfaces. Involvement of the lymphatic tissues such as the tonsils and neighbouring lymph nodes will point to involvement of echinacea, wild indigo, marigold and cleavers. Sore throats are notoriously likely to lead to remote complications elsewhere in the body and the use of remedies directed elsewhere is often indicated.

thromboangiitis obliterans see **Buerger's disease**

thrombosis ***/****
As well as being a potentially fatal condition there is likely to be previous treatment from the doctor with anticoagulant drugs. These strike a fine balance between preventing clotting and haemorrhage

and it is difficult to recommend herbal treatment that is guaranteed not to affect this balance. In cases where the risk is low or treatment non-critical, garlic, if necessary in deodorized form, may be taken freely; peripheral vasodilators like hawthorn and limeflowers may also be helpful. General attention to the arteriosclerosis is always advisable.

thrush *
Actually a ubiquitous organism, *Candida albicans* can proliferate out of normal bounds to give symptoms of thrush in the mouth or vagina, and more non-specific symptoms of debility if the bowel is the principal site. Restoration of general vitality is an initial priority as the condition almost always itself follows a breakdown in vital resistance, and rest and convalescent remedies are usually essential. Specific herbal treatment might include the use of marigold, echinacea, gum myrrh and, where indicated, either bitters or aromatic digestives. Topical treatment of mucosal surfaces may involve marigold, gum myrrh, arbor-vitae, and tannin-rich astringent herbs, in a mouthwash or douche.

thyroid disease **/***
The herbalist will always look at the wider scene, seeing the thyroid glands as much a victim as a master of events. This makes specific recommendations difficult: however, kelp is an almost universally applicable thyroid tonic, potentially applicable to both hypo- and hyperthyroidism.

tinnitus *
If caused by congestion in the middle ear, it can potentially be treated as a catarrhal problem, with appropriate herbs backed by steam inhalations to help penetrate the Eustachian tubes (see **ear problems**). If the cause is in the nervous mechanism of the inner ear, the prospects are less good, but ginkgo is worth a try, and there may be other clues to follow up.

tonsilitis see **throat problems**

travel sickness *
Ginger, preferably fresh root, chewed in advance of travel is almost specific. Although commercial motion sickness treatments are often

derived from constituents of henbane and other members of the deady nightshade group these plants are potentially dangerous and should not be used as substitutes.

ulcer, mouth *

Often arising out of a wider debility they frequently respond best to a broad-based systemic approach with restorative remedies and associated techniques applied as appropriate. Topical applications may include astringent tannin-rich herbs and marigold in aqueous solutions. See **gum disease**.

ulcer, peptic ***

Ulcers of the stomach or duodenum may be linked to a wide variety of digestive disturbances and dietary reactions and these should be pursued as a priority. Healing of any ulceration may be improved with the use of liquorice, Iceland moss, meadowsweet, comfrey root and slippery elm. Duodenal ulceration is by definition harder to affect topically than gastric.

ulcer, venous **

Caused by breakdown in the tissues of the lower leg as a result of chronically poor circulation, usually linked with varicose veins. It is notoriously slow to heal and treatment is primarily that of expert nursing and physiotherapy: internal use of circulatory stimulants and of those stimulants used in the treatment of varicose veins is indicated. Topical application of comfrey and tannin-rich herbs may, assuming compatibility with other dressings, be effective.

urinary infections **

May involve infection of the urethra (urethritis), bladder (cystitis), prostate (prostatitis) or kidney (pyelonephritis). With the exception of the latter, it is usually a simple and effective option to use urinary antiseptic herbs like uva ursi, buchu, juniper, kava kava (*Piper methysticum*), boldo (*Peumus boldo*), saw palmetto, shepherd's purse, golden rod (*Solidago virgaurea*), heather flowers (*Calluna vulgaris*), and pipsissewa (*Chimaphila umbelata*). Involvement of the kidney in any way makes the stakes much higher and many of the urinary antiseptics are likely to further irritate the organ. This should be left to expert hands.

urinary stones ✲✲

There are many diuretic herbs that were used to help dilute and possibly flush through small stones and gravel. These include parsley piert (*Alphanes arvensis*), pellitory (*Parietaria* spp.) gravel root (*Eupatorium purpurea*), stone root (*Collinsonia canadensis*), eryngo (*Eryngium maritimum*), and wild carrot. It is unlikely that actual stone breakage actually occurred after such treatment and large stones have always presented severe problems for which surgery or ultrasound may be necessary.

urticaria see **nettlerash**

vaginal problems ✲✲

Hormonal factors are often implicated in a breakdown of normal vaginal defences against infection and these should always be attended to with the appropriate internal treatment (see **menstrual problems**). General health may also be compromised, especially with thrush (see above) and this will also determine treatment. There may also be concurrent urinary infection or signs of more general pelvic inflammation. Topically, herbs may be applied in a douche form: they may include periwinkle (*Vinca major*), marigold, arbor-vitae, witch hazel and beth root.

varicella see **chicken pox**

varicose veins ✲

Internal herbal remedies such as horse chestnut, golden seal, lime-flowers and stone root (*Collinsonia canadensis*) may supplement exercises and other measures. Marigold, stone root and horse chestnut may also be applied topically.

venereal disease ✲✲✲✲

It is against the law in the UK to treat this condition without referral to a doctor, or when available a special clinic.

vertigo ✲✲✲

Dizziness may follow damage to the balance organs near the inner ear from a variety of causes: arteriosclerosis, high blood pressure, Ménière's syndrome, migraine, epilepsy or middle-ear problems. Expert diagnosis is essential and then treatment may be directed at the underlying cause if known.

vomiting **/***
If not too long-standing, this may be treated with such remedies as ginger, lemon balm, chamomile, peppermint and black horehound. Persistent vomiting may herald more serious conditions and should be diagnosed urgently, before severe fluid and electrolyte depletion occur.

warts *
Notoriously variable in their response to treatment, it may often be possible to shift them by regular repeated (2–3 times a day) application of the milky sap of fresh dandelion root over many days. Other such treatments include the orange sap of fresh celandine and the tincture of arbor-vitae. There may be clues that lead to internal treatment as well, especially if warts are common.

whooping cough ***
One of the few ways to loosen this distressing cough is by using liquorice and elecampane and/or mullein flowers: an expert medical herbalist might also use lobelia but as this is a restricted herb and as many patients are young children this must not be attempted by the inexperienced.

A Traditional Physiology

Although there are a number of coherent physiological systems outside that of developed medical science,[1] there is still surviving one system of traditional medicine, in the Far East (China, Japan, Korea and surrounding countries), that is particularly sophisticated. The following is a brief review of its main landmarks, as passed through Chinese texts and practice, to provide one example of the principles outlined in the review of physiology earlier in this volume.[2]

It is a most fascinating example. For a physiologist the imagery and associations are unusual; for a physiologist in the consulting room, they are powerful and evocative, offering a treasure-house of potential connections across all levels of human experience that normal medical science could never equal. Although foreign, there is much here that will repay attention.

In China, most insights into the workings of the human body, mind and spirit were the result of intuition and subjective experience. These in turn arose out of the conviction that the world was a whole. Just as one would never try to separate the weather from the seasons, from the activity of hot, cold and moist air, and from the effects of topographical features, so the Chinese would never attempt to take one observation about the human body out of context. Instead of isolating and dissecting individual constituents, they were concerned with events that occurred together. Such events would be linked by this relationship and would be seen to have a *mutual influence* on each other. From close observations of frequent occurrences one might eventually induce a *pattern* and predict with varying degrees of precision the implication of such patterns as they recur.

Ideas of health and ill health were thus built on symptoms, sensations and suppositions, linked together into patterns forged through human experience over centuries. The body was a shifting web of influences. Physiology was a qualitative rather than a quantitative exercise in which precisely measured fragments would be seen to have an infinitesimal half-life.

It does not seem a very precise basis for medical science: more like wandering over a new landscape with a book of rules rather than a map; or, in fact, like weather forecasting! Much that is handed down from Chinese medical history is cosy dogma: there is little sign of a tradition of radical reappraisal, of 'individual seekers after truth'. But this is true of all early traditions. In their struggle for survival early humans prospered in relation to the fitness of their behaviour to their circumstances. Chinese medicine interests Westerners today because it has, through several millennia, served billions of people moderately well, and seems to have touched upon some fundamental truths in the process.

There have been huge obstacles in the way of comprehending Chinese medicine in modern Western terms. These have come from viewing quite different ideas through Western spectacles. Chinese thought starts and ends, like the seminal text, the *I Ching*, with *change*. Everything is process, all being is in the process of becoming, nothing is fixed. Anatomical, concrete statements are rarely made. Objects are seen as transitory phenomena, as genuinely relative.

Such ideas fit well with a physiological, functional view of the human being. But they also mean that notions such as *yang*, *yin* and *qi* need to be understood. They also demand that the Westerner be particularly careful in translating words and concepts. The immediate problem with most books about Chinese medicine is that translation is very sloppy. Words like 'liver', 'spleen', 'blood', 'element' and 'organ' are used interchangeably for Western and Chinese phenomena.

One of the most rigorous authorities on Chinese texts, Professor Manfred Porkert, has insisted on creating new terms (usually of Latin origin) to translate from the Chinese. In this text we will be taking a less formidable route, and denoting Chinese concepts by words starting with capital letters, thus *Function* (a more accurate term than 'Organ', as will be come clear), *Liver* and *Spleen*.

Essential Qualitative Standards (or how to classify experience)

The following are two universally accepted standards of quality through which all experienced and observed phenomena are assessed in Oriental thought.

YANG

The *active* aspect of any phenomenon. All that is:

> dispersive
> transforming
> expanding and developing
> setting into motion
> centrifugal
> aggressive
> indeterminate (yet determining)

The implication of the last point is that what is *yang* is not able to be perceived directly, but it entirely determines that which can.

YIN

The *structive** aspect of any phenomenon.[3] All that is:

> condensing
> completing and confirming

---

*From the Latin *struere*: to form concretely (as in 'structure').

sustaining and preserving
reposing
centripetal
responsive
determinate (yet awaiting determination)

The last point is that that which is *yin* is directly perceivable but it is always in the process of being changed by influences that cannot be perceived.

At any position or in any event there will always be a blend of the active and the structive, a blend, moreover, that is always shifting in time and when viewed from different perspectives. Such relativity is intrinsic to Chinese thought and allows it to monitor the infinitely variable without difficulty.

To take a simple example. In the West, a table is an object, fixed and substantial (or at most a Platonic idea, similarly fixed). In the Chinese view that structure is merely its transitory structive, *yin*, aspect: it also forms a relationship with the people who use it and has an influence on the room in which it stands. Moreover, these active, *yang*, aspects of its existence were determined when its *yin* aspect changed from being a tree, and when it changes again to a heap of ash or a children's playhouse! Thus each table becomes a different entity to each individual human being and at each moment in time, its active aspect always reflecting the position of its structive and *vice versa*: it becomes an experience.

The example is simple. Most phenomena, especially as they affect human beings, do not have such a sharp separation between active and structive. In practice there is usually a gradation of *densities* and *activities*, constantly shifting.

Energetics

This is where the difference between modern Western and Oriental views of nature is at its most profound. In the West, the a priori assumption is that each fragment of the universe is complete unto itself, with no need for an underlying configurating principle. Attempts to involve such a force are reserved for the highest level of speculation or simply blind religious belief, and usually involve a clumsy third polarity in the tradition of Aristotle. The idea that the whole pattern might after all be the main determinant of the position and nature of its constituents has generally been rejected. The Western mind has not taken to wandering across a shifting landscape without maps. With the isolation, safe in heaven, of a separate divinity, contemplation of His works could then be allowed to proceed as yet another discrete activity.

The findings of modern science itself have already shown the limits of such thinking. Oriental thought and medicine provide a coherent cosmology built up entirely from the other point of view: underlying all phenomena there is a configurative moving spirit that precisely determines these phenomena. As the phenomena are manifestations of that energy, the energy can thus be termed 'configurational'. Configurational energy in China is referred to as qi.[4]

QI

Qi is:

> an energetic phenomenon of definable quality (i.e. *qi* is marked by what it *does*);

manifest in all movement;

in movement itself, between different levels of its own density;[5]

its *yang* aspect is movement within movement;

its *yin* aspect is the manifestation of observable phenomena.

Qi may thus be discussed as having two senses: firstly as the underlying configurative principle, and secondly as an agency with many facets, linked to the phenomena in question.

In terms of physiology, these facets of *qi* include the following concepts:

> *gu qi:* The energy derived from food, extracted by the *Spleen* (under the influence of *yuan qi*) from material passed to it by the *Stomach*; passed from the *Spleen* to the *Lungs*.

> *ta qi:* The ambient *qi* derived from inspired air (akin to the Greek *pneuma* or Indian *prana*), taken into the *Lungs*.

> *xian tian zhi qi:* Congenital *qi*: that derived from the parents and stored in the *Kidney* for use through life; unlike the other two above which constitute 'acquired *qi*', this is innate or prenatal *qi*. Considered to be beyond replenishment in life; much health advice in China is devoted to right living so as not to dissipate it beyond repair.

> Such concepts are remarkably similar to the description by Hans Selye[6] of 'general adaptation energy', the basis of one's capacity to adapt to and thus resist stresses, largely centred on the adrenal cortex.

> *yuan qi:* Catalytic *qi*, the active aspect of constitutional *qi*, that plays a central role in the initiation of other energetic processes, e.g. the formation of *gu* and *zong qi* and *xue*.

> This can be seen in part as an energetic correlate to the massed potential of the body's enzymes.

> *zong qi:* Derived from the interaction of *gu*, *ta* and *yuan qi* in the *Lungs*, it is the first product of acquired *qi* usable by the body. It nourishes the *Heart* and *Lungs* (it manifests particularly in speech and voice respectively). It specifically governs *rhythmic movement*, such as respiration and heartbeat, and is seen to be the basis of the vital 'hum' that separates the

601 Energetics

living from the corpse. It is stored in the chest, specifically within the *Pericardium*.

It may be seen as energetically encompassing the functional expression of haemoglobin in the body.

zhen qi: The product of the combination of *zong, gu* and *yuan qi* within the *Lungs*; as such it is the most refined form of *qi* and the final form used by the body. It streams to form *ying qi* and *wei qi* and is in practice indistinguishable from them.

ying qi: Nourishing *qi* circulating in intimate association with *xue*; it is seen to provide sustenance to the tissues and their functions, helping in the transformation and distribution of food essence. It is the *yin* stream of *zhen qi*.

wei qi: A highly active aspect of *qi* circulating in the peripheral areas of the body and within the body's cavities, regulating skin and sweat-gland function and being in the forefront of defence against external pathogenic influences. Thus it is most apparent when grappling with infections and the effects of climatic stress: being very *yang* it feels hot or unpleasant, and it is seen to be the basis of fever, acute local pain, shivering, coughing, vomiting, etc. It is closely associated with the *Lungs*. It is the active stream of *zhen qi*.

There are also more *yin* manifestations of *qi*.

jing ('essence'): The primal organic material, reflected in biological processes and instinctive behaviour; provides the capacity for growth and biological development; associated with the *slow* movement of organic change; it is the *yin* aspect of congenital *qi*, though able to be replenished by the *yin* aspect of *gu qi*: the food essences; stored in the *Kidneys* (sometimes seen to manifest as the sperm); a resource used by the *Lungs* in dealing with external stresses (comparable to Selye's adaptation energy, like congenital *qi*).

xue (or *Blood*): The densest, most *yin*, manifestation of *qi*; the *yin* accompaniment of *ying qi*, and also nourishing; derived from *gu qi* by the action of *yuan qi* on the marrow; stored in the *Liver* when the body is at rest; passed round by the *Heart* and kept in its channels by the *Spleen*; it is said to 'moisten'.

Xue can be appreciated as incorporating both what the West knows as blood and the subjective effect of that fluid, warming, pulsing and nourishing. As the *yin* aspect of *qi*, it can be seen as a deeper, slower, more profound response to change, a response that is by definition slower to reverse as well. It is, for example, the organic change that leads to observable pathologies. It also requires therapy acting on a more *yin* (i.e., *somatic*) level to influence it. In the Chinese context this involves either deeper needling with acupuncture, or as this begins to border on the potent or dangerous, the use of *herbal remedies* and *diet* (both of which are seen to be more *yin*).

> *jin – ye:* Both arise in the *Spleen* from food and drink and are sent to the *Lungs* for distribution; *jin* fluids are the more rarefied or *yang*, thus they are warm and nourish the skin and muscles; they flow with, as the *yin* aspect of, *wei qi*; *ye* fluids are more viscous or *yin*, and lubricate the joint cavities, marrow, brain and the '*secretion*' of (actually the sense organ associated with) each *Function*; they flow with, and are the *yin* aspect of *ying qi*.

These are only the major manifestations of *qi* in the human being. Like all Chinese concepts, these speculations arise out of subjective experience and the phenomena they describe can only be meaningful in that context. In other words, these entities are *felt*, or at most intuited, not measured. This is certainly the case of the last energetic concept we shall consider here.

> *shen:* Pure action (*yang*) – an entirely speculative concept; the ultimate conceivable configurative influence; a particularly human feature, associated with human consciousness, the ability to think, remember and aspire to the heights; stored in the *Heart*.

An essential part of the definition of many of these energetic phenomena is that they are all relatively substantial. The relativity is significant, of course: some are more substantial than others, but they are all 'real' in the Western sense. And as far as the human being is concerned, they circulate in predictable channels.

The movement of *qi* in the body is not only through meridians but through the tissues generally (especially *wei qi* and *jin*). This movement has caused much confusion in the West as it appears to have very little to do with modern concepts of fluid motion; even *xue*, a concept used to account for the production of blood, was perceived to flow in the meridians rather than through anything resembling the arteriovenous circulation.

It may be argued that the circulation referred to is conjectural, having no bearing on the movement of 'real' fluids. This would however insist on a division in nature where the Oriental view was that there could be none. *The credibility of Chinese physiology must therefore rest on an eventual compatibility between the two views of fluid movement.*

Fortunately, a closer look in the West at circulation in the interstitial areas (the actual environment of the body's cells) has shown that 'real' circulation is not just in the classic arteriovenous form.[7] Rather than there being defined flow patterns associated with the movement of blood through the capillaries, there arises a more diffuse field subjected to *oceanic currents* (see also 'Circulation' on pp. 86–94). The nature of such currents, with both fixed and variable elements like in any ocean of fluid, opens up a possibility of flow conforming with meridianal concepts.

The Five Phases
(*wu xing*)

These probably arose very early in Chinese history but they make their earliest appearance in literature (associated with astronomy, calendrical science, political divination and alchemy) at the time of the Warring States over 2,200 years ago. The system became established in the Han dynasty with widespread (often profuse) correlations, including the accretion of much portent lore. It has tended to become a formalized system, with abstract concepts removed from the rigorous reappraisal of experience. This is unfortunate for at best it can provide an excellent practical exercise into the study of change and process in nature.

The key to the successful application of the concepts of the five phases seems to be constantly to refer them to personal experience, to work upwards from simple observations, rather than downwards from theoretical constructs. They should be seen as guiding principles rather than measurable classifications, to provide a framework for ordering experience rather than limiting it.

Other terms have been used to translate *wu xing*. 'The five elements' is the most frequent, but it sadly confuses what are images of change with the static entities of Western thought. Porkert precisely but inelegantly refers to them as 'evolutive phases'. Needham describes them as 'fundamental processes'.

Each will be described in turn on the following pages. For another perspective on their relationship, see 'The Cycle of Activity', on pp. 164–70.

The Twelve Functions
(*zang fu*)

Many names are used for these, notably 'Organs', 'Officials' and 'Orbs'. 'Organ' is an inappropriate word to refer to what is a sphere of influence rather than a structure, and in any case furthers the confusion with the anatomical organ already too prevalent. 'Official' reminds us that these physiological entities were evolved with reference to the functionaries of an imperial court. 'Orb' is Porkert's inspired choice, well capturing the scope of involvement of each *zang fu*, but it sounds unfamiliar to the English ear. As this is a physiological review we will use a neutral word, *Function*, with capital first letter, to encompass both latter senses.

The same convention will be used for the individual names of each *Function* to differentiate it from its namesake in modern times. As will be seen, the *Spleen* is a very different concept from the spleen, for example, and it will be important to be reminded of that fact.

The *Functions* are the physiological manifestations of the five phases. They are divided into six pairs, each with one *yin Function* (*zang*) and one *yang Function* (*fu*), yoked together.

It is said that the *yin Functions*, each named for a solid organ, *store* without letting anything drain off (therefore they are full but never filled), while the *yang Functions*, each named for a hollow organ, *transmit* but do not store (therefore they are filled but can never be full). The *yin Functions* are the more condensed and are further from the exterior; the *yang Functions* are the more active and are nearer the exterior. Each *Function* in turn has its own *yin* aspect (storing role) and *yang* aspect (active role).

The following are the descriptions of each *Function* within its phase. Porkert refers to such descriptions as 'orbisiconography', the pictures of the orbs.*

An attempt is also made to link the pathological syndromes of each *Function* with herbal remedies in the Anglo-American tradition. The Chinese obviously have many herbal remedies of their own for each of their defined syndromes and reference may be made to a number of books on the subject for more information about them.[8] Translating any such group of conditions into an indication for Western herbal medicines is not automatic or easy. It may even not be justified, except perhaps as part of the wider effort in this text, *to extend insights into the clinical application of one tradition of herbal remedies, chosen as an archetype for many others.* The suggestions made are based on personal clinical experience, including some with the Chinese herbs themselves, as well as on discussion among those working with both Chinese and Western herbal medicine in the USA: they should not be taken as authoritative.

Wood (*mu*)

Wood is that quality in nature which is:

>solid yet workable and supple
>alive
>growing (bridging earth and heaven)
>spreading outward

---

*To shed light on the concepts described, an attempt is made to provide correspondences with modern medical phenomena. This is an exercise fraught with dangers. The links chosen will not, however, be anatomical, but functional. The implication will not be that such modern phenomena are literally the *Functions* concerned. Rather it will be: 'In its operation this phenomenon manifests the quality being discussed.'

and which is associated with:

> the taste of sourness
> spring
> midnight
> the colour green
>
> the East
> animal smells (goatish, urine, sour sweat)
> a windy climate

The Wood phase is one of the two equinoctial phases, where there is a balance between opposites. Thus its climatic expression, wind, arises out of the conflict between hot and cold air. As the only phase named for a living entity, it encompasses that vital aspiration which is growth – from lifelessness to fulfilment. It is also an inherently changeable phase (as is the influence of wind on Chinese medicine), fluctuating between one state and its opposite.

YIN FUNCTION: LIVER (*gan*)

- mediates the qualities of Wood in the living being
- is the 'general' (plans allocation of resources)
- rules flowing and spreading (gentle diffusion of activity and substance)
- is the source of calm distribution (e.g. is seen to harmonize emotions)
- stores *xue* at rest; restores it to the *Heart* on exertion (if physically fit, less if not)
- controls bile secretion (with the *Gall-bladder*)
- rules the sinews (and the capacity for muscular activity)
- manifests in the following ways:

> as the feeling of anger or frustration (if it is overcharged)
> in the nails
> in the eyes
> in the sound of shouting (or a loud voice)
> in tears (or strong emotion)
> in the radial pulse: second position left side

608   A Traditional Physiology

in the state of the sinews and muscles
as a greenish tinge to the complexion

• is that activity which is supported by moderate levels of acrid
  remedies, and in excess is relieved by sourness (or astringency)

Essentially a *Function* of *circulation*, of distribution, operating
particularly to marshal the body's energies for the rigours of
change, helping to maintain calm equilibrium of internal movement
in flux and stress (it is only when it is disturbed that the system
becomes sensitive to wind, the meteorological metaphor for changeable stresses).

It is supported in its capacity to ride change by its 'mother'
Function, the *Kidneys*, and its energetic manifestation *jing*, so to a
large extent it reflects the status of these latter factors. It is particularly linked with *muscular exertion* and *emotional arousal*.

YANG FUNCTION: GALL-BLADDER (*dan*)

• *yang* aspect of, and coupled to, the *Liver*
• rules decision-making (directs the activities of the other *Functions*)
• stores and secretes bile produced by surplus *qi* of the *Liver* (and
  sends it downwards)

This is a slightly anomalous *Function*, one of six 'irregular'
Functions; it also has aspects of the *yin Functions* generally in that
it is named for a storage organ. It is the only *yang Function* that
participates in the assimilation of food but not in its ingestion and
transportation.

Possible correspondences

To see the *Liver* in Western terms it is important to see it as even
more of a process than the other *Functions*. Within its orbit will
come those mechanisms that maintain *balance between activity
and rest*, between the processes of mobilization and consolidation,

in the face of stressors. This balance is considered in more detail in the section 'Balancing Activity and Rest', on pp. 122–6.

Of its many functions, the only ones that could be said to involve its namesake are the variable mobilization and the storage of carbohydrate reserves as liver *glycogen* as a short-term calorific reserve for muscular activity.

The position of the *Liver* in the generative cycle is between *Kidneys* and *Heart*. With all three groups of correspondences taken together it is easy to see an association with the *sympathetic arousal* of 'fright, fight, flight' in the move from the adrenal reservoir of the *Kidneys* (linked with fear) through the mobilization and muscular functions of the *Liver* (with its emotional concomitant of anger), to the final manifested activity of the *Heart*. This last stage might conceivably flow more smoothly if the body is fit: many of the symptoms of unfitness resemble those expected of a stuck *Liver*!

This link with the arousal of exercise is reinforced by another. The *Liver* is said to store *xue* when the body is at rest, and to send it to the *Heart* when it is active. Although blood as such is just one facet of the concept *xue* the resemblance to the role of the *venous sinusoids* in sympathetic arousal is extraordinary.

In terms of the central nervous system possible correspondences lie in the functional activities of the *reticular activating system* and *cerebellum*, respectively concerned as these are with co-ordinating arousal and moderating muscular response.

Pathophysiology

Disturbances of these *Functions* are generally those of their excessive activity rather than of their depletion. They are particularly vulnerable to the effects of sudden or pent-up strong emotions (and not only anger and frustration) which destabilize their activities and lead to what are described as 'congestions' in the *Liver*. This manifests as a typical rising 'heat' to affect the upper part of the body and also to give rise to symptoms classified as 'internal wind' (with some of the qualities described under the heading 'Wind' in the chapter 'Traditional Pathology', on pp. 142–3).

The heat symptoms include headaches, vertigo, tinnitus, red eyes, frequent nose bleeds, dry mouth, bitter taste, fits of anger and hypertension.

The 'internal wind' symptoms include spasm, muscle pains, cramps, paralysis, convulsions, twitching and vertigo.

The *Liver* is also vulnerable to deficiency in the core reserves of the body, i.e. the *Kidney*, and 'rising heat' symptoms are thus liable to follow general debility.

Herbal approach

The 'rising heat' and 'internal wind' symptoms can be tackled by *relaxant* and/or *vasodilatory* remedies like chamomile (*Matricaria recutita*), yarrow (*Achillea millefolium*), limeflowers (*Tilia europoea*), cramp bark (*Viburnum opulus*) and hawthorn (*Crataegus oxyacantha*).

Where they follow debility suitable *tonic* remedies assume a priority.

Fire (*huo*)

Fire is that quality in nature which is:

> heating, warming, attracting
> burning, destructive
> ascending
> blazing and illuminating

and which is associated with:

> the taste of bitterness
> summer
> midday
> the colour red
> the South
> scorched smells
> hot climate
> the number 7

611   The Twelve Functions

This is the most dramatic of the phases, the one where fulfilment occurs in the seasonal cycle. As the source of heat, Fire is closely associated with the concept of life and vitality and is usually conceived as standing astride the other phases drawing them together, co-ordinating them, and in human terms almost justifying their existence.

As a reflection of its pre-eminent position in human terms the Fire phase is manifested in the body by a double pair of *Functions*.

YIN FUNCTION I: HEART (*xin*)

· mediates the qualities of Fire in the living being
· is the 'sovereign ruler' (provides the clearest insights and the most enlightened direction)
· rules *xue* and its channels (thus includes the dynamic aspects of blood circulation)
· stores *shen* and rules it (thus is the centre of *mental activity*)
· maintains individual integrity (as one in the whole: distorts towards ego)
· manifests in the following ways:

> as the feeling of pleasure
> in the face
> in the tongue
> in the sound of laughter (and a cheerful voice)
> in sweating (as a mark of healthy exertion)
> in the radial pulse: first position left side
> in the state of the meridians and channels
> as a reddish tinge to the complexion

· is that activity which is supported by moderate levels of saltiness, and in excess is relieved by 'sweetness' (e.g. a simple peasant diet)

The essence of this *Function* is perhaps best understood through one's experience of it. The *Heart* is dominant when one feels 'on top of the world', when things all seem to fit together well, when one's mental and physical faculties are at their peak, when one is happy. At such times the circulation of blood, as well as the more experiential *qi*, *xue* and body fluids, are at peak performance, and all the body's tissues are well perfused. It is the *Heart* that dominates when one is physically fit and exercising: there is increased circulation, a free flow of sweat, a clear head, and a sense of well-being. The *Heart* can be disturbed, of course, with more localized heat and less pleasure; it is also seen to be manifested in the operations of the ego.

YIN FUNCTION II: PERICARDIUM (*xin bao*)

- has a manifestation closely linked to that of the *Heart*
- is the 'official ambassador' (representing the kingdom abroad)
- is the origin of joy and pleasure (and, persistently, social and sexual communication)
- manifests in the radial pulse: third position right side (or superficial *Heart* position)

This is a somewhat undefined *Function*, with a tantalizing overlap, in some clinical practice, with the *yang* aspect of the *Kidneys*, *Kidney Fire* (*ming-men huo*), the primal source of body heat. It is also the *Function* most associated with the relationships between an individual and the outside world: those with family, friends, work and home. Its health is sometimes judged on the ease with which an individual makes a place in the world.

It may perhaps be seen most as the manifestation of Fire on the surface, that which surrounds, like the organ for which it is named, the internal Fire functions.

YANG FUNCTION I: SMALL INTESTINE (*xiao-chang*)

- *yang* aspect of, and coupled to, the *Heart*
- rules the separation of pure from impure (the ability to *select*)

YANG FUNCTION II: TRIPLE HEATER (*san jiao*)

- *yang* aspect of, and coupled to, the *Pericardium* (and linked to *ming-men huo*, as above)
- regulates the movement of fluid
- rules the *qi* of all other *Functions*
- source of both *ying qi* and *wei qi*

This *Function* has the least connection with any anatomical entity, and so forces a purely functional and, in fact, experiential, appraisal. It seems to be the perceived *pattern* of relationships between all the *Functions*, a *network* of pathways marking both activity and flow through the living system.

Essentially the body is felt to divide into three geographical layers, with approximate boundaries at the diaphragm and the umbilicus. The upper *jiao* is the most rarefied (active or *yang*), the lower *jiao* the most congested and condensed (*yin*). Within these layers the focal points of the major *Functions* can be determined along with the vortex of activity associated with each. The *Triple Heater* provides the framework within which these *Functions* interact and the channels along which fluids and energies flow between them. It also provides an elaboration of the relationship between heat and fluid flow in the living being, the smelting, distillation and condensation of life.

The *Triple Heater* is an early *systems analysis* of the functions of the body, mind and spirit. Like all Chinese physiology it is a concept based on introspection and intuition elaborated by cumulative clinical experience. It is a fascinating and valuable insight. An attempt to sketch its main features is made in Fig. 17 on p. 615.

Possible correspondences

The *Heart*, *Pericardium* and *Triple Heater* all have obvious correspondences with the circulatory system but just as obviously are not tied to the usual modern definitions. Thus although the *Heart* refers to the heart that anyone would recognize, it does not concern itself with the control of heartbeat (a function of the *Lungs*), and it also encompasses most of the functions of the *cerebral cortex* (one

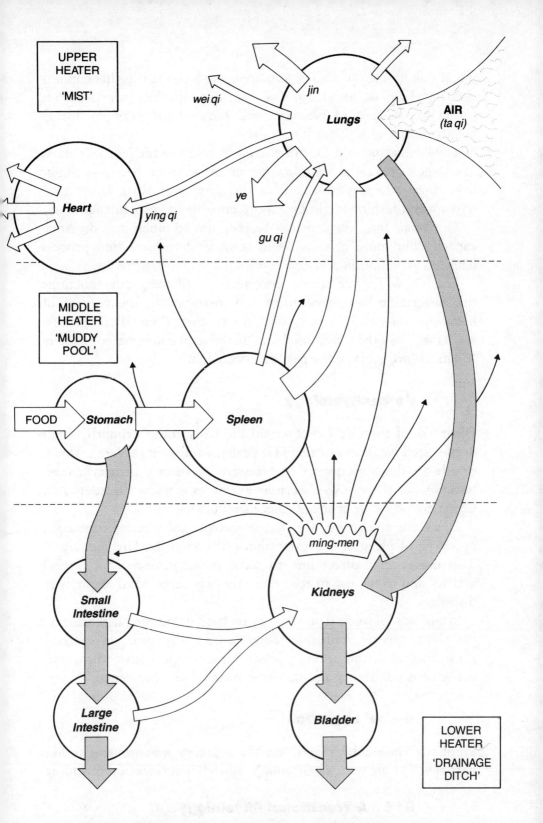

Fig. 17 The Triple Heater System: a diagrammatic view

might emphasize the *association areas* of the cortex in this connection). Making an additional link with the net effect of *endorphins* (providing feelings of pleasure, and released for example during healthy exercise) is difficult to resist.

The *Pericardium* on the other hand seems to be the *Function* most in charge of *personal relationships*, an association that casts doubt over some attempts to link it to the aorta and other anatomical structures (blushing might be a more tangible correspondence!).

The *Small Intestine* can best be seen not so much in a digestive capacity but more broadly as in control of the selection process between *assimilation* and *rejection*.

The *Triple Heater* clearly encompasses all the many functions that determine *heat generation* and *distribution*, the control of *metabolic rate*, and, in fact, *the regulation of all metabolic processes*, as well as other emotional and affective phenomena not usually so linked (probably to the patient's detriment).

Pathophysiology

Disorders of the Fire *Functions* in the body result primarily from deep-seated weakness or debility, perhaps following severe trauma, or else are the consequence of excessive intellectual activity! Manifestations of the *ego* were seen as examples of these disorders in a China bound by strict social responsibilities.

One route to disturbance that was envisaged was the formation of a type of phlegm or catarrh that obstructed the Fire *Functions*. This opens up a direct link to some manifestations of catarrhal activity and to the use of remedies otherwise applied to respiratory disorders.

Symptoms of such disturbances include palpitations, tension in the chest, mental confusion, forgetfulness, insomnia; in extreme form, mental disturbance; in lesser yet more pervasive form, self-confidence, sociability and stable personality are threatened.

Herbal approach

Emphasis should be placed on the *relaxing nervous tonics* like oatstraw (*Avena sativa*), St John's wort (*Hypericum perforatum*), vervain (*Verbena officinalis*) with possible supplementation by vitamin B complex and even the oil of evening primrose (*Oenothera biennis* spp.).

Earth (*tu*)

Earth is that quality in nature which is:

> fertile
> nourishing
> solid and stable
> restful (still and unmoving)
> central (the source, 'earthing')
> recurrent ('ashes to ashes')

and which is associated with:

> the taste of subtle sweetness (simple foods, 'fruits of the earth')
> late summer
> mid-morning
> the colour yellow
> fragrant smells (particularly of ripe, sweet fruits)
> damp climate, and thunder
> the number 5

This was originally not a phase at all but that position from which the other phases were recognized; this was *terra firma*, our world, the one thing in life that most felt able to be sure of. It has universal connotations with 'mother earth' (*Gaia*), all that is nourishing or supportive, warm and damp, and fertile. The most evocative human image of the Earth phase is mother's milk.

YIN FUNCTION: SPLEEN (*Pi*)

- mediates the qualities of Earth within the living being
- rules transformation and transportation (processing and distribution)
- is the primary digestive function ('foundation of post-natal energies')
- directs movements upwards (main antigravitational and supportive influence on the tissues and also moves food energies up to the *Lungs*)
- rules the flesh and limbs
- stores *ying qi* (the nourishing *qi* in the meridians)
- governs *xue* (keeps it and the fluids in their proper channels)
- manifests in the following ways:

> as the feeling of sympathy (empathy, contemplation, maternalism)
> in the lips (their state of fullness)
> in the mouth
> in the sound of singing (or a sing-song voice)
> in the saliva
> in the radial pulse: second position right side
> in the state of nourishment of flesh and limbs (body shape)
> as a yellow tinge to the complexion

- is that activity which is supported in moderate levels by sweetness (cereals, vegetables and herbal saponins), and in excess is relieved by bitterness (bitter digestive stimulants)

This is in some ways an anomalous *Function* (reflecting its special associations with the Earth phase), being a particularly *yin Function*, storing a *yin* form of *qi* (*ying qi*), yet also being a sphere of continuous transition it has the qualities of a *yang* or active *Function* (hence perhaps one paradoxical function claimed for it: 'the storage of ideas'). It is the *Function* associated primarily with *assimilation*, of influences and energies as well as material (a reliance on sugar in the diet and an excessively sweet tooth would be seen as a compensation for any sort of inadequate assimilation). As an Earth *Function* it also reflects the state of one's attachment to the 'earth', the motherlode, one's mother.

YANG FUNCTION: STOMACH (*wei*)

- is the yang aspect of, and is coupled to, the *Spleen* ('sea of food and fluid')
- rules receiving and digestion of food
- initiates the process of separation and selection of pure from the impure (pure to *Spleen*, impure to *Small Intestine*)
- is in charge of downward movement (contrast with *Spleen*)

Possible correspondences

On a broad physiological level the *Spleen* incorporates much of the role of the liver and endocrine pancreas. In the former anabolic metabolism and the processing of food nutrients are particular inclusions; the role of the pancreas in maintaining blood sugar and distributing it and calorific energy to the tissues is also obviously relevant. All other body functions concerned with these matters would also come under the influence of this *Function*.

Linking the control of metabolic functions to the spleen, which is in fact a component of the reticulo-endothelial and blood cell systems (and which is not essential to life), has often seemed puzzling. One possible explanation is a clinical one; diseases that we now understand as essentially liver diseases, are classically diagnosed by a palpable (thus enlarged) spleen, due to congestion of the spleen's blood flow through the liver. Any early physician would have been forgiven for associating an enlarged spleen with a syndrome of disturbed digestive and metabolic functions.

The *Spleen* has another interesting portfolio: the confinement of circulating energies into their channels and the maintenance of structural integrity. Although the blood circulation is not the only aspect of energetic movement, functions that contain it and prevent oedema must be considered as coming under the influence of the *Spleen*. These include those factors that maintain the *integrity of the vascular wall*, the production by the liver of *plasma proteins*, and most notably the semi-solid *interstitial gel* that maintains the *shape* of the body's connective tissues and also prevents the free flow of fluid through the interstitial spaces (in response to gravity, for example). *Spleen* dysfunction is seen as one of three main causes of oedema in Chinese medicine (possibly equated to liver disease, starvation or other loss of plasma proteins, or capillary and connective tissue disturbances: all modern interpretations that fit well with the wider concept of the *Spleen*).

The other causes of oedema are failure of the *Lungs* to pass condensed *fluids* to the *Kidneys* (left-heart failure?) and failure of the *Bladder* in eliminating fluids from the body (right-heart failure and kidney disease?).

A further correspondence is possible. A common feature in both main roles for the *Spleen* is the mechanism for actively passing material across cell boundaries. The processes of *active transport* and *facilitated diffusion* across the cell wall, and the basic *sodium pump* that fuels these and is also important in maintaining fluid status within and without the cell: all these may be seen as manifestations of *Spleen qi*. It is clear that wherever solids move in biological systems water moves behind: although the *Spleen* would be seen to be concerned with the fate of the 'dry', its effect on the 'wet', the body fluids, follows automatically.

In terms of the central nervous system, the *Spleen* corresponds to that faculty dominant in moments of quiet contemplation, parental warmth, peace: the *limbic system* has been suggested as mediating this capacity.

The *Stomach* is one of the few Chinese concepts that corresponds closely with the modern understanding of the organ. Nevertheless, it includes more than food handling: much that was covered in the earlier discussion of the process of *accommodation* would be incorporated in this entity, as would the process of *selection* between assimilation and rejection (as a prelude to the work of the *Small Intestine*).

Pathophysiology

As the functions most involved with digestion and assimilation it is not surprising that they are particularly vulnerable to poor or deficient diet, whether through excess or deficit.

The *Spleen* is uniquely susceptible to 'damp' (see the chapter 'Traditional Pathology') and also to the effects of extended emotional stress.

The symptoms of disturbance generally are those of disturbances in assimilation, with a particular emphasis on 'dampness' and 'mucus' symptoms. When 'cold-damp' there may be the following: congested nauseous dyspepsia, abdominal distension, fluid stools, Candidiasis, and what have been described in the Western herbal tradition as 'catarrhal' conditions. When the pathological influence is classified as 'damp-heat', there are symptoms of liver disease, jaundice, gall-bladder troubles, headaches, disturbances of blood-sugar control (hypoglycaemia or else late-onset diabetes) and the many consequences that may be linked to these.

Herbal approach

For 'cold-damp' conditions warming *aromatic digestives* are indicated like angelica (*Angelica archangelica*), cardamom (*Amomum cardamomum*), fennel (*Foeniculum vulgare*), aniseed (*Pimpinella anisum*), or elecampane (*Inula helenium*).

For 'damp-heat' conditions the *bitters* are specifically indicated.

Metal (*jin*)

Metal is that quality in nature which is:

> mouldable (solidity derived from liquidity)
> hard and strong (incisive)
> responsive to heat (but generally cold)
> conductive (hence basis for modern communications)

lustrous (brilliant, glossy, splendid)
protective (as in armour and weaponry)

and which is associated with:

the taste of acridity (as in smelting fumes)
autumn
the colour white
the West
the smell of raw flesh (and fish)
dry climate
the number 9

The Metal phase is another equinoctial phase. It is the season of decaying, where the growth of previous stages is crystallized, and all excessive material is stripped away. It is the bare pale branches of autumn trees. The counter to flinging off the colourful and active, however, is that what is left becomes increasingly potent, able when tapped to generate great energy.

YIN FUNCTION: LUNGS (*fei*)

- mediates the qualities of Metal within the living being
- is the 'prime minister' (in charge of energy allocation)
- is the source of that energy distributed *rhythmically* by breath-ing
- rules *qi* (where *qi* is movement, quickening, the vital hum; also where *qi* is air)
- is the site of *zong qi* and *chen qi* production (point where external and internal *qi* meet)
- directs movement outwards (disseminates *qi*, especially *wei qi*, and *fluid vapour*, to the skin)
- is descending and liquefying (condensing *vapour* down to the *Kidneys* as the 'upper origin of water')
- moves and adjusts water flow (like a distillation flask: hot and cold – vaporization and condensation – out and in)
- manifests in the following ways:

as the feeling of sorrow (which then depresses its activity)
in the nose
in the sound of crying (or an aggrieved voice)
in nasal secretions
in the radial pulse: first position right side
in the skin and body hair (also sweat glands)
as a white tinge to the complexion

- is that activity which is supported by moderate levels of sourness
  (e.g. fruit and vitamin C), and in excess is relieved by acrid remedies

This is the *Function* most involved in the *defence* against, and
reaction to, external pathogenic influences, especially 'cold' ones
(this would include most that we would call infections), and fever
and inflammation are activities which come within its orbit. Also
seen as the source of the 'quickening' that underlies biological life
(*zong qi*), the site of the interaction between innate vitality (the
constitutional *qi* centred on the *Kidneys*), and that from outside:
earthly (*gu*) and heavenly (*ta*) *qi*, as witnessed most dramatically in
the infant's first breath.

YANG FUNCTION: LARGE INTESTINE (*da-chang*)

- *yang* aspect of, and coupled to, the *Lungs*
- rules elimination from the body
- continues separation of pure from impure

Possible correspondences

The *Lungs* can be seen to incorporate all defence mechanisms in
the living being, both physiological and psychological, like the suit
of armour the concept was modelled on. Thus would be included
the *inflammatory* and *fever* mechanisms (notably manifested by
sweating, shivering and pallor, all obviously linked), the collective
phagocytes, and, of course, the functions of the *mucociliary escalator* and the *cough reflex*. The persistent use of fruit and vitamin
C as an aid to these protective measures is presaged here.

As the moderator of all rhythmic activity in the body, it is illuminating to see how the concept of the *Lungs* is elaborated in what is now understood of the *respiratory centres* in the brain stem. In brief, this consists firstly of two brain centres, initiating inspiration and expiration respectively, that alternate activity (by a simple switching mechanism). The inspiratory centre is however powered by a third, a powerful drive unit, the apneustic centre, that seems to display a constant activity. This is held in check only by a feedback centre, the pneumotaxic centre, receiving information from the inspiratory/expiratory couple. The apneustic centre acts in a way often associated with the *Lungs*, namely like a constant generator. This is also a quality in general associated with the whole *brain stem* (someone with destruction of the brain above the brain stem can still survive in a primal, driven way: basic functions like breathing, heartbeat, digestion, even vomiting and crying, will be maintained, all at somewhat exaggerated levels). These phenomena illustrate the concept of the *Lungs* very well.

Tissues with an inherent rhythmicity can likewise be considered. Both *cardiac* and *smooth muscle* contract spontaneously without outside stimulation, at a pace determined by the properties of each cell. The basis of this spontaneous pulsation is the cell's outer membrane being leaky to mineral ions!

It is significant to note that in clinical terms heart arrhythmias were seen more to be disturbances of the rhythmic functions of the *Lungs* than of the *Heart*.

The linkage of *Large Intestine* to *Lungs* is particularly fascinating. In one sense coupling the two organs most in contact with the outside world, most manifesting innate rhythms, one taking in substance, the other eliminating waste, one above, one below, makes for neat symmetry. On the other hand herbal practitioners persistently find associations between disorders of the respiratory system (catarrh, asthma), disorders of the bowel (constipation, irritable colon, inflammatory bowel disease) and those of the external manifestation of the *Lungs*, the skin (eczema, allergic eczema).

There are intriguing themes in personality assessment too. While the Earth phase is equated with motherhood, the Metal phase is associated with fatherhood. The *Lungs* are also seen to be disturbed when there is a tendency to hide one's emotion behind a protective shell (a suit of metal armour). Finally the *Large Intestine* has been linked with that spectrum of human qualities that moves from honour to lofty coldness!

Pathophysiology

The Metal *Functions* are particularly concerned with maintaining rhythmic activities in the body and are thus uniquely vulnerable to the effects of disturbances in the normal balance or rhythm of life: irregular habits, changing shift work, jet-lag, extremes of temperature and chronic imbalances in homoeostasis itself all put special stress on these *Functions*.

Such strains will tend to deplete the lungs and bowel and lead to increasing dryness in them, with dry non-productive coughing and irritation, asthmatic tendencies, dry mouth and throat, hoarseness and loss of voice, even blood coughing on the one hand, constipation being the archetypal symptom on the other. The tendency of lung diseases to end the life of the very old and infirm, as well as the near-epidemic incidence of tuberculosis were both explained in these terms.

Apart from depletion the Metal *Functions* could also be affected by congestion, the Chinese equivalent of 'catarrh' with symptoms of more productive coughing, fevers, pulmonary congestion (such as follows heart failure), respiratory and nasal congestion.

Herbal approach

For dry, depleted conditions mucilaginous and tonic remedies are indicated, to act either as *relaxing expectorants* or *bulk laxatives*. Liquorice (*Glycyrrhiza glabra*), comfrey (*Symphytum officinale*), linseed (*Linum usitatissimum*) are among many of this type.

For congested catarrhal states, the *stimulating expectorants* may be applied such as garlic (*Allium sativum*), aniseed (*Pimpinella anisum*) and squills (*Urginea maritima*). Liquorice may be applied here as well, and the professional herbalist in Britain would be drawn particularly to using lobelia (*Lobelia inflata*), not usually available on general sale. In former times *emetics* would have been another strategy.

Water (*shun*)

Water is that quality in nature which is:

> soaking and sinking (as in waterlogged)
> cold (often equated with ice)
> yielding and fluid
> tending to stillness (finding the lowest level, the 'watercourse way')
> deep and dark (hidden, latent, full of potential)
> necessary for buoyancy (i.e. supportive of vitality)
> dissolving

and which is associated with:

> the taste of saltiness (salinity)
> winter
> late afternoon
> the colours blue and black
> the North
> the smells of rotting and putrefaction
> cold climate
> the number 6

The Water phase represents the time in the cycle of least activity, when life withdraws to its minimum reserves. Yet these reserves, like the seed or rootstock, are also the most powerful, and *the ultimate source of new life*, and its constitutional reserves. We thus have the paradox of the most still and apparently lifeless phase being the most packed with life. One is reminded that right living in Taoist terms is compared to the way of water: not resisting the way we are meant to go.

YIN FUNCTION: KIDNEYS (*shen*)

- mediates the qualities of Water within the living being
- is the 'root of life' (stores the constitutional energy received from one's parents)

- is the store of will
- source of introversion, hibernation, latency (the winter seed)
- stores *jing*
- rules birth and development (including that of other *Functions*)
- rules the bones and produces the marrow (which includes the brain and spinal cord)
- is the 'door of respiration' (the ultimate receptor of inspired *qi* from the *Lungs*)
- is the source of both *yin* and *yang* (Water and Fire)
- in its *yang* aspect it is known as *ming-men huo* (Life Gate Fire), sometimes identified with the right kidney, and has the following roles:

> source of body heat
> source of body power
> fuels the *Triple Heater*
> fuels the *Spleen* and *Stomach*
> co-ordinates the reproductive system

- thus rules water (and its movement through the body)
- manifests in the following ways:

> as the feeling of fear (which stimulates it to most activity)
> in the hair on the head
> in the ears (and hearing)
> in the sound of moaning (or a sad dull voice)
> in sputum
> in the radial pulse: third position on the left (and also right) side
> in the bones, teeth, joints and marrow
> as a black hue to the complexion

- is that activity which is supported by moderate levels of bitterness, and in excess is relieved by saltiness

This *Function* is very much the body's central resource. It combines a domination over the body's *fluids* (a metaphor for the more *yin* energies of the body, a concept that comes close to incorporating all modern physiology!) with the 'inner fire' that makes all movement possible.

The activities of this *Function*, or *Kidney qi*, have been visualized as arising out of the heating of the *yin Kidneys* (Water) and *jing*, by the *yang Kidneys* (Fire). This view has been challenged by other theorists who prefer to keep all Fire *Functions* in their proper place: there is thus in practice an interesting confusion between *ming-men huo* and the *Pericardium*.

YANG FUNCTION: BLADDER (*pang-guang*)

- *yang* aspect of, and coupled to, the *Kidneys*
- site of confluence of both *yang* and *yin* fluids (eliminating the latter)
- rules fluid elimination

Possible correspondences

Although the *Kidneys* clearly do not tie closely to any single organ, there is much to be said for linking them to the embryonic *genital ridge*, the tissue that evolves to form both the gonads (testes or ovaries) and the adrenal cortex, both glands that will secrete *steroidal hormones*. The steroidal hormones include those governing reproduction, fluid control, and the ability to maintain life (adaptability) in the face of stress. Such physical templates can do little justice to a notion that remains largely inarticulate, the source of life, but they are at least one of its facets.

In the context of the central nervous system the *Kidneys* have possible reflections in the properties of the human *basal ganglia*: their neural circuitry is unusually centripetal, their functions furthest from the black-box pattern of much of the rest of the brain (stimulus in – response out). Although of moderate proportion in animal brains they are substantial in the human and with their clear influence over intentionality in muscle movement have seriously been postulated as the seat of the will.

The *Bladder* is more clearly linked to the modern idea of the kidneys as well as to the urinary system. The non-steroidal hormones *ADH* and *renin-angiotensin* also have close functional affinities.

Pathophysiology

As the source of constitutional reserves almost all problems affecting the Water *Functions* are of depletion. In Chinese medicine such a prospect followed prolonged abuse, illness, profligacy or stress. (Excessive sexual activity was a recurring *leitmotif* in Chinese explanations.) Such depletions were seen as essentially terminal, and more widely as a general mark of ageing.

The depletion could either be primarily of *yang* energies, with pale complexion, aching loins, impotence, frequency of urination and weakness, especially in the legs; or of *yin* energies, where the weakness is associated with paradoxical signs of heat in the body.

Herbal approach

This is one area where Chinese herbs are difficult to replace. One of their *yang* tonics is fenugreek (*Trigonella foenum-graecum*) which is used and understood in the West, but others like Du Zhong (*Eucommia ulmoides*) are not equatable with Western herbs.

Similarly, it is difficult to replace Gou Qi Zi (*Lycium chinensis*) or Di Huang (*Rehmannia glutinosa*) as Kidney *yin* tonics.

Circadian Rhythms

As all Chinese concepts are always in the process of change, and as the sum of all such changes is cyclical, it is not surprising that they have a highly developed sense of the biological and associated rhythms that have only been recently investigated in the West. A summary of the latter was discussed earlier (see 'Balancing Activity and Rest', on pp. 122–26.

An interesting prospect for correspondences between Chinese *Functions* and Western physiological concepts lies in comparing the two views of the circadian cycle. Fig. 18 (see p. 000) can be linked with the Chinese division of the 24-hour day into twelve 2-hour phases, during each of which one of the *Functions* is seen to predominate. This arrangement has sometimes led to each *Function* being given a Roman numeral shorthand, as follows:

I	*Heart*	11.00–13.00	Fire
II	*Small Intestine*	13.00–15.00	
III	*Bladder*	15.00–17.00	Water
IV	*Kidneys*	17.00–19.00	
V	*Pericardium*	19.00–21.00	Fire
VI	*Triple Heater*	21.00–23.00	
VII	*Gall-bladder*	23.00–01.00	Wood
VIII	*Liver*	01.00–03.00	
IX	*Lungs*	03.00–05.00	Metal
X	*Large Intestine*	05.00–07.00	
XI	*Stomach*	07.00–09.00	Earth
XII	*Spleen*	09.00–11.00	

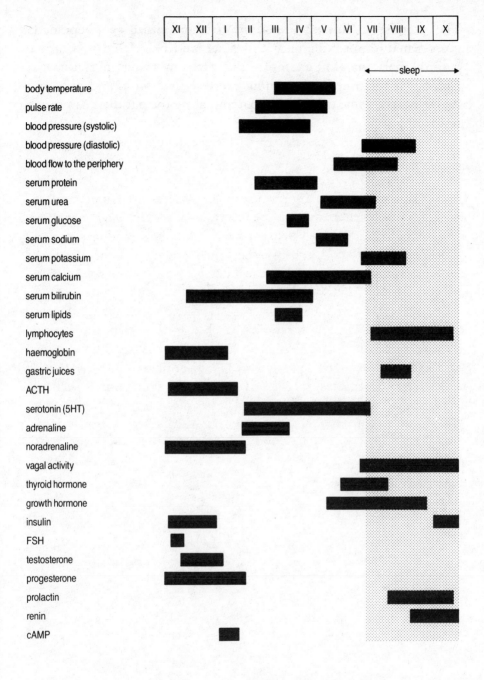

Fig. 18 Circadian rhythms: peak activities in relation to the Chinese clock

The exercise in linking *Functions* to their circadian phenomena must remain approximate at this stage and be related to Chinese cultural patterns (for example, the early morning in traditional China was the time for breathing exercises like *tai qi* and *qi gong*). Nevertheless, some time spent contemplating the parallels can prove rewarding.

Bibliographical Notes

Part I: Roots

INTRODUCTION

1 Davies, D. (1975) *Centenarians of the Andes*, Doubleday, New York.

2 Easton, J. (1799) *Human Longevity, recording the name, age, place of residence and year of the decease of 1,712 persons who attained a century, and upwards, from AD 66 to 1799*, London (quoted by William Rees-Mogg in the *Independent*, 15 Jan. 1990).

3 Turshen, M. (1984) *The Political Ecology of Disease in Tanzania*, Rutgers University Press, New Jersey. Doyal, L. and Pennell (1976) ' "Pox Britannica", health, medicine and underdevelopment', *Race and Class*, 18, p. 155.

4 Gleick, J. (1987) *Chaos: Making a New Science*, Heinemann, London. Glass, L. and Mackey, M. C. (1988) *From Clocks to Chaos: The Rhythms of Life*, Princeton University Press, New Jersey.

5 For a review of the development of the systems view a posthumous collection of the essays of one of its pioneers can be recommended: Bertalanffy, L. von (1981) *A Systems View of Man*, Westview Press, Boulder, Colorado. See also: Capra, F. (1982) *The Turning Point*, Wildwood House, London, pp. 285–332.

6 Bannerman, R., Burton, J., Wen-Chieh, C. (eds.) (1983) *Traditional Medicine and Health Care Coverage*, World Health Organisation, Geneva. WHO/UNICEF Meeting Report (1978) *Primary Health Care; Report of the International Conference on Primary Health Care, Alma Alta, USSR*, WHO, Geneva.

7 WHO meeting Report (1978) *The Promotion and Development of Traditional Medicine*, WHO Technical Report Series 622, Geneva.

8 Farnsworth, N., Anderele, O., Bingel, A. S., Soejarto, D. D., and Zhengang Guo (1985) 'Medicinal plants in therapy', *Update/Le Point-Bulletin of the World Health Organisation*, 63(6), pp. 965–81 (showing high correlation between plants used in traditional medicine and the drugs obtained from them as a demonstration of the inherent value of folk knowledge). Hiller, S. M. and Jewell, J. A. (1983) *Health Care and Traditional Medicine in China, 1800–1982*, Routledge & Kegan Paul, London.

9 Survey (July 1984) carried out in *Journal of Alternative Medicine*, Newman Turner Publ., Sussex, UK. *Alternative Medical Practices in Europe* (1987) Report No E874, Frost & Sullivan Ltd, London.

PHYSIOLOGY

1 An excellent introductory statement to what is sometimes a difficult subject may be found in a translation of a text by one of France's leading phenomenologists: Merleau-Ponty, M. (1962) *Phenomenology of Perception*, Routledge & Kegan Paul, London.

2 Quoted in 'Existence', May, R. Angel, E. and Ellenberger, H. (eds.) (1958) Touchstone, Basic Books, New York, p. 30 (with thanks to Mark Seem). A rigorous review of Nietzsche's contribution to modern thought is Martin Heidegger's four-volume work *Nietzsche*, Harper & Row, New York, 1979.

3 Bohm, D. (1980) *Wholeness and the Implicate Order*, Routledge & Kegan Paul, London.

4 Skinner, Q. (ed.) (1985) *The Return of Grand Theory in the Human Sciences*, Cambridge University Press, Cambridge.

5 Pirsig, R., (1974) *Zen and the Art of Motorcycle Maintenance*, Bodley Head, London.

6 Watt, A. (ed.) (1988) *Talking Health* RSM Publications, London.

7 Coward, R. (1989) *The Whole Truth: The Myth of Alternative Health*, Faber & Faber, London.

8 Bertallanfy, L. von (1981) *A Systems View of Man* (essays posthumously edited by Paul A. LaViolette), Westview Press, Boulder, Colorado.

9 Most of the material presented is in the public domain of physiological knowledge and few specific references will therefore be necessary. Further details of all the items touched on can be found in any good physiology text. I am personally grateful for the work of Arthur Guyton, which provided me with my main reference text, from his 3rd edition in my earliest days as a medical student, through to those days spent as a teacher of the same subject. I have no hesitation in recommending his latest edition: Guyton, A. C. (1986) *Textbook of Medical Physiology*, 7th edition, W. B. Saunders Company, Philadelphia. For a good survey of the subject of pathological changes, microbiology, virology and the immune system, the following general text can also be recommended: Taussig, M. J. (1984) *Processes in Pathology and Microbiology*, 2nd edition, Blackwell Scientific Publications, Oxford.

10 Forster, H. B., Niklas, H. and Lutz, S. (1980) *Planta Medica*, Stuttgart, 40 (4), p. 309.

11 Grabar, P. (1975) 'The "globulines-transporteurs" theory and auto-sensitisation', in *Medical Hypotheses*, 1(5), pp. 172–5. ibid. (1977) 'Les principales étapes du développement de l'immunologie', in *Annales Immunologiae*, Paris, 128C (4–5), pp. 739–51. ibid. and Escribano, M. J. (1976) *Induction de*

tolérance immunitaire par des haptènes libres non réactifs, CR Acad. Sci. [D], Paris, 282 (20), pp. 1833–6 (English abstract).

12 See especially: 'Pathogenesis of ankylosing spondylitis and rheumatoid arthritis', in Proceedings of the Second International Symposium, 14–17 April, 1987, *Brit. J. Rheumatol.* (1988), Suppl. 2, pp. 1–178. Also: Cooper, R. *et al.* (1988) 'Raised titres of anti-Klebsiella IgA in ankylosing spondylitis, rheumatoid arthritis, and inflammatory bowel disease', in *BMJ (Clin. Res.)*, 296(6634), pp. 1432–4. Russell, A. S. (1988) '*Klebsiella* and ankylosing spondylitis' in the editorial of *Clin. and Exp. Rheumatol.*, 6(1), pp. 1–2. Schorr-Lesnnick, B. *et al.* (1988) 'Selected rheumatologic and dermatologic manifestations of inflammatory bowel disease', in *Amer. J. Gastroenterol.*, 83(3), pp. 216–23. Schwimmbeck, P. L. *et al.* (1987) 'Autoimmune pathogenesis for ankylosing spondylitis (AS) and Reiter's syndrome (RS): autoantibodies against an epitope shared by HLA B27 and *Klebsiella pneumoniae* nitrogenase in sera of HLA B27 patients with AS and RS', in *Trans. Assoc. Amer. Physicians*, 100, pp. 28–39.

13 Although there are certainly some immunologists active in the area: '3rd International Symposium on Immunological and Clinical Problems of Food Allergy, October 1–4, 1986, Taormina, Italy,' in *Ann. Allergy* (1987), vol. 59(5 pt 2), pp. 1–203. Hosen, H. (1986) 'The relationship of clinical allergy and the chemical contamination of food', in *J. Asthma*, 23(4), pp. 207–9. Paganelli, R. *et al.* (1986) 'The role of antigenic absorption and circulating immune complexes in food allergy', in *Ann. Allergy*, 57(5), pp. 330–36. Walker, W. A. (1986) 'Allergen absorption in the intestine: implication for food allergy in infants', in *J. Allergy Clin. Immunol.*, 78, pp. 1003–9.

14 See *WHICH?*, January 1987, Consumers Association, London.

15 Saper, C. B. *et al.* (1985) 'Atriopeptin-immunoreactive neurons in the brain: presence in cardiovascular respiratory areas', in *Science*, 227, pp. 1047–9.

16 Vogel, G. (1971) 'The effects of drugs of plant origin on capillary permeability and the lymphatic system', in *Pharmacognosy and Phytochemistry*, Wagner, H. and Horhammer, L. (eds.), Springer-Verlag, Berlin, pp. 370–84.

17 ibid. (1977) 'Natural substances with an effect on the liver', in *New Natural Products and Plant Drugs with Pharmacological, Biological or Therapeutical Activity*, Wagner, H., and Wolff, P. (eds.), Springer-Verlag, Berlin, pp. 249–65.

18 *Amer. J. Clin. Nutr.*, suppl., Sept. 1988.

19 Driesch, H. (1927) *Mind and Body*, Methuen, London. A useful introduction to this debate is to be found in the early pages of: Sheldrake, R. (1988) *The Presence of the Past*, Collins, London.

20 Whitehead, A. N. (1938) *Adventures of Ideas*, Cambridge University Press. See also: Emmet, D. (1966) *Whitehead's Philosophy of Organism*, Macmillan, London.

21 See also: Needham, J. (1956) *Science and Civilisation in China*, Cambridge University Press, vol. 2, p. 562. Needham makes much of the possibly direct link between Leibniz's and Whitehead's organismic views and the essential framework of Chinese science and thought.

22 Thomson, D'arcy W. (1942) *On Growth and Form*, Cambridge University Press.

23 Sheldrake, R., *The Presence of the Past*.

24 Lovelock, J. E. (1987) *Gaia: A New Look at Life on Earth*, Oxford University Press.

25 For a review of such cellular dynamics see Fulton, A. B. (1984) *The Cytoskeleton: Cellular Architecture and Choreography*, Chapman & Hall, London, esp. pp. 60–63.

26 Glass, L., and Mackey, M. C. (1988) *From Clocks to Chaos: The Rhythms of Life*, Princeton University Press, New Jersey.

27 ibid., p. 9.

28 Donovan, B. T. (1988) *Humours, Hormones and the Mind*, Macmillan, London, p. 5. This is an excellent review of the many overlapping disciplines increasingly linked to endocrinology.

29 Fulder, S. (1980) *The Root of Being: Ginseng and the Pharmacology of Harmony*, Hutchinson, London, pp. 156–85.

TRADITIONAL PATHOLOGY

1 It is a matter of contention whether such views are genuinely indigenous or whether they are pervasive influences of Galenic or other systematic medicine. For example, Professor Unschuld suggests a late development, during the first millennium AD, of such concepts in China. See: Unschuld, P. U. (1985) *Medicine in China: A History of Ideas*, University of California Press, pp. 111–15; but the ubiquity and thus, at the very least, approval of the notions in even primitive communities is well attested. See: Brun, V. and Schumacher, T. (1987) *Traditional Herbal Medicine in Northern Thailand*, University of California Press, pp. 70–74. Coulter, H. L. (1973) *Divided Legacy*, vol. 1, Wehawken Book Co., Washington DC (accounts of early Greek medicine). Foster, F. M. (1978) 'Hippocrates' Latin American legacy: "hot" and "cold" in contemporary folk medicine', in *Colloquia in Anthropology*, vol. II, Whetherington, R. K. (ed.), Southern Methodist University, Dallas, pp. 3–19. Greenwood, B. (1981) 'Cold or Spirits? Choice and ambiguity in Morocco's pluralistic health system', in *Soc. Sci. & Med.*, 15B, pp. 119–135. Greenwood, B. (1984) 'Cultural factors in the perception and treatment of illness in Morocco', Ph.D thesis, University of Cambridge.

Harwood, A. (1971) 'The hot/cold theory of disease: the implication for the treatment of Puerto Rican patients', in *JAMA*, 2116, pp. 1153–8. Heyn, B. (1987) *Ayurvedic Medicine*, Thorsons, London, pp. 39–42. Khan, M. S. (1986) *Islamic Medicine*, Routledge & Kegan Paul, London, pp. 37–50. Strehlow, W. and Hertzka, G. (1988) *Hildegard of Bingen's Medicine*, Bear & Co., Santa Fe. Account of the writings of a German twelfth-century mystic and herbalist. Thomson, R. (1978) *Natural Medicine*, McGraw-Hill, New York, pp. 41–64 (Afghan traditions).

2 Helman, C. (1978) ' "Feed a cold, starve a fever" – folk models of infection in an English suburban community, and their relation to medical treatment', in *Culture, Medicine and Psychiatry*, 2, pp. 107–37. This revealing record of patients' views of disease provides powerful evidence that the concepts elaborated in this section are not merely historical.

3 See also: Porkert, M. (1983) *The Essentials of Chinese Diagnostics*, Acta Medicinae Sinensis, Zürich. Kaptchuk, T. J. (1983) *The Web that has no Weaver*, Congdon & Weed, New York. Amber, R. and Babey-Brooke, A. M. (1966) *The Pulse in Occident and Orient*, Aurora Press, New York.

4 For a detailed explanation of pulse types see Porkert, and Kaptchuk, ibid.

5 For some examples see: Dummer, T. (1988) *Tibetan Medicine*, Routledge & Kegan Paul, London, pp. 51–72. Brun, V. and Schumacher, T. (1987) *Traditional Herbal Medicine in Northern Thailand*, University of California Press, pp. 59–95. Heyn, B. (1987) *Ayurvedic Medicine*, Thorsons, London. Khan, M. S. (1986) *Islamic Medicine*, Routledge & Kegan Paul, London, pp. 51–8. Sofowora, A. (1982) *Medicinal Plants and Traditional Medicine in Africa*, John Wiley, Chichester, pp. 26–8. Tabor, D. (1981) 'Ripe and unripe: concepts of health and sickness in Ayurvedic medicine', in *Soc. Sci. & Med.*, vol. 15, pp. 439–55. Thomson, R. (1978) *Natural Medicine*, McGraw-Hill, New York, pp. 32–45. An account of Islamic medicine as practised in Afghanistan. Vogel, V. (1970) *American Indian Medicine*, University of Oklahoma Press, pp. 13–24. MacDonald, C. (1974) *Medicines of the Maori*, Collins, New Zealand.

THERAPEUTICS

1 As for example in: Brun, V. and Schumacher, T. (1987) *Traditional Herbal Medicine in Northern Thailand*, University of California Press. Cosminsky, S. and Harrison, I. (1984) *Traditional Medicine*, vol. II, 1976–81, and *An Annotated Bibliography of Africa, Latin America, and the Caribbean*, Garland Publishing Inc., New York. A valuable collection of references to all aspects of traditional health practices in the areas listed. Densmore, F. (1974, orig. 1928) *How Indians Use Wild Plants for Food, Medicine and Crafts*, Dover Publications, New York,

pp. 322–68. Farnsworth, N., Anderele, O., Bingel, A. S., Soejarto, D. D. and Zhengang Guo (1985) 'Medicinal plants in therapy,' in *Update/Le Point-Bulletin of the World Health Organisation*, 63(6), pp. 965–81. This shows a high correlation between plants used in traditional medicine and the drugs obtained from them as a demonstration of the inherent value of folk knowledge. Halberstein, R. A. and Saunders, A. B. (1978) 'Traditional medical practices and medical plant usage on a Bahamian island', in *Culture, Medicine and Psychiatry*, 2, pp. 177–208. Hand, W. D. (ed.) (1976) *American Folk Medicine: A Symposium*, University of California Press. Accounts of folk methods of health care from Spanish America, French Louisiana, and native American, black American and French Canadian cultures among others. Hamnett, M. P. and Connell, J. (1981) 'Diagnosis and cure: the resort to traditional and modern medical practitioners in the North Solomons, Papua New Guinea', in *Soc. Sci. & Med.*, 15B, pp. 489–98. Hillier, S. M. and Jewell, J. A. (1983) *Health Care and Traditional Medicine in China, 1800–1982*, Routledge & Kegan Paul, London. Imperato, P. J. (1970) 'Indigenous medical beliefs and practices in Bamako, a Moslem African city', in *Trop. Geogr. Med.*, 22, pp. 211–20. Linares Mazari, M. E. (ed.) (1986) *La herbolaria en Mexico*, UNAM, Cuarderno de Extension Academica, 36 (Mexico). MacDonald, C. (1974) *Medicines of the Maori*, Collins, New Zealand. Maclean, U. (1971) *Magical Medicine: A Nigerian Case-Study*, Allen Lane, London. Oswald, I. H. (1983) 'Are traditional healers the solution to failures of primary health care in rural Nepal?', in *Soc. Sci. & Med.*, 17 (5), pp. 255–7. Sofowora, A. (1982) *Medicinal Plants and Traditional Medicine in Africa*, John Wiley, Chichester. Soon Young Yoon (1983) 'A legacy without heirs: Korean indigenous medicine and primary health care', in *Soc. Sci. & Med.*, 17(19), pp. 1467–76. Vogel, V. (1970) *American Indian Medicine*, University of Oklahoma Press, Oklahoma.

2 *New Guide to Health; or the Botanic Family Physician*, Boston, 1835.

3 An excellent account of the history of this period and of herbal medicine in general can be found in: Griggs, B. (1981) *Green Pharmacy: A History of Herbal Medicine*, Jill Norman & Hobhouse, London.

4 Lyle, T. J. (1897) *Physio-Medical Therapeutics, Materia Medica and Pharmacy*, Salem, Ohio.

5 Thurston, J. M. (1900) *The Philosophy of Physiomedicalism*, Nicholson, Richmond, Indiana.

6 Cook, W. H. (1890) *The Science and Practice of Medicine*, Cincinnati.

7 Bates, B. (1983) *The Way of Wyrd*, Century, London. A fascinating account of a native European cosmology, based on early Anglo-Saxon writings.

8 Eliade, M. (1954) *Myth of the Eternal Return: Cosmos and History* (tr. William Trask), Arkana, London.

639   Bibliographical Notes

9 For a historical review of the development of systematic pharmacology in Chinese texts, see: Unschuld, P. U. (1985) *Medicine in China: A History of Ideas*, University of California Press, pp. 111–16 and 179–88.

10 ibid. (1986) *Medicine in China: A History of Pharmaceutics*, University of California Press, pp. 112–13.

11 As for example in: Bensky, D. and Gamble, A. (1986) *Chinese Herbal Medicine: Materia Medica*, Eastland Press, Seattle. Burang, T. (1974) *The Tibetan Art of Healing*, Watkins, London, pp. 58–75. Hasegawa, M. (ed.) (1985) *Herbal Medicine: Kampo, Past and Present*, Tsumura Juntendo, Inc., Tokyo, pp. 1–10 and 130–39. Lyle, T. J. (1897) *Physio-Medical Therapeutics, Materia Medica and Pharmacy*. Porkert, M. (1978) *Klinische Chinesische Pharmakologie*, Verlag für Medizin Fischer, Heidelberg. ibid. (1984) *Klassische Chinesische Rezeptur*, Acta Medicinae Sinensis, Zürich. Priest, A. W. and Priest, L. R. (1982) *Herbal Medication: A Clinical and Dispensary Handbook*, L. N. Fowler & Co. Ltd, London. Sofowora, A. (1982) *Medicinal Plants and Traditional Medicine in Africa*, John Wiley, Chichester, pp. 33–53. Vogel, V. (1970) *American Indian Medicine*, University of Oklahoma Press, Oklahoma, pp. 171–4 and 197–213. Webb, W. H. (1916) *Standard Guide to Non-poisonous Herbal Medicine*, Southport, UK.

12 Messegué, M. (1979) *Health Secrets of Plants and Herbs*, Collins, London.

13 Selye, H. (1956, reprinted 1976) *The Stress of Life*, McGraw-Hill, New York.

Part II: Branches

RESEARCH

1 Quoted in Judson, H. F. (1980) *The Search for Solutions*, Rinehart & Winston, New York.

2 Read particularly: Needham, J. (1956) *Science and Civilisation in China*, vol. 2: *History of Scientific Thought*, Cambridge University Press.

3 Rogers, C. R. (1961) *On Becoming a Person: A Therapist's View of Psychotherapy*, Constable, London.

4 Bateson, G. (1973) *Steps to an Ecology of Mind*, Granada, St Albans, UK.

5 Hayes, N. A. and Forman, J. C. (1987) 'The activity of compounds extracted from feverfew on histamine release from rat mast cells', in *J. Pharm. Pharmacol.*,

39, pp. 466–70. Heptinstall, S. *et al.* (1987) 'Extracts of feverfew may inhibit platelet behaviour via neutralisation of sulphydryl groups', in *J. Pharm. Pharmacol.*, pp. 459–65. Murphy, J. J. *et al.* (1988) 'Randomised double-blind placebo-controlled trial of feverfew in migraine prevention', in the *Lancet*, ii, pp. 189–92. Waller, P. C. and Ramsay, L. E. (1985) 'Efficacy of feverfew as prophylactic treatment of migraine', in *BMJ*, 291, p. 1128.

6 See: *Complementary Medical Research*, the journal of the Research Council for Complementary Medicine in London, especially vol. 1, no. 1, 1986.

7 Reason, P. and Rowan, J. (1981) *Human Inquiry: A Sourcebook of New Paradigm Research*, John Wiley, Chichester.

8 Diesing, P. (1972) *Patterns of Discovery in the Social Sciences*, Routledge & Kegan Paul, London.

9 Cooper, M. R. and Johnson, A. W. (1984) *Poisonous Plants in Britain and Their Effects on Animals and Man*, Ministry of Agriculture, Fisheries and Food, Reference Book 161, Her Majesty's Stationery Office, London.

10 ibid., p. xi.

11 See: *American Pharmacy*, vol. NS24 (3), March 1984/121, pp. 20–21.

12 Weston, C. F. *et al.* (1987) 'Veno-occlusive disease of the liver secondary to ingestion of comfrey', in *BMJ*, vol. 295, p. 183.

13 Harvey, J. and Colin-Jones, D. G. (1981) 'Mistletoe hepatitis', in *BMJ*, vol. 282 pp. 186–7.

14 MacGregor, F. B. *et al.* (1989) 'Hepatotoxicity of herbal remedies', in *BMJ*, vol 299, pp. 1156–7.

15 Fletcher Hyde, F. (1981) 'Mistletoe hepatitis', in *BMJ*, vol. 282, p. 739.

TRADITIONAL PHARMACOLOGY

1 Hansen, T. M. *et al.* (1983) 'Treatment of rheumatoid arthritis with prostaglandin E_1 precursors *cis*-linoleic acid and γ-linolenic acid', in *Scan. J. Rheumatol.*, 12, pp. 85–8. Kunkel, S. L. *et al.* (1981) 'Suppression of chronic inflammation by evening primrose oil', in *Prog. Lip. Res.*, 28, pp. 885–8. Manku, M. S. *et al.* (1983) 'Essential fatty acids in the plasma phospholids of patients with atopic eczema', in *Brit. J. Dermatol.*, 110, pp. 643–8. Wright, S. and Burton, J. L. (1982) 'Oral evening-primrose-seed oil improves atopic eczema' in the *Lancet*, ii, pp. 1120–22.

2 Wagner, H. *et al.* (1985) 'Immunstimulierend wirkende Polysaccharide (Heteroglykane) aus höheren Pflanzen', in *Arzneimittel-Forschung* (Aulendorf, Germany), 35 (11), 7, pp. 1069–75.

3 Haslam, E. *et al.* (1989) 'Traditional herbal medicines – the role of polyphenols', in *Planta Medica*, Stuttgart, 55, pp. 1–8.

4 Hattor, M. *et al.* (1982) *Chem. Pharm. Bull.*, 30, p. 1338.

5 Fairburn, J. W. (ed.) (1976) 'The anthraquinone laxatives', in *Pharmacology*, 14, Suppl. 1, pp. 7–101.

6 Chan, H. and But, P. (1986) *Pharmacology and Applications of Chinese Materia Medica*, vol. 1, World Scientific, Singapore.

7 Sticher, O. (1977) 'Plant mono-, di-, and sesquiterpenoids with pharmacological and therapeutical activity', in *New Natural Products and Plant Drugs with Pharmacological, Biological or Therapeutical Activity*, Wagner, H. and Wolff, P. (eds.), Springer-Verlag, Berlin, pp. 137–76. Herz, W. (1971) 'Sesquiterpene lactones in Compositae', in *Pharmacognosy and Phytochemistry*, Wagner, H. and Horhammer, L. (eds.), Springer-Verlag, Berlin, pp. 64–92.

8 Forster, H. B., Niklas, H. and Lutz, S. (1980) *Planta Medica*, 40, 4, p. 309.

9 Szelenyi, I. *et al.* (1979) 'Pharmacological investigations with compounds of chamomile. III. Experimental studies of the ulcerprotective effect of chamomile', *Planta Medica*, 35, pp. 218–27.

10 Croteau and Fagerson, *Phytochemistry*, vol. II.

11 Shibata, S. (1977) 'Saponins with biological and pharmacological activity', in *New Natural Products and Plant Drugs with Pharmacological, Biological or Therapeutical Activity*, Wagner, H. and Wolff, P. (eds.), pp. 177–96. Takeda, K., (1972) 'The steroidal sapogenins of the Dioscoreaceae', in *Progress in Phytochemistry*, vol. 3, Rheinhold, L. and Liwshitz, Y. (eds.), John Wiley, Chichester, pp. 287–334.

12 Vogel, G. (1971) 'The effects of drugs of plant origin on capillary permeability and the lymphatic system', in *Pharmacognosy and Phytochemistry*, Wagner, H. and Horhammer, L. (eds.), Springer-Verlag, Berlin, pp. 370–84.

13 For a seminal discussion of much of this material, see: Fulder, S. (1980) *The Root of Being: Ginseng and the Pharmacology of Harmony*, Hutchinson, London, pp. 156–85. The following review of literature on Asian remedies will also provide interesting source material: Appleby, J. H. (1987) *A Selective Index to Siberian, Far Eastern, and Central Asian Russian Materia Medica*, Wellcome Unit for the History of Medicine, Oxford.

14 Fletcher Hyde, F. (1978) 'The origin and practice of herbal medicine', in *Mims Magazine*, pp. 127–36.

15 Akabas, M. *et al.* (1988) 'A bitter substance induces a rise in intracellular calcium in a subpopulation of rat taste cells', in *Science*, 242, p. 1047.

16 Schmid, W. (1966) 'Pflanzliche Bitterstoffe', in *Planta Medica*, suppl. 34.

17 With due acknowledgement to: Gibaldi, M. (1977) *Biopharmaceutics and Clinical Pharmacokinetics*, Lea and Febiger, Philadelphia.

18 Messegué, M. (1979) *Health Secrets of Plants and Herbs*, Collins, London.

PRACTICAL MATTERS

1 *British Herbal Pharmacopoeia* (1990), British Herbal Medicines Association, Bournemouth, UK.

2 The material has been extracted from a number of sources as well as from the author's own experience, notably: Davis, H. *et al.* (1949) *Bentley's Textbook of Pharmaceutics*, Ballière, Tindall and Cox, London; and the course material for the School of Herbal Medicine (Phytotherapy), Bucksteep Manor, Bodle Street Green, Hailsham, written by its principal, Hein Zeylstra.

REMEDIES

1 Wren, R. C. (1907) (rewritten Williamson, E. M. and Evans, F. J. (1988)) *Potters New Cyclopaedia of Botanical Drugs and Preparations*, C. W. Daniel Co., Saffron Walden, UK.

2 Autore, G., Capasso, F. and Mascolo, N. (1987) 'Biological screening of Italian medicinal plants for anti-inflammatory activity', in *Phytother. Res.*, 1, 1, pp. 28–31. Phillipson, J. D. and Anderson, L. A. (1984) 'Herbal remedies used in sedative and antirheumatic preparations; part 2', in *Pharm. J.*, July 28, pp. 111–15.

3 Tamm, C. H. (1977) 'Recent advances in the field of antibiotics', in *New Natural Products and Plant Drugs with Pharmacological, Biological or Therapeutical Activity*, Wagner, H., and Wolff, P. (eds.), Springer-Verlag, Berlin, pp. 82–136. Tschesche, R. (1971) 'Advances in the chemistry of antibiotic substances from higher plants', in *Pharmacognosy and Phytochemistry*, Wagner, H. and Horhammer, L. (eds.), Springer-Verlag, Berlin, pp. 274–89.

4 Stoessl, A. (1970) 'Antifungal compounds produced by higher plants', in *Recent Advances in Phytochemistry*, vol. 3, Steelink, C. and Runeckles, V. C. (eds.), Appleton-Century-Crofts, New York, pp. 143–80.

5 Cordell, G. A. (1977) 'Recent experimental and clinical data concerning anti-tumour and cytotoxic agents from plants', in *New Natural Products and Plant Drugs with Pharmacological, Biological or Therapeutical Activity*, Wagner, H., and Wolff, P. (eds.), Springer-Verlag, Berlin, pp. 54–81. Herz, W. (1971)

'Sesquiterpene lactones in Compositae', in *Pharmacognosy and Phytochemistry*, Wagner, H. and Horhammer, L. (eds.), pp. 64–92. Sticher, O. (1977) 'Plant mono-, di-, and sesquiterpenoids with pharmacological and therapeutical activity', in *New Natural Products and Plant Drugs with Pharmacological Biological or Therapeutical Activity*, Wagner, H. and Wolff, P. (eds.), pp. 137–76.

Appendixes

A TRADITIONAL PHYSIOLOGY

1 Notably those of the Indian sub-continent, see especially: Keswani, N. H. (ed.) (1974) *The Science of Medicine and Physiological Concepts in Ancient and Medieval India*, All-India Institute of Medical Sciences, New Delhi. Review of Ayurvedic and Unani texts.

2 I am particularly grateful for my contacts with Professor Manfred Porkert and his work: Porkert, M. (1974) *The Theoretical Foundations of Chinese Medicine*, MIT Press, Cambridge, Massachusetts. ibid. (1983) *The Essentials of Chinese Diagnostics*, Acta Medicinae Sinensis, Zürich. The work of the following other eminent sinologists should also be mentioned: Larre, Fr. C., Schatz, J. and Rochat de la Vallée, E. (1986) *Survey of Traditional Chinese Medicine*, Institut Ricci, Paris. Needham, J. (1956) *Science and Civilisation in China*, vol. 2, Cambridge University Press. Unschuld, P. U. (1985) *Medicine in China: A History of Ideas*, University of California Press.

3 See: Porkert (1974).

4 For a fascinating discussion of the nature of *qi*, see that between Manfred Porkert and Fritjof Capra at the Traditional Acupuncture Foundation Conference in Washington in 1983, reported in *Journal of Traditional Acupuncture*, VII, 2, pp. 15–20, TAF, American City Building, Columbia.

5 'Each birth is a condensation, each death a dispersal': Kaptchuk, T. (1983) *The Web that has no Weaver*, Congdon & Weed, New York. An inspiring and accessible book on Chinese medicine.

6 Selye, H. (1956 reprinted 1976) *The Stress of Life*, McGraw-Hill, New York.

7 Granger, H. J., Guyton, A. C. and Taylor, A. E. (1975) *Circulatory Physiology II: Dynamics and Control of the Body Fluids* W. B. Saunders Co., Philadelphia.

8 Notably: Bensky, D. and Gamble, A. (1986) *Chinese Herbal Medicine: Materia Medica*, Eastland Press, Seattle. Porkert, M. (1978) *Klinische Chinesische Pharmakologie*, Verlag für Medizin Fischer, Heidelberg. ibid. (1984) *Klassische Chinesische Rezeptur*, Acta Medicinae Sinensis, Zürich. Shih-Chen, L. (1973) *Chinese Medicinal Herbs*, Georgetown Press, San Francisco. Yeung, Him-che (1983) *Handbook of Chinese Herbs and Formulas*, vols. I and II, Him-che Yeung, Los Angeles.

General Index

abortifacient 256, 439
abscesses 490, 492
absinthe 436–7
absinthin 437
absorption 46
acacia gum 374
accommodation 29, 43
accommodative responses 43
acetic acid 270, 369, 378
acetylcholine 449
  receptors 125
acetylcoenzyme A 81, 84
achilleine 399, 401
achillin 299, 399
acid 267–72
  eliminating 111–12
  stomach 320
acidosis 340
aconitic acid 399
acrid components 301
acrid principles 224
acrid remedies 41, 319
  as antiseptic 198
  digestive-tract effects 320
  metabolic activity 83–4
  and phagocytic activity 78
acrid taste 192–3
ACTH 237, 506, 509
active principle 261
active transfer 47
active transport 336, 620
acupuncture 603
  point 40, 262
acute conditions, heroic treatment 395–6
adaptability 309
adaptogenic remedies 128, 228, 247, 309, 505
additives 220
adenine 331
adenosine 88
ADH 107, 237, 628

ADP 80–81
adrenal cortex 127, 506, 509
adrenaline 81–3, 123–4, 331
aesculin 287
agar-agar 103, 275, 374
age 341, 344–5
ageing 533
aglycones 108, 281, 287, 289
agropyrene 465
Aids 57, 69, 207
air 114–15, 155
alantoic acid 477
alantol 477
alantolactone 477
albumin 339
alcohol 89, 220, 494
  metabolic effect 340
aldosterone 108, 127, 509–10
algin 275
alkaloids 322, 327–31, 463, 467, 516
  acrid 317
alkaloids *see also* under group name
allantoin 545
  regeneration 547
allergic reactions 98
allergy 70, 74, 106, 226, 503
allicin 301, 414
alliin 414
allopathy 64, 155
almonds 219, 222, 314
aloe-emodin 445
alteratives 202, 214, 486–504
amarogentin 435
amaropanin 435
amaroswerin 435
amenorrhoea 451, 461, 521–2, 525
American Medical Association 153
amino-acids 84, 107
aminophylline 331
ammonia 84

association areas 38, 616
asthma 173, 206, 277, 624–5
  allergic 449
  azulenes for 300
  liquorice for 508
  plant drug block 125
  thyme for 483
  treatment 408
astringents 43, 283
  in immune disturbance 78
ATP 80–81
atropine 262, 329
  alkaloids 125
aucubin 503
autoantibodies 71, 73
autoimmune disease 59, 73–4, 117
  alteratives for 486
  digestives for 226
  liquorice for 509
autoimmunity 70–71
autonomic nervous system 89, 123–6, 159, 162
avenacosides 511
avenasterol 511
avenine 511
aversion of harmful influences 42
Avicenna 17
azulenes 295, 299–300, 399, 437

B-lymphocytes 68–9
bacteria 54
balchanolide 437
balsam 268
balsamic resins 304–5
baptisine 525
barbiturates 340
barks 360
Bateson, G. 237
baths 380–81
Beach, W. 158
beeswax 375, 385
beetroot 308
behaviour 23
Belaiche, P. 246
benzaldehyde 314, 484
benzoic acid 268, 271–2, 304
benzopyrone 286
benzylisoquinolines 330
berberine 331, 440
bergapten 287, 472, 536
beta-blockers 90
betain 488
betaine 541

betulin 495
bile 48, 100, 103–6
  black 106
  flow 323, 325, 496
  problems 105
bile salts 103
bile–bowel axis 103, 444
biliary disease, bitters for 429
biliousness 106
bilirubin 507
bioavailability 244–5, 332
biochemistry 30
bioflavonoids 271, 292–3
bisabolol 295, 300, 449
bitter digestives 181
bitter glycosides 543
bitter principles 321–7, 548
bitter remedies 41, 43, 52, 62, 429–47
  appetite increase 323
  for bile flow 105–6, 325
  chemical category 295
  digestive secretion increase 323–4
  for fevers 66
  for gentle provocation 213
  in immense disturbance 78
bitter taste 190–91
  receptors 322–3
bitters 226
bland taste 193–4, 464
blepharitis 463
blistering 62
blood, poisoning 490
blood flow 88, 90, 318
  regional 338
  and tissue availability 346
blood pressure 90
  high 108, 125
  hormonal control 108
blood–brain barrier 339
blood-letting 155
blood-sugar levels 48
bloodstream 91–2
body
  constants maintenance 127
  cooling 183
  function 23
  heating 182
  herbal effects on 243
  language 27
  response to stimulation 260
  rhythms 118–26
  temperature 64, 83

boils 490, 492, 535
bone healing 546
Boot, J. 155
borneol 295, 298, 427, 454, 482
bowel 99
  disease 106, 285, 416
  flora 74, 76, 103, 337, 341
  garlic for 417
  infections 549
  secretions 323
  toxicity thesis 117
  wall damage 76–7
  see also Twelve Functions, the
bradykinin 59, 88, 449
brain stem 237, 624
bran 100–101
breast-feeding 339
breathlessness 277
British Herbal Pharmacopoeia 350, 391
British Medical Association 154
bronchitis 60, 116, 206
  chronic 483
brown fat 83
brucellosis 59, 60
Brunner's glands 323, 324
bufadenolides 311
bulbs 360
Burnet, F. 71
burns 98, 490, 514

cadinene 437, 516, 536
caffeine 32, 108, 220, 331
  and noradrenaline 125
calamenene 516
calcitonin, secretion 323
calcium 49, 101, 311, 472, 511
calcium phosphate 110
calcium urate 110
calor 58
campesterol 531
camphene 295, 399, 419
camphor 295–8, 399, 427, 463, 477
canadine 331, 440
cancer *see* tumours
candidiasis 207, 212
Cannon, W. B. 159
capillaries 87, 92, 107
  fragility 98, 292
  lung 115
capsaicin 317, 319
capsanthin 421
capsorubin 421

capsules 378–9
carbohydrates 81, 272–5, 374
carbon dioxide 53, 92, 111–12, 114
carboxylic acids 267
carbuncles 490
cardenolides 311
cardioactive glycosides 310–13, 341
carminatives *see* aromatic digestives
carotene 513, 541
carotenoid pigments 295
carotenoids 543
carrageen 275
carrier
  capacity 336
  mechanisms 47
Cartesian split 118
carvacrol 295, 482, 536
carvone, 295, 427
caryophyllene 427, 437, 488
cascarosides 445
castine 523
catabolism 80–82
catalpol 538
catarrh 52, 116, 475
  eliminatives for 214
  persistent 66
  ribwort for 503
  therapy 408
catechol 283
cathartics 102
caulosapogenin 525
cayenne plaster 62
cell
  cleaning 96–7
  culture 245–6
  function 119
  health 246
  membrane 33
  vital activity 121–2
cell-to-cell communication 34
Celsus 58
Centre for Complementary Health Studies,
    University of Exeter 236
cereals 101, 219
cerebellum 610
cerebral cortex 614
cetraric acid 549
chamaelirin 520
chamazulene 299
chatarinine 454
chemical messengers 127
chemoreceptor centre 237

651   General Index

chest infections, ginger for 420
chilblains 469
childbirth 525–7
  complications 537
childhood
  acute condition treatment in 395–6
  colic 450
  coughs 483
  fevers 451, 453
  respiratory congestion 503
chill phase of fever 64
Chinese medicine 596–7
Chinese pharmacology 183–94
Chinese physiology 605–29
Chinese tonic remedies 527–41
chloramphenicol 341
chlorophyll 52
cholagogues 61, 78, 85, 101, 103, 105, 202
  gentle 213
cholera 57, 63
choleretics see cholagogues
choleric 106
cholesterol 48, 51, 84, 103, 105, 375
  myrrh for 502
choline 459, 531
chondroblasts 545
chronic disease 206–7
chrysaphenol 444
chrysophanic acid 445
cineol 295, 298, 399, 516
cineole 300, 456
cinnamaldehyde 413
cinnamic acid 268, 304
cinnamyl acetate 413
circadian rhythms 630–32
circulation 30, 86–94
  disorders 79
  effects of garlic 416
  mechanisms 88
  oceanic currents 604, 87–8
circulatory stimulants 53, 61, 93, 178, 227, 395
  for chronic conditions 396–8
  for fevers 67
cirrhosis 207
citral 295, 298, 452
citric acid 268, 271
citrin 292
citronellal 295, 298, 452
citronellol 298
clinical effects, measurement 242–4
clinical research 236–9
clonal elimination hypothesis 71

clotting factors 287
cocaine 39
cochineal 288
codeine 237, 262, 331
coeliac disease 50, 339
coffee 125, 285
Coffin, A. 154
colchicine 262
colchicinen 328
cold 34, 397
  common 56
  and illness 135–6
'cold' illness 203, 226
cold-damp
  and illness 138–9
  remedies 423–7
colic 276, 411
  in infants 426
  therapy 450
colitis 60
  mucous 290
  ulcerative 61, 71, 74, 226
colloids 373
colon, cancer 100, 103
colonic irrigation 99–100
comminution 368
complement 59, 68
conditioned reflex 40
conjunctivitis 463, 469, 509
consolidine 545
constipation 102, 105–6, 256, 290, 342, 624–5
contra-indications 257
contraceptives, oral 341
control functions 118–31
convalescence 202, 209, 217–23
convulsions 173, 450
Cook, W. H. 122, 126, 159–63, 208
Cooper, M. R. 250
copaene 516
corms 360
coronary arteries 90, 537
corpus luteum 523–4
costunolide 437
cough 173, 180, 483
  in cleaning the lung 115
  dry 116
  productive 478
cough reflex 623
coughing 475
  reduction 485
coumarins 286–7, 402, 413, 424, 449, 506
counter-irritation 62, 178, 269, 317, 333

cranberry 271, 300–301
creams 383–4
creatinine 107
   clearance 345
Crohn's disease 207, 226, 460
cross-reactivity 74
Culpeper, N. 174
Curtis, A. 158
cyanide 313, 336
cyanogenic glycosides 313–15, 399, 402, 485, 517
cycle of activity 164–70
cymene 295, 516
cymol 295, 482
cynoglossine 545
cystitis 108, 471

damianin 516
dammaradienol 477
damp-heat 226, 429
   and illness 138–40
D'arcy Thomson, W. 120
de Quincey, T. 237
death-cap mushroom 442
decoction 370–71
defence functions 68
deficiency syndromes 226
dehydration 464
demulcent action 276
Department of Health 149
depression 448, 517
   oats for 512
   St John's wort for 513
   tonic foods 221
depuratives 202, 214, 486
dermatitis 60
detoxification 81, 157
   techniques 99
di-homo-gamma-linoleic acid (GLA) 269
diabetes 47, 51, 71, 206, 325, 346, 539
diallyl disulphide 414
dianthron 513
diaphoretics 66, 94, 114, 177, 202, 395–6, 398
diaphragm 115
diarrhoea 173, 179, 180, 274, 276, 397, 469
   cooling remedy 441
   peppermint for 457
   tannin remedies 285
diazepams 454–5
dicoumarol 287
Diesing, P. 241
diet 209, 219–20
diffusion 47

digestion 46
   inadequate 77, 78
digestive stimulants 61, 400
digestive tract 276, 334–7
   angelica for 411
   aromatic digestives for 423–7
   comfrey for 547
   garlic for 417
   liquorice for 508
   relaxants 451
digitalis glycosides 104, 109
digoxin 262, 313, 340
Dioscorides 235
diosgenin 307, 534–5
diosphenol 298
disaccharides 272
discrimination 29, 38
distal tubule 107
distillation 372–3
disulphides 301
diterpenes 295, 322
diuretics 61, 108, 193, 202, 342, 464–73
   mild 213
   osmotic 108
   saponins 308
diurnal rhythms 123
diverticulitis 100–101, 460
Doctrine of Signatures 194
dodecanol 536
dolor 58
dosage 344–5
double-blind clinical trial 239
douches 381, 441, 483, 490, 526
Driesch, H. 120
dropsy 90–91, 109, 310, 433–4
drugs 104, 215–16
dryness and illness 141–2
duodenum
   mucosa 323
   muscle tone 323
   ulcer 125
dysentery 274, 469
dysmenorrhoea 421, 513, 521–2, 525, 527
   hops for 461
   peppermint for 458
   wormwood for 438
dyspepsia 276
   nervous 173
   therapy 441
dysphagia 276

ear-drops 381–2

earth 166–70
Earth 617
earth mother 167
Easton, J. 5
echinacea 54, 58
echinacein 488
echinacin 488–9
echinacoside 488
echinalone 488
echinidine 545
ecosystem 16, 54
eczema 61, 206, 299, 449, 494, 624
  alteratives for 486
EFAs 269
effector lymphocytes 69
efficacy of herbs 234–9
egg 219, 221
El-Rhazes 17
electrical pulse 34
elemene 531
elements 155
elephantiasis 98
Eliade, M. 165
elimination 202
eliminative 214
elixirs 375
ellagic acid 283
embolism 90
embrocations 62, 383
embryo 131
emesis 95
emetics 157, 202, 476, 625
emetine 331
emmenogogue 256, 473
emodin 444, 445
emollient action 276
empyema 59
emulsions 374–5
endocarditis 74
endoplasmic reticulum 121
endorphins 616
enemas 382
energetics 600–629
energy production 80
entero-hepatic circulation 245, 341–2
enuresis 433, 513
enzymes 46, 80
eosinophils 60
ephedrine 328
epilepsy 475
Epstein-Barr infection 207, 209, 212
equisetonin 467

ergometrine 330
ergotamine 262, 330
ericolin 470
eriodictyol 292
ethers 300, 369
eucalyptole 427
eugenol 281–2, 399, 413
exercise 97, 124–5, 218–19
exhaustion 448
exorphins 76
expectorants 43, 53, 78, 202, 320, 475–85, 500
  relaxing 116, 194, 479–83, 503, 508, 546, 625
  stimulating 116, 476–8, 625
  warming 116, 476–8
expression, drug 372
extracts, solid 380
eye, diseases 463
eye-drops 382
eyebath 426, 451, 509

faradiol 480
farnesene 295, 449
farnesol 437
fasting 221, 337
fat, brown see brown fat
fatigue 211–12, 397
  tonic foods 221
fatigue syndromes 226
fats,
  assimilation 48
  catabolism 81
fatty acids 81
feeling 38
fenchone 295, 424, 463
fertility 521
fever 63–7, 156–7, 180
  childhood 451, 453
  cooling remedies 428–63
  heroic treatment 395–6
  management 65–7, 200
  sweating in 113–14
fibre 105, 100–101, 274
  natural 101
fibroblasts 488, 545
fibroids 207
filariasis 98
Fire 155, 611–12
first-pass effect 245, 246, 340
fish 219, 221
fish poisons 306
fish senses 35
flap mechanism 96

flatulence 276, 411
flavolignans 442
flavones 291–4
flavonoids 291–4, 463, 467
flavonols 292
flavonones 292
flowers 354
fluid
   extracts 375–6
   movement 604
   retention 108, 110
follicle-stimulating hormone (FSH) 524
food
   acid 112
   additives 104, 340
   allergies 75, 212, 226
   immunological challenge 324
   intolerance 74–6, 211
   neurosis 76
   overconsumption 89
   poisonous 250–51
   quality 144
   and remedy absorption 336–7
   restorative 219–20
   as tonic 221–3
Food and Drug Administration 149
food poisoning 549
foreign body reaction 59
formic acid 269–70, 497
formulae 391
fracture, bark 360
Friar's Balsam 272
friedelin 477
'fright, fight, flight' 89, 112, 124, 610
frigidity 541
fructose 84
fruit 105, 360
FSH 123
fucosterin 515
fucoxanthin 515
Fuller, B. 8
fumaric acid 268
fumaroprotocetraric acid 549
Function 607
functional adjustments 203
functional assay 243
fungus 54
furanocoumarins 410, 472, 536

Gaia 121, 617
galactose 84
galacturonic acid 274

Galen 17, 174–5, 177, 180, 203, 235
galiosin 493
gallbladder 105
   see also Twelve Functions, the
gallic acid 283
gallstones 105–6
gangrene, garlic for 416
gargles 382–3, 483
gas exchange 114
gastric acid 323
gastrin 323
gastritis 60
gastrointestinal motility 337
genistein 292
genital ridge 628
gentiamarin 435
gentiin 435
gentiopicrin 435
gentiopicroside 435
gentisin 292, 435
geraniol 295, 298, 452, 459
germacranolides 437
germanium 414
giant cells 60
gingerol 419
ginsenin 530, 532
ginsenosides 530–31
GLA 269
glandular fever 463
   convalescence 217
Glass, L. 121
globicin 437
glomerulonephritis 71
glomerulus 107
glucagon 48
   secretion 323
glucocorticoids 127, 130
glucokinins 414
glucoquinone 497
glucose 47, 84, 107
glucosilinates 315
glucovanilline 465
glucuronate 341
gluten 50, 250, 511–12
glycerins 376
glycerol 369
glycolytic pathway 81
glycymarin 506
glycyrrhizin 506–7
gobosterin 491
goitre 316
Golgi bodies 121

IgA 42, 69, 74
IgD 42, 69
IgE 42, 69, 76
IgG 69
IgM 69
immune response 70
immune system 67–79, 226
  garlic for 416
  integration 127
immunity, mechanisms 69–70
immunodeficiency 207
impotence 541
incontinence 469
Indians, native American 151
indole alkaloids 330, 511
infants, colic 426
infections 54, 57
  alteratives for 486
  bacterial 490
  chest 413
  chronic 58
  fungal 457
  garlic for 415–17
  lung 74
  myrrh for 501
  urinary 74, 466, 469, 471
  viral 395, 490
inflammation 58, 180, 318
  alteratives for 486
  chronic, bitters for 429
  cooling remedies 428–63
  gentian for 435
  liquorice for 509
  as opportunity 60
inflammatory process 178
inflammatory response 61
influenza 57
infusion 369–70
ingestion 29, 43
inhalants 383
inhalations
  fennel 426
  relaxant 451
inhibition, competitive 336
inositol 465
insomnia 457
  hops for 460
  St John's wort for 513
insulin 47, 123
  secretion 323
integration 32, 126–9, 228
intelligence 38

intercellular fluid 96
intercellular matrix 87
interferons 68, 488
intracellular matrix 121
intrinsic factor, secretion 323
inulin 49, 353, 477, 488, 545
iodine 316, 463, 515
ipecac alkaloids 331
iridoid glycosides 321, 538
iridoids 299
iron 49, 84, 101, 472, 497
irritable bowel 101, 103, 460, 513,
    624
  see also bowel
irritant, in volatile oils 302–3
isoflavones 292
isolichenin 549
isoprene 294
isoquinoline alkaloids 330
isosafrol 536
isothiocyanates 315
isovalerianic acid 399, 454
isovaleric acid 436
ivain 399

jaundice 105, 464
  therapy 441
jellies 384
jet-lag 625
johimbine 330
Johnson, A. W. 250

kaempferol 292, 399, 531
kallidin 88
kaolin 285
keto-acid precursors 84
khellin 287
kidneys 107–12
  excretion 342, 345–6
  failure 98, 340
  stones 496
  see also Twelve Functions, the
Kneipp, S. 381
Krebs cycle 81, 271
Kuppfer cells 68

lactic acid 68, 111
lactones 321
laetrile 315
lager 97
lanolin 375, 385
lavendulyl 437

laxatives 61, 78, 202, 224, 430
  anthraquinone 102, 257, 289, 444–6
  bulk 101, 256, 625
  excessive use of 100–101
  osmotic 271
  stimulating 102
lead 469
learning 38
lecithin 48, 84
leeches 155
Leibniz, G. W. 120
lemon juice 106, 326
leprosy 59, 60
leukotrienes 59
Li Tung-Yuan 170
lice 446
lichen acids 549–50
lichenin 549
ligustilide 536
limbic system 35, 127, 620
limonene 295, 298, 424, 452, 456
linalool 295, 298, 452, 459, 482
linctuses 376
liniments 62, 383
Linnaeus, C. 352
linoleic acid 268
lipid-solubility 335, 338–9
lipoproteins 48
liquiritigetol 292, 506
liquorice 502
liver 49, 72, 104
  anabolism 82
  bicarbonate production 323
  bitter digestives for 181
  bitters for 429
  dandelion for 432–3
  disturbances 98
  function 531
  inflammation 105
  integration 127
  metabolic functions 84
  metabolism 341
  plasma protein levels 339
  poisons remedy 442–3
  thyme for 483
  see also Twelve Functions, the
lotions 383
Lovelock, J. 121
lozenges 379
lunar cycle 130
lung disease, angelica for 411
lung infections, garlic for 417

lungs 52
  see also Twelve Functions, the
luparenol 459
luparol 459
lupulin 459
luteinizing hormone 523
luteolin 399, 449
Lyle, T. J. 159
lymph flow stimulation 97
lymph nodes 211
lymphadenopathy 97, 463, 494
lymphatic pump 96
lymphatic system, capillaries 96
lymphatics 78, 96–8, 202, 486, 494
lymphocytes 60, 69, 97
  see also T-cells
lymphokines 68, 76, 488
lysergic acid diethylamide (LSD) 330
lysine 329
lysosomes 46
lysosyme 68

M-plates 74
Macer Floridus de Viribus Herbarum 426
maceration 371
Mackey, M. 121
macrophage 58, 60, 68, 488
  response 246
magnoflorine 525
malabsorption syndrome 50, 346
malic acid 268
maltol 531
manganese 472
mannitol 465–6, 538
maps, information evaluation 241
marc 369
marigold 54
massage 92, 97
mastitis 463
matricin 299
maturation 130
ME *see* myalgic encephalomyelitis
Medawar, P. 235
medicinal plant properties 234–9
Medicines Act 1968 238, 252
melaena 543
melancholic 106
mels 377
membrane barrier 338–9
membrane receptor 34, 69
memory 38
memory lymphocytes 69

physiomedicalism 153
physostigmine 330
phytates 101
phytic acid 49
phytosterols 467
pills 379
pilocarpine 262, 295, 298, 399, 424, 427, 449, 454
pinene 516
piperidine alkaloids 329
piperitone 456
Pirsig, R. 18
pituitary gland, 107, 127
pituitary hormone activity 523
pK 335
placebo effects 240
placental membrane 339
plague 63
plant
    classification 352–3
    drug extraction 369–73
    drying 367
    poisonous 249–50
    storage 368
    structure 354–64
    underground structure 360
plasma cells 69
plasma protein 339
plasma proteins, low levels 98
plasmin 59
plasters 385–6
poisoning 250
poisons 178
    for infections 63
polio 57
polyacetylenes 489, 492
polybasic acids 267–8
polymorphonuclear leucocytes 68
polyphenols 282
polysaccharides 272–3
    immuno-stimulating 273
Popper, K. 235
Porkert, M. 597, 605
porridge 101, 221
posology 63
post-viral syndrome 204, 207, 212
    convalescence 217
potassium 31, 33, 109–10, 312, 433–4, 465, 503
potatoes 219, 221
poultice 62, 386
    comfrey 546
powders 379–80, 386
prana 45

pregnancy 255–7
premenstrual tension 110, 523–4
prescribing 205
primary defences 42
Primary Health Care 11
proazulenes 449
process patterns 26
processes of living 25
processing 80–85
progesterone 108, 123
prolactin 123
prolapse 173
properdin-complement pathway 68
prostaglandins 59, 76, 289, 545
    inhibition 419
prostate, hypertrophy 519
prostatitis 471, 520
protein 81
    for emulsions 374
protein binding 339–40, 345
protoalkaloids 328
protoberberines 331
protocetraric acid 549
protopanaxadiol 531
protopanaxatriol 531
protopine 331
proximal tubules 107
prunasin 484
psilocybin 330
psoriasis 71, 206, 494, 545
psychoneuroimmunology 24
puberty 130
PUFAs 268–9
pulegone 456
pulse 201, 211
purine alkaloids 331
pyorrhoea 490
pyrexia 63
pyridine alkaloids 329
pyrogallol 283
pyrogen 64
pyrrolidine alkaloids 329
pyrrolizidine 545
pyrrolizidine alkaloids 329, 480

qi 600–602
qi gong 632
qi tonics 223, 528
quality control 348–87
quercitol 292
quercitrin 399, 402, 449
quinidine 536

quinine 343
quinoline alkaloids 330
quinolizidine alkaloids 329

radiation damage 98
rationalism 14
Raynaud's disease 206, 226, 404
reabsorption 50
reaction 29, 42, 46, 228
reactive responses 43
Reason, P. 240
receptors 34
recovery time 204
rectum 334
red blood cells 93
references 394
reflex 39
regeneration 59
rehmannin 538
rejection 29, 45, 53, 228
    disorders 79
relaxants 182, 247, 447–63
    in volatile oils 303
remedy
    absorption 332–7
    adaptogenic 532
    Chinese tonic 527–41
    cooling 428–63
    distribution 338–40
    excretion 341–3
    'Harmony' 308, 509
    healing 542–50
    as herbal remedy 391
    hormonal 505–41
    metabolism 340–41
    relaxant 611
    warming 395–427
removal 31, 228
renaline 330
renin 123
renin-angiotensin system 108, 628
reproduction 32, 130–31
research policy 240–48
reserpine 330
resin 43, 62, 224, 268, 399, 419, 470, 488
    as antiseptic 198
    chemistry 304–5
    in immune disturbance 78
    in myrrh 501
resistance
    subdued 201
    vital 200

respiratory centres 624
respiratory system 114–17, 277
response 27, 39
    healing 258
    patterns 40
rest 124–5, 218
restorative remedies 220–23, 228
reticular activating system 610
rheinanthrone 289
rheumatism 206, 496
    liquorice for 509
rheumatoid arthritis 62, 71, 74
    and lung infections 214
rhinitis 60
    allergic 408
rhizomes 360
rhythm 121, 128, 160, 164
rice 219
    brown 101
ricinine 328
ridentin 437
Rogers, C. R. 236
Rome, medical traditions 150
root vegetables 219, 221
roots 360
rotenone 292
Rowan, J. 240
Royal Society of Medicine Colloquia 21
rubber 295
rubefacients 62, 178, 281, 316, 317
rubor 58
rutin 293, 402, 456, 499

sabinene 399, 427
safety 249–54
safrol 536
Saint's triad 105
salicylates 399
salicylic acid 268, 279–81
saliva 271
salpingitis 61, 521
salty taste 188–9
santanolides 437
santolinyl 437
santonin 437
sapogenin 306, 534
saponins 131, 191, 465, 467
    chemistry 305–9
    steroidal 306–7, 353, 518, 526
saprophytes 56
sarcoidosis 60
sarsapogenin 307

Index of
Botanical
Names

Garcinia hanburii 305
Gaultheria procumbens 279, 495, 583
Gentiana lutea 292, 321, 434
Geranium maculatum 589
Geum urbanum 281
Ginkgo biloba 322, 560, 590
Glechoma hederacea see *Nepeta hederacea*
Glycyrrhiza glabra 192, 222, 262, 292, 307, 308,
    501, 505, 558, 563, 566, 568, 569, 571, 572,
    574, 575, 577, 582, 585, 589, 591, 593, 625
Glycyrrhiza uralensis 510, 534
Gnaphalium uliginosum 478, 575
Gossypium herbaceum 256
Gratiola officinalis 313
Grindelia spp. 561
Guaiacum officinale 299, 304, 584, 588

Hamamelis virginiana 384, 547, 569, 570, 575,
    592
Harpagophytum procumbens 582, 584
Heliotropium europaeum 252
Helleborus niger 313
Helleborus viride 313
Hordeum vulgare 50, 222, 250, 466
Humulus lupulus 204, 321, 322, 458, 568, 577,
    583
Hydrangea arborescens 519, 586
Hydrastis canadensis 256, 322, 330, 439, 573,
    574, 575, 592
Hydrocotle asiatica see *Centella asiatica*
Hyoscyamus niger 125, 252, 328, 561, 591
Hypericum perforatum 221, 253, 512, 569, 579,
    581, 583, 588, 616
Hyssopus officinalis 484, 565, 566, 568

Inula helenium 223, 303, 477, 563, 568, 574, 585,
    593, 621
Ipomoea jalapa 252
Ipomoea purpurea 252

Jateorrhiza palmata 322
Juglans regia 535
Juniperus communis 256, 298, 471, 584, 591

Krameria triandra 570, 575

Laburnum anagyroides 329
Lactuca virosa 321, 484
Lamium album 581
Lavandula officinalis 576, 583
Leonurus cardiaca 559, 573, 576, 581
Ligustrum lucidum 541

Linum usitatissimum 102, 222, 256, 289, 314,
    379, 386, 563, 568, 570, 585, 625
Liquidamber orientalis 305
Lobelia inflata 157, 252, 307, 329, 561, 563, 568,
    585, 593, 625
Lophophora williamsii 330
Lycium chinensis 529, 540

Malaleuca leucadendron 198, 300
Mandragora officinarum 252
Manihot esculenta 314
Marrubium vulgare 322, 568
Marsdenia condurango 560
Matricaria chamomilla see *Matricaria recutita*
Matricaria recutita 182, 204, 256, 273, 295, 299,
    314, 446, 448, 562, 566, 567, 568, 571, 572,
    577, 581, 582, 583, 589, 593, 611
Melissa officinalis 182, 298, 451, 566, 571, 577,
    593
Mentha pulegium 256
Mentha x piperita 182, 198, 204, 295, 456, 566,
    567, 568, 571, 577, 583, 593
Menyanthes trifoliata 582, 588
Mitchella repens 526, 579, 581
Monarda punctata 282
Monotropa uniflora 279
Morinda officinalis 535
Morus alba 539
Myrica cerifera 157, 574
Myristica fragrans 300, 425
Myroxylon balsamum 271, 305
Myroxylon pereirae 305

Nasturtium officinale 317
Nepeta hederacea 222, 503, 565, 567, 575, 589

Oenethera biennis and spp. 222, 269, 586,
    616
Ophiopogon japonicus 541
Origanum vulgare 256

Paeonia lactiflora 539
Panax ginseng 192, 223, 306, 307, 308, 509, 528,
    529, 569, 577, 578, 586
Panax quinquefolium 530, 541
Papaver somniferum 237
Parietaria spp. 592
Passiflora incarnata 182, 329, 456, 577
Petroselinum crispum 112, 270, 291, 300, 472,
    581, 584, 586
Peumus boldo 574, 591
Phellodendron amurense 441

671   Index of Botanical Names

List of Common Plant Names

To find references to the common names of herbs mentioned in this book, look up their botanical names and then use the Index of Botanical Names.

aconite *Aconitum* spp.
agnus-castus *Vitex agnus-castus*
agrimony *Agrimonia officinalis*
alder buckthorn *Rhamnus frangula*
aloes *Aloe vera*
angelica *Angelica archangelica*
angostura *Cusparia angustura*
aniseed *Pimpinella anisum*
arbor-vitae *Thuja occidentalis*
arnica *Arnica montana*
artichoke *Cynara scolymus*
asafoetida *Ferula foetida*
asparagus root *Asparagus cochinchinensis*
autumn crocus *Crocus sativa*
avens *Geum urbanum*

Ba Ji *Morinda officinalis*
Bai Shao *Paeonia lactiflora*
Bai Zhu *Atractylodes macrocephala*
balm *Melissa officinalis*
balm of Gilead *Populus gileadensis*
barberry bark *Berberis vulgaris*
barley *Hordeum vulgare*
bayberry *Myrica cerifera*
bearberry *Arctostaphylos uva-ursi*
beggar's buttons *Arctium lappa*
belladonna *Atropa belladonna*
benzoin *Styrax* spp.
beth root *Trillium erectum*
birch *Betula* spp.
birth root *Trillium erectum*
bistort *Polygonum bistorta*
bittersweet *Solanum dulcamara*
black haw bark *Viburnum prunifolium*
black sampson *Echinacea angustifolia*
blackberry leaf *Rubus fructicosus*

bladderwrack *Fucus vesiculosus*
blessed thistle *Cnicus benedictus*
bloodroot *Sanguinaria canadensis*
boldo *Peumus boldo*
boneset *Eupatorium perfoliatum*
borage *Borago officinalis*
bottlebrush *Equisetum arvense*
broccoli *Brassica oleracea*
broom *Cytisus scoparius*
bryony *Bryonia alba*
buchu *Barosma betulina*
buckbean *Menyanthes trifoliata*
buckthorn, California *Rhamnus purshiana*
buckwheat *Fagopyrum esculentum*
burdock *Arctium lappa* and spp.

cabbage *Brassica oleracea*
cajaput *Melaleuca leucadendron*
calabar bean *Physostigma venenosum*
calendula *Calendula officinalis*
caraway *Carum carvi*
cardamom *Amomum cardamomum*
carrot *Daucus carota*
cascara sagrada *Rhamnus purshiana*
cassava *Manihot esculenta*
cassia *Cinnamomum cassia*
catechu *Acacia catechu*
cayenne *Capsicum minimum*
celandine, greater *Chelidonium major*
celery *Apium graveolens*
centaury *Erythraea centaurium*
chamomile, German *Matricaria recutita*
chamomile, Roman *Anthemis nobile*
chamomile, wild *Matricaria recutita*
charlock *Sinapsis arvensis*
chaste tree *Vitex agnus-castus*

checkerberry *Mitchella repens*
cherry bark, wild *Prunus serotina*
chickweed *Stellaria media*
chicory *Cichorium intybus*
chilli *Capsicum minimum*
chiretta *Swertia chirata*
cinchona bark *Cinchona* spp.
cinnamon *Cinnamomum zeylanicum*
cinnamon, Chinese *Cinnamomum cassia*
cleavers *Galium aparine*
clivers *Galium aparine*
clover, red *Trifolium pratense*
cloveroot *Geum urbanum*
cloves *Eugenia caryophyllata*
cocoa *Theobroma cacao*
coffee *Caffea arabica*
cohosh, black *Cimicifuga racemosa*
cohosh, blue *Caulophyllum thalictroides*
cola *Cola vera*
colophony *Pinus palustris*
coltsfoot *Tussilago farfara*
columbo *Jateorrhiza palmata*
comfrey *Symphytum officinale*
condurango *Marsdenia condurango*
corn silk *Zea mays*
cotton-root bark *Gossypium herbaceum*
couch grass *Agropyron repens*
cowslip *Primula vera*
cramp bark *Viburnum opulus*
cranesbill *Geranium maculatum*
cudweed *Gnaphalium uliginosum*
curled dock *Rumex crispus*

Da Zao *Zizyphus jujuba*
daisy *Bellis perennis*
damiana *Turnera diffusa*
dandelion *Taraxacum officinale*
Dang Gui *Angelica sinensis*
Dang Shen *Codonopsis pilulosa*
datura *Datura stramonium*
deadly nightshade *Atropa belladonna*
devil's claw *Harpagophytum procumbens*
dill *Anethum graveolens*
dock, yellow *Rumex crispus*
dragon's blood *Daemonorops* spp.
Du Zhong *Eucommia ulmoides*

echinacea *Echinacea angustifolia*
elderflower *Sambucus nigra*
elecampane *Inula helenium*
eryngo *Eryngium maritimum*
eucalyptus *Eucalyptus* spp.

euphorbia *Euphorbia hirta*
evening primrose *Oenethera biennis* and spp.
eyebright *Euphrasia officinalis*

false unicorn root *Chamaelirium luteum*
fennel *Foeniculum vulgare*
fenugreek *Trigonella foenum-graecum*
feverfew *Tanacetum parthenium*
figworth *Scrophularia nodosa*
flax *Linum usitatissimum*
foxglove *Digitalis* spp.
frankincense *Boswellia* spp.
fumitory *Fumaria officinalis*

gamboge *Garcinia hanburii*
Gan Cao *Glycyrrhiza uralensis*
garlic *Allium sativum*
gentian *Gentiana lutea*
ginger *Zingiber officinale*
ginkgo *Ginkgo biloba*
ginseng *Panax ginseng*
ginseng, American *Panax quinquefolium*
golden rod *Solidago virgaurea*
golden seal *Hydrastis canadensis*
golden thread *Coptis chinensis*
gotu kola *Centella asiatica*
Gou Qi Zi *Lycium chinensis*
gravel root *Eupatorium purpurea*
grindelia *Grindelia* spp.
ground ivy *Glechoma hederacea*
guelder rose *Viburnum opulus*

hawthorn *Crataegus* spp.
heather *Calluna vulgaris*
hedge hyssop *Gratiola officinalis*
Hei Zhi Ma *Sesamum indicum*
heliotrope *Heliotropium europaeum*
hellebore, black *Helleborus niger*
hellebore, green *Helleborus viride*
helonias root *Chamaelirium luteum*
hemlock *Conium maculatum*
henbane *Hyoscyamus niger*
hops *Humulus lupulus*
horehound, black *Ballota nigra*
horehound, white *Marrubium vulgare*
horse chestnut *Aesculus hippocastanum*
horsemint *Monarda punctata*
horseradish *Cochlearia armoracia*
horsetail *Equisetum arvense*
Hu Lu Ba *Trigonella foenum-graecum*
Hu Tao Ren *Juglans regia*
Huang Qi *Astragalus membranaceous*

hydrangea *Hydrangea arborescens*
hyssop *Hyssopus officinalis*

Iceland moss *Cetraria islandica*
Indian pipe *Monotropa uniflora*
Indian snakeroot *Rauwolfia serpentaria*
ipecacuanha *Cephaelis ipecacuanha*
Irish moss *Chondrus crispus*

jaborandi *Pilocarpus microphyllus*
jalap *Ipomoea jalapa*
jimson weed *Datura stramonium*
johimbe *Corynanthe yohimbi*
jujube *Zizyphus jujuba*
juniper *Juniperus communis*

kale *Brassica oleracea*
kava-kava *Piper methysticum*
kelp *Fucus vesiculosus*
knitbone *Symphytum officinale*
kohlrabi *Brassica oleracea*
kola *Cola vera*
kombe *Strophantus kombe*

laburnum *Laburnum anagyroides*
lady's mantle *Alchemilla vulgaris*
lavender *Lavandula officinalis*
lemon balm *Melissa officinalis*
lettuce, wild *Lactuca virosa*
life root *Senecio aureus*
lignum-vitae *Guaiacum officinale*
lily-of-the-valley *Convallaria majalis*
limeflowers *Tilia europoea* and spp.
linden flowers *Tilia europea* and spp.
linseed *Linum usitatissimum*
lion's tooth *Taraxacum officinale*
liquorice *Glycyrrhiza glabra*
liquorice, Chinese *Glycyrrhiza uralensis*
lobelia *Lobelia inflata*
lycium *Lycium chinensis*

Ma Huang *Ephedra sinica*
Madagascar periwinkle *Catharanthus rosea*
madder *Rubia tinctoria*
Mai Men Dong *Ophiopogon japonicus*
maize *Zea mays*
male fern *Dryopteris felix-mas*
mandrake *Mandragora officinarum*
manioc *Manihot esculenta*
marigold *Calendula officinalis*
marjoram *Origanum vulgare*
marshmallow *Althaea officinalis*

may apple *Podophyllum peltatum*
maybush *Crataegus* spp.
mayflower *Crataegus* spp.
meadow saffron *Crocus sativus*
meadowsweet *Filipendula ulmaria*
milfoil *Achillea millefolium*
milk thistle *Carduus marianus*
mistletoe *Viscum album*
monk's pepper *Vitex agnus-castus*
morning glory *Ipomoea purpurea*
motherwort *Leonurus cardiaca*
mouse-eared hawkweed *Pilosella officinarum*
mugwort *Artemisia vulgaris*
mulberry *Morus alba*
mullein *Verbascum thapsus*
mustard, black *Brassica nigra*
mustard, white *Sinapis alba*
myrrh *Commiphora mol-mol*

nasturtium *Tropaeolum majus*
nettle *Urtica dioica*
nightshade *Atropa belladonna*
Nu Zhen Zi *Ligustrum lucidum*
nutmeg *Myristica fragrans*

oak *Quercus robur*
oak galls *Quercus robur*
oats *Avena sativa*
onion *Allium cepa*
Oregon grape *Berberis aquifolium*
ouabain *Strophantus gratus*

paeony *Paeonia lactiflora*
parsley *Petroselinum crispum*
parsley piert *Aphanes arvensis*
partridge berry *Mitchella repens*
passionflower *Passiflora incarnata*
pearl barley *Hordeum vulgare*
pellitory *Parietaria* spp.
pennyroyal *Mentha pulegium*
pepper *Piper nigra*
peppermint *Mentha x piperita*
periwinkle, common *Vinca major*
periwinkle, Madagascar *Catharanthus rosea*
Peru balsam *Myroxylon pereirae*
pewterwort *Equisetum arvense*
pheasant's eye *Adonis vernalis*
pilewort *Ranunculus ficaria*
pine *Pinus* spp.
pipsissewa *Chimaphila umbelata*
plantain, English *Plantago lanceolata*
plantain, rat's tail *Plantago major*

pleurisy root *Asclepias tuberosa*
poison oak *Rhus toxicodedron*
poke root *Phytolacca decandra*
poplar *Populus* spp.
prickly ash *Zanthoxylum americanum*
psyllium seeds *Plantago psyllium*
pumpkin seeds *Cucurbita maxima*
purple coneflower *Echinacea angustifolia*

quassia *Picrasma excelsa*
quebrach *Aspidosperma quebracho-blanco*
quickset *Crataegus* spp.
quillaia *Quillaia saponaria*

radish *Raphanus sativus*
ragwort *Senecio jacobaea*
rapeseed *Brassica napus*
raspberry leaves *Rubus idaeus*
red clover *Trifolium pratense*
rehmannia *Rehmannia glutinosa*
Ren Shen *Panax ginseng*
rhatany *Krameria triandra*
rhubarb *Rheum* spp.
ribwort *Plantago lanceolata*
rosemary *Rosmarinus officinalis*
rue *Ruta graveolens*

sabal *Serenoa serrulata*
sage *Salvia officinalis*
Sang Shen *Mori alba*
sarsaparilla *Smilax* spp.
saw palmetto *Serenoa serrulata*
scullcap *Scutellaria laterifolia*
scurvy grass *Cochlearia officinalis*
scutch *Agropyron repens*
self-heal *Prunella vulgaris*
senna *Cassia angustifolia*
sesame seeds *Sesamum indicum*
seven barks *Hydrangea arborescens*
Sheng Di Huang *Rehmannia glutinosa*
shepherd's purse *Capsella bursa-pastoris*
Shu Di Huang *Rehmannia glutinosa*
Siberian ginseng *Eleutherococcus senticosus*
silver birch *Betula* spp.
skunk cabbage *Symplocarpus foetidus*
slippery elm *Ulmus fulva*
snakeroot *Polygala senega*
soap bark *Quillaia saponaria*
soapwort *Saponaria officinalis*
southernwood *Artemisia abrotanum*
spindle-tree *Euonymus europaeus*

squaw root *Caulophyllum thalictroides*
squaw vine *Mitchella repens*
squills *Urginea maritima*
St John's wort *Hypericum perforatum*
sticky-willie *Galium aparine*
stinging nettle *Urtica dioica*
stone root *Collinsonia canadensis*
storax *Liquidamber orientalis*
strophanthus *Strophantus kombe*
sundew *Drosera rotundifolia*
sweet flag *Acorus calamus*
sweet violet *Viola odorata*

tansy *Tanacetum vulgare*
thyme, common *Thymus officinalis*
thyme, wild *Thymus serpillum*
Tian Men Dong *Asparagus cochinensis*
Tolu balsam *Myroxylon balsamum*
tormentil *Potentilla erecta*
turnip *Brassica rapa*

uva-ursi *Arctostaphylos uva-ursi*
valerian *Valeriana officinalis*
vervain *Verbena officinalis*
violet *Viola odorata*

wahoo *Euonymus atropurpureus*
wake robin *Trillium erectum*
wall germander *Teucrium chamaedrys*
wallflower *Cheiranthus cheiri*
watercress *Nasturtium officinale*
white bryony *Bryonia alba*
white deadnettle *Lamium album*
white horehound *Marrubium vulgare*
whitethorn *Crataegus* spp.
wild carrot *Daucus carota*
wild cherry bark *Prunus serotina*
wild indigo *Baptisia tinctoria*
wild lettuce *Lactuca virosa*
wild thyme *Thymus serpyllum*
wild yam *Dioscorea villosa*
willow *Salix* spp.
wintergreen *Gaultheria procumbens*
witch hazel *Hamamelis virginiana*
wolfberry *Lycium chinensis*
wood betony *Stachys betonica*
wormwood *Artemisia absinthium*

yarrow *Achillea millefolium*
yellow dock *Rumex crispus*
yellow root *Hydrastis canadensis*
yohimbe *Corynanthe yohimbi*